Illustrated Principles of Exercise Physiology

Kenneth Axen, PhD
Clinical Associate Professor
Department of Rehabilitation Medicine
New York University School of Medicine

Kathleen V. Axen, PhD, CDN
Professor
Department of Health and Nutrition Sciences
Brooklyn College of CUNY

Illustrated by Kenneth Axen, PhD

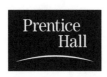

Prentice Hall

Upper Saddle River, New Jersey 07458

Library of Congress Cataloging-in-Publication Data

Axen, Kenneth.
    Illustrated principles of exercise physiology / Kenneth Axen and Kathleen V. Axen ;
illustrated by Kenneth Axen.
        p. cm.
    Includes bibliographical references and index.
    ISBN 0-13-040022-X
        1. Exercise—Physiological aspects. I. Axen, Kathleen V. II. Title.

QP301.A95 2000
612′.-044-dc21

00-048365

Publisher: Julie Alexander
Executive Editor: Greg Vis
Acquisitions Editor: Mark Cohen
Production Editor: Marianne Hutchinson
Production Liaison: Larry Hayden
Director of Manufacturing and Production: Bruce Johnson
Managing Editor: Patrick Walsh
Manufacturing Manager: Ilene Sanford
Creative Director: Marianne Frasco
Cover Design Coordinator: Maria Guglielmo
Marketing Manager: Tiffany Price
Editorial Assistant: Melissa Kerian
Interior Design and Composition: Pine Tree Composition
Printing and Binding: Banta Company

Prentice-Hall International (UK) Limited, *London*
Prentice-Hall of Australia Pty. Limited, *Sydney*
Prentice-Hall Canada Inc., *Toronto*
Prentice-Hall Hispanoamericana, S. A., *Mexico*
Prentice-Hall of India Private Limited, *New Delhi*
Prentice-Hall of Japan, Inc., *Tokyo*
Prentice-Hall Singapore Pte. Ltd.
Editora Prentice-Hall do Brasil, Ltda., *Rio de Janeiro*

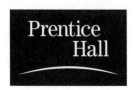

10 9 8 7 6 5 4 3 2 1
ISBN 0-13-040022-X

Dedicated with love to
Laurel, Christine, Marie, and Nils

Acknowledgments

We are deeply grateful to Mark Cohen for providing us with the opportunity to create this book and for his uncompromising dedication to the integrity of the work.

We thank Larry Hayden (and the staff at Prentice-Hall Publishers) and Marianne Hutchinson (and the staff at Pine Tree Composition) for the beautiful layout and typography, exquisite cover design, and their indefatigable efforts in actualizing this book. We also thank Kathy Whittier, Sue Morris, and Steve Martel for their meticulous attention to detail, and Fred D. Baldini for his positive review of our initial proposal.

We are particularly indebted to our readers, whose thoughtful comments improved the clarity, accuracy, and readability of our text. Our readers (listed alphabetically) were Christine Axen (high school sophomore), Christopher Dunbar, PhD (exercise physiologist), François Haas, PhD (respiratory physiologist and lifelong research associate), Marshall Hagins, MA, PT (physical therapist and dance injury specialist), Jacob I. Hirsch, MD (cardiologist and first mentor), Brian Lehrer, MA, PT (physical therapist and Ironman triathlete), Simon Ressner, PE (architectural engineer and firefighter), Roseanne Schnoll, PhD, RD (nutritionist), and Anthony Sgherza, PhD, PT (physical therapist and athletic trainer).

Preface

Our goal was to create a clearly written, beautifully illustrated overview of the principles of exercise physiology that would be an ideal book for a one-semester, undergraduate course in exercise physiology, as well as a useful prerequisite text for more advanced exercise-related courses. The text evolved from extensive lecture notes that were prepared while teaching undergraduate and graduate courses in exercise physiology in the Department of Physical Therapy at Long Island University, and graduate courses in nutrition and exercise in the Department of Health and Nutrition Sciences and the Department of Physical Education and Exercise Science at Brooklyn College, CUNY.

The text was designed to follow a logical progression, to provide a reasonable reading assignment for each lecture, and to emphasize the basic concepts of exercise physiology. These features enable our book to be used as a primary text in the hands of a knowledgeable instructor or as a supplemental review book that is compatible with any existing exercise physiology textbook.

Writing style

Instead of providing a broad compendium of information, we adopted the concise writing style utilized by scientific journals. This permitted us to cover the major topics in exercise physiology while eliminating ancillary material that drives students to skip and skim.

Following the philosophy of our previous book, we use the topics we cover as vehicles to explain basic principles, to promote quantitative reasoning, and to teach the mechanistic thinking required to understand the fundamentals of exercise physiology. Rather than avoiding graphs and equations, for example, some figures were specifically designed to teach students how to interpret information presented in graphical and algebraic form.

Illustrations

Our book contains 350 original, elegant, pen-and-ink illustrations that were hand-drawn by one of the authors. The ability of the author and illustrator to communicate via the corpus callosum produced a book with unparalleled correspondence between text and figures and unprecedented coherency among its illustrations.

The wide variety of drawings are clearly labeled in plain English and are related to one another through the use of extensive cross-referencing, recurring icons, and consistent color symbolism. Nearly two-thirds of the illustrations are completely new and have no counterpart in any of the existing exercise physiology books. The clarity, legibility, and simplicity of our line drawings make them an ideal source of transparencies for lectures. Our experience with our previous book has shown that students bring their lightweight, inexpensive books to class and actively take notes on the figures during lectures.

Pedagogical features

In accordance with our premise that color contains information that can be used to teach exercise physiology, we developed a logical coloring scheme in which colors are chosen according to functional, anatomical, or artistic considerations. The colors are indicated on each figure by a simple, unobtrusive code that enables the reader to color every illustration without referring to a legend.

This unique feature of our book enables relevant information to be presented in three different ways—once in a concisely written text, once nonverbally as a memorable diagram that can be colored, and once in a conversational figure legend that bridges the gap between the text and figures. Because some information can only be seen when the figure is colored, the act of coloring enables the reader to appreciate this information as it emerges and to fully realize the point of the illustration.

Coloring Instructions

Colors are coded as a lowercase letter that appears on the figure or as a subscript to a label; a code that is used for a particular shape (icon) applies to all like icons in that figure. The code for each of the fourteen colors used in this book appears at the bottom of even numbered pages. The symbols "–" and "+" are used to indicate application of color with light and heavy pressure, respectively. Try using the side of the lead to cover areas with light-pressure color; light-pressure background color can be applied over previously colored areas to save time.

We used thirteen inexpensive (Berol Verithin) colored pencils that were purchased in an art supply store. The colors included three blues: **a**zure (sky blue), **b**lue (true blue) and **n**avy (indigo blue); two yellows: **c**anary (canary yellow) and **y**ellow (yellow ochre); and one each of **gr**ay (light grey), **g**reen (grass green), blac**k**, **o**range (orange ochre), **p**ink, **r**ed (crimson red), **t**an (golden brown), **v**iolet (or lavender), and **w**hite (do not color).

Color each illustration as instructed in the figure legend, which guides you through the processes depicted in the figure in the proper sequence. Use the colors that are indicated because they have been chosen to convey information (see inside cover).

Some examples of our coloring scheme are:

- green (meaning "go") is the color of sodium, sodium channels, and excitatory neurotransmitters. Therefore, depolarization, muscle contraction, and the QRS complex of the ECG are also green to indicate that these processes are mediated by an influx of sodium into cells.

- red (meaning "stop") is the color of potassium, potassium channels, and inhibitory neurotransmitters. Therefore, repolarization, muscle relaxation, and the T wave of the ECG are also red to indicate that these processes are mediated by an efflux of potassium out of cells.

- arterial blood is red, capillary blood is violet, and venous blood is blue to indicate their corresponding oxygen content. Therefore, the oxyhemoglobin dissociation curve is depicted as a line divided into segments of different colors, including black (severely hypoxemic blood), navy (mildly hypoxemic blood), blue (mixed venous blood), violet (capillary blood), and red (arterial blood).

When the book is fully colored, it will serve as a useful study tool for review.

Contents

Acknowledgments — iv

Preface — v

Coloring Instructions — vi

1 Bioenergetics — 1

Principles of energy transfer 2
Forms of energy 3
Units of chemical and thermal energy 3
Units of work 3
Conversion between calories and joules 5
Power 5
Entropy 5
Efficiency of energy transfer 6
Free energy 6
Free energy changes 7
Exergonic and endergonic reactions 7
Standard free energy 7
Coupling of exergonic and endergonic reactions 8
Adenosine triphosphate (ATP) 8
Role of ATP as an energy carrier 9
Activation energy 10
Effect of enzymes on chemical reactions 10
Enzyme kinetics 11
Effect of temperature on reaction rate 12
The Q_{10} effect 12

2 Metabolism — 13

Anabolism and catabolism 15
Energy sources 15
Structure of carbohydrates 15
Disaccharides 15
Polysaccharides 16
Digestion and absorption of carbohydrates 17
Glucose uptake by cells 18
Glycogen 18
Glycogen synthesis 20
Glycogenolysis 20
Glycolysis 22
Oxidation and reduction 23
Production of $NADH + H^+$ in glycolysis 24
Anaerobic glycolysis 24
Krebs cycle 25
Electron transport chain 26
Chemiosmotic-coupling mechanism 26
Dependence of the Krebs cycle on oxygen 29
Aerobic glycolysis 29
Anaerobic production of ATP 29

Energy yield of anaerobic and aerobic metabolism 29
Gluconeogenesis 29
Pathway of gluconeogenesis 33
Summary of carbohydrate metabolism 33
Metabolism of fat 35
Digestion and absorption of fat 37
Storage of triglyceride 38
Synthesis of fat 38
Circulating lipids 40
Lipolysis 40
Oxidation of fat 40
Ketogenesis 41
Metabolism of fat during exercise 41
Metabolism of protein 42
Digestion and absorption of protein 42
Metabolism of amino acids 42
Gluconeogensis from amino acids 43
Fate of the amino group 44
Effect of exercise on protein metabolism 45
Summary 45

3 Energy systems

47

ATP-PCr system 48
Glycolysis 50
Glycolytic system 50
Effect of glycogen breakdown on glycolysis 50
Lactic acid formation 52
Isozymes of lactate dehydrogenase 53
Oxidative system 53
Functional differences among energy systems 54
Anaerobic and aerobic components of ATP production 55
Oxygen consumption during exercise 56
Oxygen deficit 57
Excess postexercise oxygen consumption (EPOC) 57
Effect of exercise intensity on oxygen consumption 57
Factors that influence $\dot{V}O_2$max 57
Effect of exercise intensity on blood lactate levels 58
Lactate threshold (LT) 60
Physiological fuel value of nutrients 61
Energy content of nutrients 62
Direct calorimetry 62
Thermal equivalent for oxygen 63
Indirect calorimetry 64
Respiratory quotient (RQ) 65
RQ for carbohydrate 65
RQ for fat 66
RQ for protein 66
Nonprotein RQ 67
Effect of protein breakdown on urinary nitrogen 68
Effect of exercise intensity and duration on fuel utilization 68
Respiratory exchange ratio (R) 69
Components of energy expenditure 70
Resting metabolic rate (RMR) 72
Thermic effect of feeding (TEF) 73
Thermic effect of exercise (TEE) 73

Efficiency of exercise 73
Economy of exercise 75
METs 75

4 Skeletal muscle   79

Structure of skeletal muscle 80
Sarcomere 80
Structure of actin and myosin filaments 81
Interaction between actin and myosin filaments 82
Effect of sarcomere length on muscle force 83
Neural control of muscle contraction 85
Innervation of skeletal muscle 85
Structure and function of nerve fibers 86
Action potentials in nerve fibers 86
Transmission of action potentials in nerve fibers 87
Neuromuscular junction 87
Excitation-contraction coupling 88
Twitch 90
Types of muscle contractions 91
Effect of external load on muscle contraction 91
Motor unit 93
Spatial and temporal summation 94
Contractile and metabolic properties of muscle fibers 95
Muscle fiber types 96
Contractile properties of slow-twitch and fast-twitch motor units 96
Fatigability of slow-twitch and fast-twitch muscle fibers 97
Types of fatigue 97
Relative distributions of muscle fiber types 99
Distribution of muscle fiber types in elite athletes 99
Recruitment patterns of motor units 99
Components of a reflex arc 100
Reflex control of skeletal muscle contraction 100
Muscle spindles 101
Stretch reflex 101
Golgi tendon organs 102
Golgi tendon reflex 102
Summary of factors that influence muscle force 102

5 Cardiovascular system   103

Components of the cardiovascular system 104
Action potentials in cardiac muscle fibers 105
Cardiac muscle contraction 106
Effect of initial fiber length on cardiac muscle contraction 106
Effect of external load on cardiac muscle contraction 108
Electrical activity of the heart 109
The electrocardiogram (ECG) 110
Autonomic control of cardiac function 112
Cardiac cycle 113
Pressure and volume changes during the cardiac cycle 114
Ejection fraction 116
Effect of heart rate and stroke volume on cardiac output 117
Stroke work 119
Double product 121
Measurement of blood pressure by sphygmomanometry 121
Mean arterial pressure and pulse pressure 122
Systemic circulation 123

Types of blood vessels   124
Functional differences among types of blood vessels   125
Determinants of vascular resistance   126
Mechanisms that regulate the caliber of arterioles   127
Autoregulation   128
Model of the systemic circuit   129
Regulation of arterial blood pressure   129
Baroreceptor reflexes   130
Capillary fluid shift mechanism   131
Kidney-body fluid mechanism   132
Cardiovascular reflexes during exercise   133
Cardiac function curves   134
Factors that modify the cardiac function curve   136
Vascular function curves   137
Mean systemic pressure   138
Determinants of mean systemic pressure   139
Resistance to venous return   141
Equating cardiac function and vascular function curves   141
Regulation of cardiac output during exercise   142

6   Respiratory system   145

Gas exchange in the lung   147
Diffusion constants for oxygen and carbon dioxide   148
Geometry of the pulmonary membrane   148
Tracheobronchial tree   148
Partial pressure gradients   149
Partial pressures of oxygen and carbon dioxide   149
Dynamics of gas exchange in the lung   152
Oxygen carriage by blood   153
Oxyhemoglobin dissociation curve   154
The a-$\bar{v}$ O_2 difference   155
Fick equation   156
Factors affecting the oxyhemoglobin dissociation curve   158
Carbon dioxide carriage by blood   159
Blood pH   160
Acid-base disturbances   161
Compensated acid-base disturbances   161
Pulmonary ventilation   161
Effect of alveolar ventilation on arterial blood gases   162
Hypoventilation and hyperventilation   163
Mechanics of breathing   164
Respiratory muscles   165
Inspiratory muscles   166
Expiratory muscles   167
Mechanical properties of the lung   167
Elastic properties of the lung   167
Resistive properties of the lung   169
Factors that affect airway resistance   170
Regulation of arterial blood gases   171
Respiratory reflexes   171
Chemoreceptor reflexes   172
Ventilatory responses to carbon dioxide and oxygen   173
Phases of the ventilatory response to exercise   174
Effect of exercise intensity on ventilation   175
Ventilatory and lactate thresholds   176
Measurement of ventilatory threshold   177

Ventilatory equivalents for oxygen and carbon dioxide   178
Blood levels of oxygen and carbon dioxide during exercise   180
Respiratory compensation   181
Pulmonary function tests   183
Lung volumes and capacities   183
Forced vital capacity and FEV_1 183
Maximum voluntary ventilation   183

7   Endocrine system   187

Endocrine glands   188
Classes of hormones   189
Mechanisms of hormone action   190
Second messenger mechanism   190
Control of gene transcription   191
Effect of exercise on hormone release   193
Pituitary gland   194
Anterior pituitary hormones   195
Growth hormone   197
Thyroid hormone   197
Adrenocorticotropic hormone   198
Glucocorticoids   198
Mineralocorticoids   199
Antidiuretic hormone   201
Catecholamines   203
Androgens and estrogens   204
Pancreatic hormones   204
Insulin   204
Glucagon   206
Effect of exercise on secretion of metabolic hormones   206
Endocrine regulation of glycogenolysis and gluconeogenesis   206
Endocrine regulation of lipolysis   207
Maintenance of plasma glucose levels during exercise   207
Overview of endocrine regulation of fuel flux during exercise   208
Insulin-independent uptake of glucose by skeletal muscle   208
Exercise and diabetes mellitus   208
Postexercise endocrine effects   210

8   Temperature regulation   211

Heat production   213
Heat exchange between the body and the environment   214
Radiation   214
Conduction   216
Convection   217
Evaporation   218
Factors that influence evaporation   219
Regulation of body temperature   220
Room temperature control system   220
Body temperature control system   221
Thermoreceptors   222
Temperature regulatory center   222
Thermoregulation in cold stress   223
Thermoregulation in heat stress   224
Effect of ambient temperature on mechanisms of heat loss   225
Sweat glands   226
Effect of sweat loss on body fluids   226
Responses to sweat loss   227

Heat acclimatization   228
Environmental factors that predispose to hyperthermia   228
Wet bulb globe temperature   228
Heat illness   229

9   Training for strength and endurance   231

Specificity of training   233
Cross-training   233
Trainability and the overload principle   234
Reversibility principle   235
Principles of muscle training programs   235
Assessment of muscle strength   236
Muscle strength training programs   238
Dynamic strength training   238
Static strength training   239
Isokinetic strength training   239
Muscular adaptations to resistance training   239
Metabolic adaptations to resistance training   241
Neural adaptations to resistance training   242
Aerobic training   244
Use of heart rate to guide training intensity   245
Use of rating of perceived exertion to guide training intensity   245
Use of blood lactate levels to guide training intensity   247
Effects of aerobic training   247
Effects of endurance training on $\dot{V}O_2$max   247
Cardiac adaptations to endurance training   248
Effect of endurance training on capillary density   248
Effect of endurance training on blood volume   249
Circulatory and thermoregulatory effects of expanded blood volume   250
Respiratory adaptations to endurance training   250
Mitochondrial adaptations to endurance training   250
Effect of endurance training on O_2 uptake   252
Effect of endurance training on endocrine response to exercise   252
Effect of endurance training on fuel utilization   253
Effect of endurance training on blood lactate levels   253
Longitudinal changes with endurance training   254

10   Nutrition   257

Nutrients   258
Nutrient requirements   258
Dietary Reference Intake   260
Factors affecting nutrient requirements   260
Nutritional support of exercise performance   260
Nutritional supplements   260
Characteristics of a healthful diet   260
Dietary assessment   261
Energy requirements   261
Carbohydrate intake   262
High carbohydrate diets   262
Form of dietary carbohydrate   263
Effect of dietary carbohydrate on glycogen storage   263
Glycogen loading   264
Carbohydrate intake before and during exercise   265
Postexercise carbohydrate intake   267
Fat intake   268
Polyunsaturated fatty acids   269

Essential fatty acids   269
High fat diets   270
Dietary sources of fat   271
Protein intake   271
Essential amino acids   272
Protein requirements   273
Assessment of protein requirements   274
Protein requirements for endurance exercise   275
Protein requirements for strength training   275
Upper limit for protein intake   275
Vitamins   276
Vitamin requirements   276
Antioxidants   276
Excessive vitamin intake   276
Mineral requirements   277
Mineral supplementation   278
Excessive mineral intake   278
Fluid requirements   279
Composition of fluid replacement   279
Nutritional supplements as ergogenic aids   280
Evaluation of nutritional ergogenic aids   280
Creatine monohydrate   281
β-hydroxy β-methylbutyrate   281
Conjugated linoleic acid   282
Ginseng   282
Coenzyme Q   283

11   Body composition and weight control   285

Obesity   286
Adipose tissue   286
Regional distribution of body fat   289
Waist-to-hip ratio   289
Measurement of body fat   290
Densitometry   290
Skinfold thickness   293
Bioelectrical impedance analysis   294
Other indirect techniques of assessment   295
Body weight   295
Body Mass Index   296
Changes in body weight   296
Energy balance   296
Regulation of energy intake   297
Leptin   297
Estimation of daily energy requirements   298
Changes in energy balance   298
Effect of exercise on weight loss   299
Effect of diet on weight loss   300
Very low carbohydrate diets   300
Effect of energy deficit on weight loss   301
Causes of obesity   302
Genetic etiology of obesity   302
Developmental origin of obesity   302
Environmental causes of obesity   303
Underweight   303

About the Authors   306

Figures

1 Bioenergetics

1.1 Energy conversions 2
1.2 Conservation of energy 2
1.3 Forms of energy in exercise 3
1.4 Determination of mechanical work from force and distance 3
1.5 Quantification of mechanical work 4
1.6 Equivalent expressions for mechanical work 4
1.7 Conversion between calories and joules 5
1.8 Entropy 6
1.9 Efficiency of energy transfer 6
1.10 Exergonic and endergonic reactions 7
1.11 Coupling of exergonic and endergonic reactions 8
1.12 Adenosine triphosphate (ATP) 9
1.13 Role of ATP as an energy carrier 9
1.14 Activation energy 10
1.15 Effect of enzymes on reaction rate 11
1.16 Enzyme function 11
1.17 Enzyme kinetics 12
1.18 Effect of temperature on enzyme-catalyzed reactions 12

2 Metabolism

2.1 Metabolic pathway 14
2.2 Energy transfer from fuel to muscle 14
2.3 Anabolism and catabolism 15
2.4 Structure of glucose 16
2.5 Conversions between monosaccharides and disaccharides 16
2.6 Digestion of starch 17
2.7 Stages of starch digestion 17
2.8 Absorption of monosaccharides into the blood 18
2.9 Glucose uptake by cells 19
2.10 Structure of glycogen 19
2.11 Glycogen synthesis 20
2.12 Glycogenolysis 21
2.13 Glycogenolysis in liver and muscle 21
2.14 Glycolysis 22
2.15 Oxidation and reduction 23
2.16 Hydrogen carriers 24
2.17 Anaerobic glycolysis 25
2.18 Krebs cycle 26
2.19 Hydrogen carriers in the Krebs cycle 27
2.20 Structure of a mitochondrion 27
2.21 Electron transport chain 28
2.22 Aerobic glycolysis 30
2.23 Anaerobic and aerobic production of ATP 31
2.24 Substrates for gluconeogenesis 32

2.25 Cori cycle 32
2.26 Gluconeogenesis 33
2.27 Overview of carbohydrate metabolism 34
2.28 Structure of fatty acids 35
2.29 Esterification 35
2.30 Lipolysis and esterification 36
2.31 Absorption of fat 37
2.32 Storage of dietary fat in adipose tissue 38
2.33 Triglyceride flux in muscle and adipose tissue 39
2.34 Forms of fat in the blood 39
2.35 β-oxidation 40
2.36 Metabolism of fatty acids 41
2.37 Structure of amino acids 42
2.38 Structure of branched-chain amino acids 42
2.39 Peptide bond 43
2.40 Overview of protein metabolism 43
2.41 Alanine shuttle 44
2.42 Overview of metabolism 45

3 Energy systems

3.1   Energy systems 48
3.2   Use of PCr to regenerate ATP 49
3.3   Use of ADP to regenerate ATP 49
3.4   Modulation of rate-limiting enzymes 51
3.5   Factors that promote lactic acid formation 52
3.6   Oxidative system 53
3.7   Maximal rates and durations of ATP production 54
3.8   ATP supply during maximal exercises of different durations 55
3.9   Oxygen uptake during exercise 56
3.10 Fates of lactate 58
3.11 Effect of exercise intensity on oxygen consumption 59
3.12 Effect of exercise intensity on blood lactate levels 59
3.13 Determinants of blood lactate levels 60
3.14 Lactate production and removal 61
3.15 Physiological fuel value of nutrients 62
3.16 Direct calorimetry 63
3.17 Thermal equivalent for oxygen 64
3.18 J valve 64
3.19 Principles of open-circuit spirometry 65
3.20 Respiratory quotient 66
3.21 Use of nonprotein RQ to determine fuel utilization 67
3.22 Effect of exercise intensity and duration on fuel utilization 68
3.23 Metabolic and nonmetabolic production of CO_2 69
3.24 Effect of lactic acid formation on respiratory exchange ratio 70
3.25 Effect of lactic acid formation on blood levels of bicarbonate 71
3.26 Components of total daily energy expenditure 71
3.27 Nomogram for body surface area 72
3.28 External work during cycle ergometry 73
3.29 External work during inclined treadmill exercise 74
3.30 Energy cost of walking 74
3.31 Economy of exercise 75
3.32 Effect of body mass on oxygen consumption 76

3.33 METs 76
3.34 Energy cost of treadmill exercise protocols 77

4 Skeletal muscle

4.1   Structure of skeletal muscle 80
4.2   Arrangement of actin and myosin filaments 80
4.3   Sarcomere 81
4.4   Structure of actin and myosin filament 81
4.5   Effect of calcium ions on actin filament 82
4.6   Interaction between actin and myosin filaments 83
4.7   Effect of sarcomere length on filament interaction 84
4.8   Length-tension relationship of skeletal muscle 84
4.9   Organization of the nervous system 85
4.10 Innervation of skeletal muscle 86
4.11 Structure of an alpha motor neuron 87
4.12 Membrane potentials in nerve cells 87
4.13 Action potentials in nerve fibers 88
4.14 Neuromuscular transmission and excitation-contraction coupling 89
4.15 Muscle twitch 90
4.16 Types of muscle contractions 91
4.17 Effect of external load on concentric muscle contraction 92
4.18 Force-velocity characteristic of skeletal muscle 93
4.19 Motor unit 93
4.20 Spatial and temporal summation 94
4.21 Tetanus 95
4.22 Effect of muscle fiber type on twitch duration 95
4.23 Effect of motor unit type on tension and fatigue 96
4.24 Effect of muscle fiber type on force-velocity characteristic 97
4.25 Central and peripheral fatigue 98
4.26 Distribution of muscle fiber types 99
4.27 Recruitment patterns of motor units 100
4.28 Stretch reflex 101
4.29 Golgi tendon reflex 102

5 Cardiovascular system

5.1   Components of the cardiovascular system 104
5.2   Action potentials in cardiac muscle fibers 105
5.3   Relationship between action potential and twitch tension in cardiac muscle 106
5.4   Effect of fiber length on force-velocity characteristic 107
5.5   Effect of fiber length on ventricular pressures 107
5.6   Force-velocity characteristic of cardiac muscle 108
5.7   Conduction system of the heart 109
5.8   Electrical activity of the heart 110
5.9   Normal electrocardiogram 111
5.10 Chest leads 111
5.11 Autonomic innervation of the heart 112
5.12 Autonomic control of heart rate 112
5.13 Valves of the heart 113
5.14 Phases of the cardiac cycle 114
5.15 Pressure and volume changes during the cardiac cycle 115
5.16 Factors that influence stroke volume 116
5.17 Effect of myocardial contractility on ejection fraction 117
5.18 Determinants of cardiac output 118

5.19   Heart rate and stroke volume responses to exercise   118
5.20   Ventricular pressure-volume relationships during the cardiac cycle   119
5.21   Determination of stroke work   120
5.22   Effects of arterial blood pressure and stroke volume on stroke work   120
5.23   Measurement of arterial blood pressure by sphygmomanometry   121
5.24   Mean arterial pressure and pulse pressure   122
5.25   Arrangement of vascular beds in the systemic circulation   123
5.26   Arrangement of blood vessels in a vascular bed   124
5.27   Types of blood vessels   125
5.28   Functional differences among blood vessels   125
5.29   Constituents of blood   126
5.30   Effect of radius on resistance to fluid flow   127
5.31   Mechanisms that regulate the caliber of arterioles   127
5.32   Autoregulation   128
5.33   Model of the systemic circuit   129
5.34   Transduction characteristics of arterial baroreceptors   130
5.35   Block diagram of a baroreceptor reflex   130
5.36   Capillary fluid shift mechanism   131
5.37   Hemoconcentration during exercise   132
5.38   Renal circulation   132
5.39   Effect of arterial blood pressure on urine output   133
5.40   Cardiovascular reflexes during exercise   134
5.41   Redistribution of cardiac output during exercise   135
5.42   Law of the heart   135
5.43   Cardiac function curve   136
5.44   Factors that modify the cardiac function curve   136
5.45   Vascular function curve   137
5.46   Blood pressure changes during measurement of P_{ms} 138
5.47   Blood volume changes during measurement of P_{ms} 139
5.48   Effects of venomotor tone on vascular function curve   140
5.49   Mechanical and neural factors that influence P_{ms} 140
5.50   Effects of vasomotor tone on vascular function curve   141
5.51   Equating cardiac function and vascular function curves   142
5.52   Cardiovascular responses to exercise   143

6   Respiratory system

6.1   Transport of oxygen and carbon dioxide   146
6.2   Pulmonary membrane   147
6.3   Diffusion of gases across the pulmonary membrane   147
6.4   Effect of membrane geometry on diffusion   148
6.5   Tracheobronchial tree   149
6.6   Partial pressures   150
6.7   Composition of inspired air and alveolar gas   150
6.8   Partial pressure gradients for oxygen and carbon dioxide   151
6.9   Dynamics of gas exchange in the lung   152
6.10   Dynamics of gas exchange in the lung during exercise   153
6.11   Carriage of oxygen by hemoglobin   154
6.12   Oxygen saturation of hemoglobin   154
6.13   Oxyhemoglobin dissociation curve   155
6.14   Effect of oxygen uptake on a-$\bar{v}$ O_2 difference   156
6.15   Effect of blood flow and O_2 extraction on O_2 uptake   147
6.16   Factors affecting the oxyhemoglobin dissociation curve   158

6.17   Carriage of carbon dioxide by the blood   159
6.18   Acid-base disturbances   160
6.19   Compensated acid-base disturbances   161
6.20   Pulmonary ventilation   162
6.21   Effect of alveolar ventilation on alveolar PCO_2 163
6.22   Possible PCO_2-PO_2 combinations in alveolar gas   163
6.23   Effect of alveolar ventilation on alveolar PCO_2 and PO_2 164
6.24   Lung and chest wall   165
6.25   Respiratory muscles   165
6.26   Action of the diaphragm   166
6.27   Action of the external intercostal muscles   167
6.28   Elastic properties of springs   168
6.29   Elastic properties of the lung   168
6.30   Airway resistance   169
6.31   Effect of lung volume on airway resistance   170
6.32   Effect of bronchial muscle tone on airway diameter   171
6.33   Block diagram of a respiratory reflex   172
6.34   Transduction characteristics of arterial chemoreceptors   172
6.35   Block diagram of a blood gas control system   173
6.36   Ventilatory responses to carbon dioxide and oxygen   174
6.37   Phases of the ventilatory response to exercise   175
6.38   Ventilatory response to steady-state exercise   176
6.39   Determination of VT from $\dot{V}_E$ and $\dot{V}O_2$ data   177
6.40   Effect of exercise intensity on $\dot{V}O_2$ and $\dot{V}CO_2$ 178
6.41   Ventilatory equivalents for oxygen and carbon dioxide   179
6.42   Determination of VT from V_EO_2 data   179
6.43   Effect of exercise intensity on PO_2 and PCO_2 levels   180
6.44   Effect of exercise intensity on alveolar PCO_2 181
6.45   Ventilatory stimuli during exercise   182
6.46   Respiratory mechanoreceptors   182
6.47   Spirometer   183
6.48   Lung volumes and capacities   184
6.49   Helium dilution   185
6.50   Forced vital capacity and FEV_1 186
6.51   Maximum voluntary ventilation   186

7   Endocrine system

7.1   Schema of endocrine system   188
7.2   Schematic diagram of hormone action   189
7.3   Catecholamines   189
7.4   Steroid hormones   190
7.5   Second messenger mechanism of hormone action   191
7.6   Hormonal control of gene transcription   192
7.7   Time course of endocrine secretions during exercise   193
7.8   Pituitary gland   194
7.9   Anterior pituitary hormones   195
7.10   Regulation of anterior pituitary hormone secretion   196
7.11   Thyroid gland   197
7.12   Thyroid hormone   197
7.13   Adrenal gland   198
7.14   Mechanism of aldosterone action   199
7.15   Block diagram of potassium control system   200

7.16   Mechanism of ADH action   201
7.17   Block diagram of sodium control system   202
7.18   Effect of exercise intensity on ADH secretion   202
7.19   Effects of catecholamines   203
7.20   Pancreatic islets   204
7.21   Effects of hormones on blood glucose levels   205
7.22   Block diagram of glucose control system   205
7.23   Glucose uptake by skeletal muscle   206
7.24   Glucose tolerance test   207
7.25   Maintenance of plasma glucose levels during exercise   208
7.26   Endocrine regulation of fuel flux during exercise   209

8   Temperature regulation

8.1   Effect of heat flux on temperature   212
8.2   Principles of temperature regulation   212
8.3   Mechanisms of heat gain   213
8.4   Effect of physical activity on heat production   213
8.5   Heat exchange between the body and the environment   214
8.6   Effect of temperature gradient on radiation   215
8.7   Radiation   215
8.8   Effect of temperature gradient on conduction   216
8.9   Effect of medium on conduction   217
8.10   Convection   217
8.11   Wind Chill Index   218
8.12   Evaporative heat loss   219
8.13   Heat Stress Index   219
8.14   Room temperature control system   220
8.15   Block diagram of room temperature control system   221
8.16   Block diagram of body temperature control system   221
8.17   Components of body temperature control system   222
8.18   Thermoregulation in cold stress   223
8.19   Effect of vasomotor tone on heat loss   224
8.20   Thermoregulation in heat stress   224
8.21   Effect of ambient temperature on heat loss mechanisms   225
8.22   Sweat glands   226
8.23   Effect of sweat loss on body fluids   227
8.24   Effect of blood volume on thermoregulation   228
8.25   Wet bulb globe temperature (WBGT)   229

9   Training for strength and endurance

9.1   Components of an exercise prescription   232
9.2   Components of muscle performance   232
9.3   Specificity of training   233
9.4   Effects of cross-training   234
9.5   Overload principle   235
9.6   Effects of strength and endurance training on muscle   236
9.7   Static dynamometry   237
9.8   Isokinetic dynamometry   237
9.9   Effect of joint angle on maximal muscle force   238
9.10   The n-RM load   238
9.11   Maximal isokinetic and isotonic contractions   240
9.12   Effect of muscle cross-sectional area on strength   240
9.13   Hypertrophy and hyperplasia   241

9.14   Effects of resistance training on ATP-PCr system   241
9.15   Effects of resistance training on glycolytic system   242

9.16   Components of muscle strength   243
9.17   Longitudinal changes with strength training   243
9.18   Neural factors that influence muscle strength   244
9.19   Use of heart rate to guide training intensity   245
9.20   Rating of perceived exertion (RPE)   246

9.21   Individual differences in RPE   246
9.22   Effect of endurance training on $\dot{V}O_2$max   247
9.23   Cardiac adaptations to endurance training   248
9.24   Effect of endurance training on capillary density   249
9.25   Effect of endurance training on blood volume   250

9.26   Effect of endurance training on the oxidative system   251
9.27   Effect of endurance training on blood levels of catecholamines   252
9.28   Effect of endurance training on fuel utilization   253
9.29   Effect of endurance training on blood lactate levels   254
9.30   Longitudinal changes with endurance training   255

10   Nutrition

10.1   Categories of nutrients   258
10.2   Nutrient requirements   259
10.3   Determination of the recommended dietary allowance (RDA)   259
10.4   Assessment of nutrient intake   261
10.5   Composition of representative diets   262

10.6   High carbohydrate diets   263
10.7   Effect of carbohydrate intake on glycogen synthesis   264
10.8   Glycogen loading technique   265
10.9   Effect of carbohydrate ingestion on blood glucose during exercise   266
10.10 Postexercise glycogen synthesis   267

10.11 Mechanism of postexercise glycogen synthesis   268
10.12 Structures of unsaturated fatty acids   269
10.13 Effect of diet composition on glycogen storage   270
10.14 Essential amino acid requirements   271
10.15 Complete and incomplete proteins   272

10.16 Protein requirements   273
10.17 Nitrogen balance   273
10.18 Effect of protein intake on nitrogen balance   274
10.19 Upper limit of protein requirement   275
10.20 Function of antioxidants   277

10.21 Mineral status   278
10.22 Water balance   279
10.23 Osmotic effects of glucose and glucose polymers   280
10.24 Effect of creatine monohydrate supplementation   281
10.25 Structure of conjugated linoleic acid   282

11   Body composition and weight control

11.1   Effect of obesity on disease risk   286
11.2   Structure of an adipocyte   287
11.3   Fat depots   287
11.4   Hypertrophy and hyperplasia of adipocytes   288
11.5   Patterns of fat deposition   289

11.6   Models of body composition   290
11.7   Effect of body composition on body density   291

11.8   Principles of densitometry   292

11.9   Effect of body composition on densitomery measurements   293

11.10   Measurement of skinfold thickness   294

11.11   Effect of body composition on bioelectrical impedance   295

11.12   Effect of energy balance on body weight   296

11.13   Mechanism of leptin action   297

11.14   Effect of exercise on composition of weight loss   299

11.15   Effect of exercise on metabolic rate during weight loss   299

11.16   Composition of weight loss and its calorie equivalent   300

11.17   Temporal changes in the calorie equivalents of weight loss   301

11.18   Factors that promote obesity   302

chapter **one.**
bioenergetics

Bioenergetics is the study of the storage, release, and utilization of energy in biological systems.

Principles of energy transfer

The *first law of thermodynamics* states that energy can neither be created nor destroyed, only transformed. Two consequences of this law are that energy can be converted from one form to another (Figure 1.1) and that the total amount of energy before a conversion is equal to the total amount of energy after the conversion (Figure 1.2).

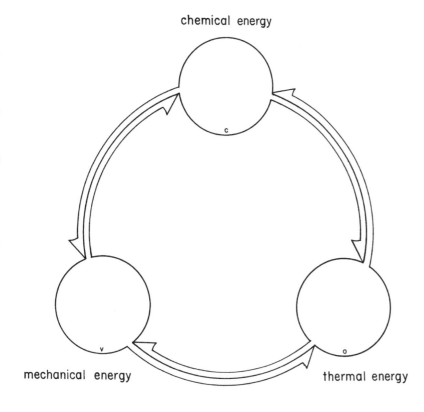

chemical energy

mechanical energy

thermal energy

Figure 1.1   Energy conversions. Color the circle labeled chemical energy and its connections to the other circles. Repeat this process for the remaining circles, noting that chemical energy (bond energy), mechanical energy (work), and thermal energy (heat) are interchangeable forms of energy.

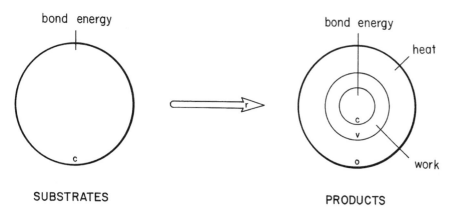

bond energy

bond energy

heat

work

SUBSTRATES

PRODUCTS

Figure 1.2   Conservation of energy. This figure illustrates the energetics of a chemical reaction in which some portion of the initial bond energy is transformed into mechanical work while another portion is dissipated as heat. Color the figure from left to right, noting that the total energy of the substrates (area of circle at left) is equal to the total energy of the products (area of circle at right). The bond energy that remains after the reaction (center, right circle) was not transformed and can therefore be regarded as usable energy for a different reaction. Compare this figure with Figure 1.1.

Forms of energy

Energy can be regarded as the capacity to do work.

Forms of energy that are relevant to exercise physiology include: (1) chemical energy that is stored or released during the making or breaking of molecular bonds; (2) thermal energy that is absorbed or released in the form of heat; (3) mechanical energy that is expended in the performance of physical work; (4) electrical energy that reflects the work needed to move charged particles against the forces produced by electric fields; and (5) radiant energy that is transmitted in the form of electromagnetic waves (Figure 1.3).

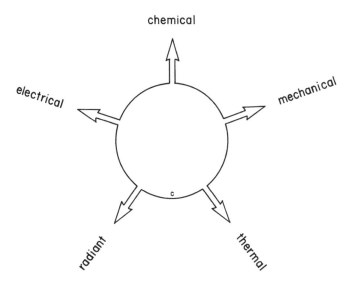

Figure 1.3   Forms of energy in exercise. Color the diagram, identifying the different forms of energy that are relevant to the study of exercise.

Units of chemical and thermal energy

Chemical energy and *thermal energy* are two forms of energy that are measured in calories, where 1 calorie (cal) is the amount of heat needed to raise the temperature of 1 g of water by 1° Centigrade (1° Celsius). One kilocalorie (kcal or Cal) is equal to 1000 calories.

Units of work

Mechanical work is determined by the vector product of force (F) and distance (d) (i.e., work = F·d, Figure 1.4). It follows from this equation that different combinations of force and distance can result in the same amount of mechanical work (Figure 1.5).

Using the terminology of the Système International d'Unités (SI units), work is measured in units of joules (J), where 1 J is the amount of work that is done when 1 Newton (N) of force acts through a distance of 1 m, i.e., 1 J = 1 Newton · meter (N·m) (Figure 1.6, left panel). A Newton, defined as the force needed to make a 1 kg mass have an acceleration of $1 \ m/s^2$, is approximately equal to 0.225 lb.

Mechanical work is also determined by the product of pressure and volume. Since pressure, defined as force per unit area, can be expressed in units of N/m^2 and volume can be expressed in units of m^3, it follows that work (in J) = pressure (P, in N/m^2) · volume (V, in m^3) = P·V (in N·m, or J) (Figure 1.6, middle panel).

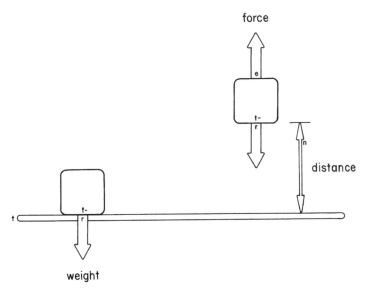

force

distance

weight

Figure 1.4   Determination of mechanical work from force and distance. Color the block at left and the horizontal surface, noting that the weight of the block is a downward force. In theory, Newton's law (F = ma) dictates that the force needed to lift an object must exceed its weight when the object is accelerated but equals its weight when the object is either being held or being lifted at a constant velocity (conditions in which acceleration is zero). Color the block at right and its arrows, noting that the force (arrow pointing up) needed to lift the block slowly (so that the effects of acceleration can be neglected) is equal to the weight of the block (arrow pointing down). Under these conditions, the mechanical work performed in lifting the block to a given height is determined by the product of the applied force (equal to the weight of the block) and the vertical distance (height), i.e., work = weight · height. Note that the weight of an object (w, in N) is given by the product of its mass (m, in kg) and the acceleration of gravity (g = 9.8 m/s^2), i.e., w = m · g.

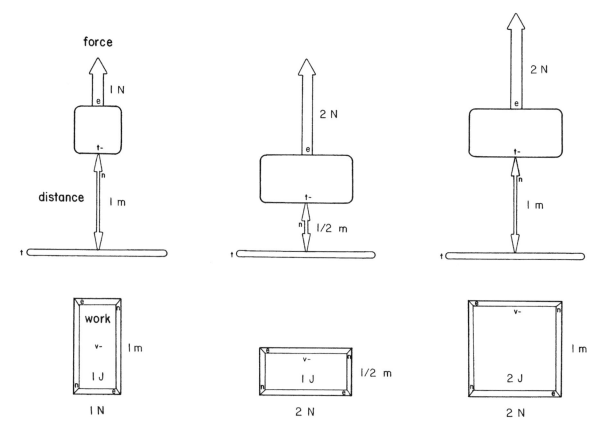

Figure 1.5.   Quantification of mechanical work. Color the block and its force and distance arrows in the upper left panel, noting that these conditions are identical to those shown in Figure 1.4. Color the edges of the rectangle in the lower left panel, noting that its horizontal dimension (base) is equal to 1 N (the force used to lift the block) and its vertical dimension (height) is equal to 1 m (the distance the block was lifted). Color the interior of the rectangle, noting that its area is 1 N · m = 1 J, the amount of work performed when a force of 1 N acts through a distance of 1 m. Because the area of a rectangle can be calculated by the product of its base (force, in N) and height (distance, in m), observe that the area of this rectangle is a quantitative measure of the mechanical work associated with this force and this distance. Color the 2 N block in the middle panel, its arrows, and the edges of the rectangle beneath it. Color the interior of the rectangle, noting that the same amount of work (the same area) is performed when twice the force (2N) acts through half the distance (½ m). Repeat the process for the conditions shown in the right panel, in which the 2 N block is lifted to a height of 1 m. Color the interior of the corresponding rectangle, noting that twice as much work (twice the area) is performed when twice the force (2N) acts through the same distance (1 m). These examples explain why area in a force-distance diagram can be regarded as a quantitative measure of work.

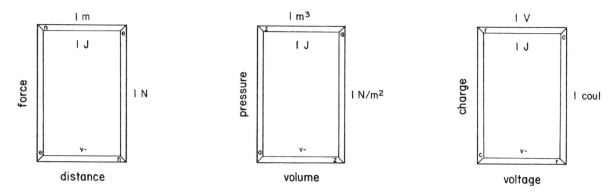

Figure 1.6.   Equivalent expressions for mechanical work. Color the edges and areas of each of the rectangles, noting that work can be quantified from the area in a force-distance diagram (left panel), a pressure-volume diagram (middle panel), or a charge-voltage diagram (right panel). One coulomb is the quantity of charge transferred in 1 second under conditions in which there is a constant current of 1 ampere, i.e., 1 ampere = 1 coul/s. Compare this figure with Figure 1.5.

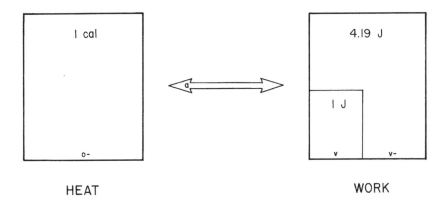

HEAT   WORK

Figure 1.7 Conversion between calories and joules. Color the rectangle labeled heat, noting that its area corresponds to 1 cal. Color the horizontal arrow and the rectangle labeled work, noting that its area corresponds to 4.19 J; identify the smaller rectangle whose area corresponds to 1 J. Note that the areas of the two large rectangles are equal, indicating that 1 cal of heat and 4.19 joules of work are equal amounts of energy. Compare this figure with Figure 1.1.

Mechanical work is also determined by the product of charge, which is measured in coulombs (coul), and voltage, which is measured in volts. Since 1 volt is equal to 1 J/coul, it follows that work (in J) = charge (q, in coul) · voltage (V, in volts) = q · V (in J) (Figure 1.6, right panel).

Conversion between calories and joules

One calorie is approximately the same amount of energy as 4.19 joules (Figure 1.7). This conversion factor, 4.19 J/cal, enables a given amount of energy in the form of heat (in cal) to be translated into an equal amount of energy in the form of work (in J), and vice versa.

Power

Power is defined as the rate at which work is performed and is expressed in units of watts (1 watt = 1 joule per second). Thus, the average power (in watts) associated with the performance of a given amount of work can be calculated by dividing the amount of work (in joules) by the time in which the work was performed (in seconds), i.e.,

$$power = work/time$$

In accord with this definition, power output increases when the same amount of work is performed in less time or when more work is performed in the same amount of time. Because work can be expressed as the product of force and distance (Figure 1.4), it follows that

$$power = force \cdot distance/time$$

Because velocity is given by distance divided by time, i.e., velocity = distance/time, this term can be replaced by velocity, i.e.,

$$power = force \cdot velocity$$

Thus, an alternative expression for power is the product of force and velocity. In accord with this definition, power output increases when more force is exerted at the same velocity, or when the same force is exerted at a higher velocity. During cycling, for example, more power would be needed to pedal at the same cadence against a higher resistance (higher force at the same velocity) or to pedal at a higher cadence against the same resistance (same force at a higher velocity) (Figure 3.28).

Entropy

Entropy is a term that is used to quantify the amount of disorder or randomness in a system. The *second law of thermodynamics* states that every energy transfer increases the entropy of the universe. For example, molecules of ice, which are rigidly arranged in a lattice structure, have more order and therefore less entropy than molecules of water that move about independently (Figure 1.8). Thus, the transition from ice to water is accompanied by an increase in entropy.

Although living organisms increase the order of their internal environments and thereby decrease their entropy, they do so by employing heat-dissipating mechanisms that increase the entropy of their external environment. Because the decrease in entropy of the internal environment leads to an even greater increase in the entropy of the external environment,

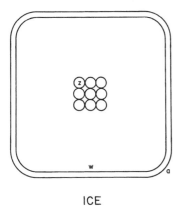

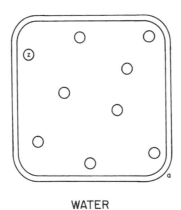

ICE   WATER

Figure 1.8   Entropy. Color and count the molecules of ice (left panel) and water (right panel). Note that the molecules of ice have more order and therefore less entropy than the same number of molecules of water.

the total entropy of the universe increases and the second law of thermodynamics is satisfied.

Efficiency of energy transfer

The second law of thermodynamics is the reason that physical and chemical processes naturally proceed in the direction in which the final products of a reaction contain less usable energy than the initial reactants (substrates). It also explains why the conversion of energy from one form to another is not perfect. As a result, every energy exchange releases some energy in an unusable form, usually as heat.

Efficiency is a term that is used to denote the ratio of the usable energy derived from a reaction (useful energy output) to the energy supplied by the initial substrates (energy input) (Figure 1.9). The efficiency of an energy transformation is calculated by dividing the useful energy output by the energy input, and expressing the ratio as a percent, i.e., efficiency (%) = (useful energy output) · 100/(energy input).

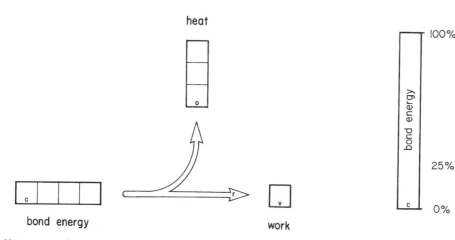

Figure 1.9   Efficiency of energy transfer. This figure illustrates the energetics of a chemical reaction in which bond energy (energy input) is transformed into mechanical work (useful energy output) and heat. Begin at the left by coloring the four-box rectangle that quantifies the initial bond energy of the substrates. Color the arrow that indicates the reaction, the three-box rectangle labeled heat, and the one-box square labeled work. Color the bar graphs at right, noting that the total amount of energy before the reaction (bond energy, bar graph at left) is equal to the total amount of energy after the reaction (work plus heat, bar graph at right). Compare the two bar graphs, noting that one-quarter of the energy input is transformed into useful work while the remaining three-quarters of the energy input is dissipated as heat. The efficiency of this reaction (calculated by dividing the useful energy output by the energy input and expressing the ratio as a percent) is therefore 25%. Compare this figure with Figure 1.2.

Free energy

The usable energy that is stored in the chemical bonds of molecules is called the *free energy;* it is measured in units of kcal per mole and symbolized by G. Free energy pertains to

that portion of the initial bond energy that actually ends up being transformed into a useful form of energy, such as that used to perform mechanical work or to form a new molecular bond. Although it is difficult to determine the absolute amount of free energy in a particular molecule, it is easy to determine the change in free energy that occurs during the course of a chemical reaction.

Free energy changes

Since the products of spontaneously occurring physical and chemical processes contain less free energy than the initial substrates, reactions naturally proceed in the direction that enables them to go from a state of higher free energy to one of lower free energy, i.e., down their free energy gradient. Therefore, a comparison of the free energy of the products and substrates can be used to predict the direction in which a reaction would naturally proceed.

The difference between the free energy of the final products and the initial substrates is called the free energy change (symbolized by ΔG) and is derived by subtracting the free energy of the substrates from the free energy of the products, i.e., $\Delta G = G_{products} - G_{substrates}$.

In accord with this definition: (1) ΔG is negative when the products have less free energy than the substrates (energy is released during the reaction); (2) ΔG is zero when the prod-ucts have the same amount of free energy as the substrates (the reaction is in equilibrium); and (3) ΔG is positive when the products have more free energy than the substrates (energy is absorbed during the reaction).

Exergonic and endergonic reactions

Reactions that are associated with a decrease in free energy (ΔG is negative) are termed *exergonic reactions*, whereas reactions that are associated with an increase in free energy (ΔG is positive) are termed *endergonic reactions* (Fig. 1.10).

Exergonic reactions occur spontaneously and release energy into their surroundings. In contrast, endergonic reactions do not occur spontaneously because they require an input of energy from their surroundings.

Standard free energy

The *standard free energy* change (symbolized by $\Delta G°$) for a given reaction is the free energy change measured in a laboratory under what are called standard conditions. Standard

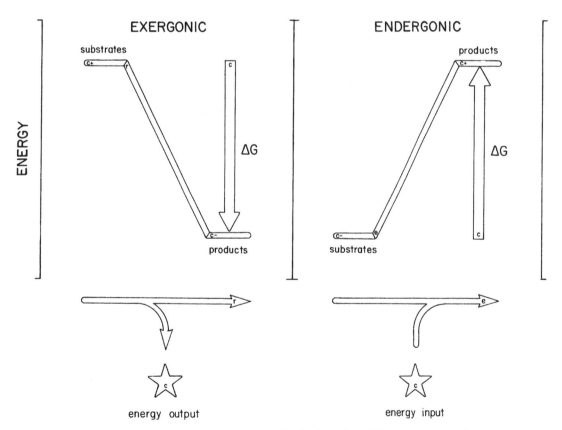

Figure 1.10   Exergonic and endergonic reactions. Color the lines from left to right, noting that an exergonic reaction (left panel) is associated with a decrease in free energy and that an endergonic reaction (right panel) is associated with an increase in free energy. Color the vertical arrows that indicate the free energy change (ΔG) associated with the two reactions, noting that the arrow points down in the exergonic reaction (ΔG is negative) and up in the endergonic reaction (ΔG is positive). Color the arrows at the bottom of each panel, noting that exergonic reactions release energy (energy output, indicated by star) into their environment, whereas endergonic reactions absorb energy (energy input, indicated by star) from their environment.

conditions entail a temperature of 25°C, a pressure of 1 atmosphere, a pH of 7.0, and concentrations of substrates and products that are maintained at 1 mol/L. Although standard conditions differ markedly from physiological conditions, categorizing reactions in terms of their standard free energy changes provides a means of comparing the energetics of different reactions.

For example, since the standard free energy changes ($\Delta G°$) are additive in any sequence of consecutive reactions, biochemical pathways consisting of a series of reactions can potentially proceed as long as the algebraic sum of the individual $\Delta G°$ values is negative. Stated another way, the overall pathway must be exergonic even though some of its intermediate steps might be endergonic.

Coupling of exergonic and endergonic reactions

Energy that is released during exergonic reactions can be used to drive endergonic reactions that are coupled to them.

Since humans maintain an essentially constant body temperature, energy is transferred between chemical reactions by a common intermediate that links the two reactions. Two chemical reactions have a common intermediate when: (1) they occur sequentially; and (2) a product of the first reaction is a substrate for the second reaction (Figure 1.11).

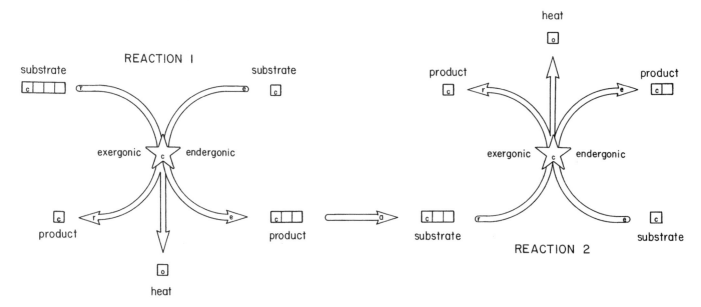

Figure 1.11 Coupling of exergonic and endergonic reactions. Begin in the upper left corner by coloring the four-box rectangle of initial bond energy (substrate at left). Color Reaction 1 (at left) in which an exergonic reaction is coupled to an endergonic reaction. Color the star that symbolizes the energy released during the breaking of bonds, the square labeled heat, and the products of this reaction. Observe that the three-box product of Reaction 1 is also a substrate for Reaction 2 (at right). Color Reaction 2, noting that a different exergonic reaction is coupled to a different endergonic reaction. Color the star that symbolizes the energy released during the breaking of bonds and the square labeled heat. Because some energy is dissipated as heat during every energy exchange, the products of reactions always contain less usable energy than the substrates. For this reason, the efficiency of a reaction is always less than 100%. Compare this figure with Figure 1.9.

Adenosine triphosphate (ATP)

ATP is made up of a molecule of adenosine to which three phosphate groups are attached. The energy that is carried by ATP is stored between the bonds of its phosphate groups. The various energy-requiring functions of the body—such as muscle contraction, the absorption of nutrients, and the synthesis of cellular structures—all use the energy stored in ATP.

ADP (adenosine diphosphate) is produced when one terminal phosphate group of ATP is removed and AMP (adenosine monophosphate) is formed when both terminal phosphate groups of ATP are removed (Figure 1.12).

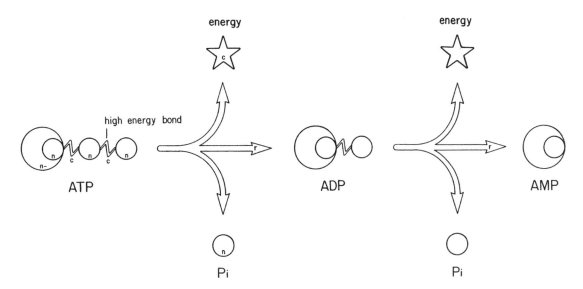

Figure 1.12   Adenosine triphosphate (ATP). Begin at the left by coloring the molecule of ATP, noting the high-energy bonds between the phosphate groups. Color the arrow at left which indicates the reaction in which ATP is broken down to adenosine diphosphate (ADP) and inorganic phosphate (Pi). Color the resulting ADP molecule, Pi molecule, and the star which symbolizes the energy released by this reaction. Color the arrow at right which indicates the reaction in which ADP is broken down to adenosine monophosphate (AMP) and Pi. Color the resulting AMP molecule, Pi molecule, and the star which symbolizes the energy released by this reaction. Adenosine is made up of a molecule of adenine (a purine) bound to a molecule of ribose (a five-carbon sugar).

Role of ATP as an energy carrier

The standard free energy change ($\Delta G°$) is −7.3 kcal/mol for the reaction in which ATP is broken down to ADP and Pi, and − 6.7 kcal/mol for the reaction in which ADP is broken down to AMP and Pi. Because of these large, negative values for $\Delta G°$, the terminal phosphate bonds of ATP are said to be high-energy bonds.

As a specific example, ATP, acting as a common intermediate, serves as a carrier of chemical energy between very high-energy phosphate compounds, such as phosphocreatine ($\Delta G° = -10.3$ kcal/mol), and low-energy phosphate compounds, such as glucose 6-phosphate ($\Delta G° = -3.3$ kcal/mol) (Figure 1.13).

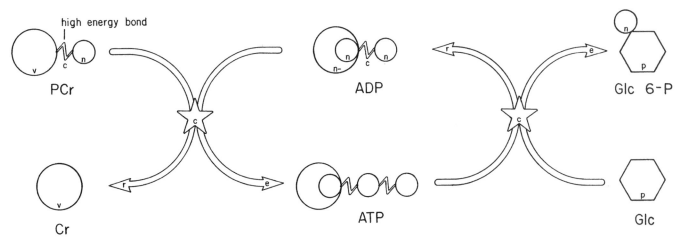

Figure 1.13   Role of ATP as an energy carrier. Color the molecule of phosphocreatine (PCr), noting its high-energy bond. Color the downward arrow of the first reaction (at left) in which PCr is broken down to free creatine (Cr) and phosphate (Pi), the star that symbolizes the energy released by this reaction, and the arrow of the coupled reaction in which this energy is used to make ATP from ADP and Pi. Color the molecules of Cr, ADP, and ATP. Color the upward arrow of the second reaction (at right) in which ATP is broken down to ADP and Pi, the star that symbolizes the energy released by this reaction, and the arrow of the coupled reaction in which this energy is used to make glucose 6-phosphate (Glc 6-P) from glucose (Glc) and phosphate. Color the molecules of glucose and glucose 6-phosphate. Compare this figure with Figure 1.11, noting that ATP acts as a common intermediate between a very high-energy phosphate donor (phosphocreatine) and a low-energy phosphate acceptor (glucose).

Activation energy

Reactions require the input of a certain amount of energy to initiate them. This energy is called the *activation energy,* and it can be viewed as an energy barrier that a molecule of sub-strate must overcome before it can enter its reaction (Figure 1.14). For this reason, the magnitude of the activation energy is an important determinant of the rate at which a particular reaction actually proceeds.

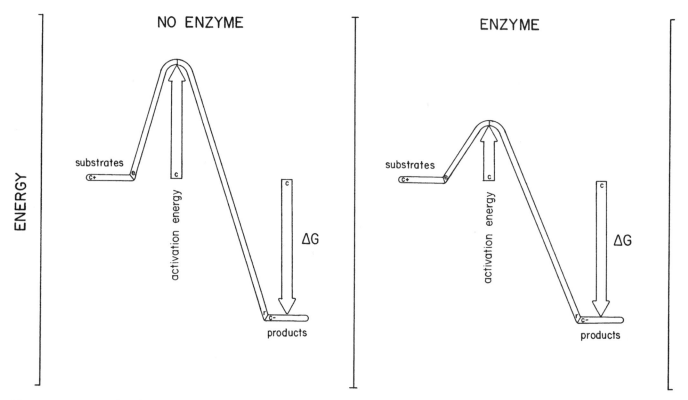

Figure 1.14 Activation energy. Color each panel, noting that the activation energy can be regarded as an energy barrier that must be overcome before a reaction can proceed down its free energy gradient. Color the upward arrows that indicate the magnitude of the activation energy and the downward arrows that indicate the magnitude of the free energy change associated with the reaction (ΔG). Note that enzymes (right panel) lower the activation energy, and thereby increase the rates of the reactions they catalyze, but do not influence the magnitude of the free energy change (ΔG = G products − G substrates). Compare this figure with Figure 1.10.

Effect of enzymes on chemical reactions

Enzymes are proteins that function as catalysts, which are substances that increase the rate of a chemical reaction without being changed by the reaction (Figure 1.15). Enzymes contain active sites that bind with specific molecules; these active sites physically hold the substrates in positions that facilitate the reaction (Figure 1.16).

This function of enzymes lowers the activation energy and thereby greatly accelerates the reactions that they catalyze. However, enzymes do not influence the directions of reactions, the final concentrations of the substrates and products, or the free energy changes (Figure 1.14).

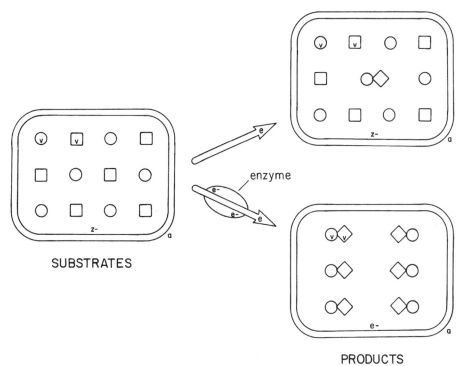

Figure 1.15   Effect of enzymes on reaction rate. Color and count the molecules of substrate, which consist of six circular and six square molecules with no bonds between them (left panel). Color the arrows that indicate the passage of the same amount of time, and the products of the reaction that occurred during this period. Observe that only one circular molecule spontaneously bonded with one square molecule in the absence of the enzyme (upper right panel). Also observe that six circular molecules bonded with six square molecules in the presence of the enzyme (lower right panel). Color the backgrounds in each condition, noting that the enzyme greatly accelerated the reaction.

SUBSTRATES

PRODUCTS

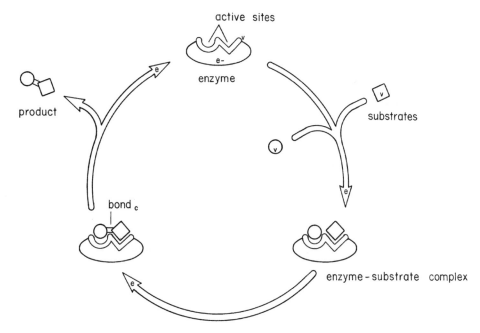

Figure 1.16   Enzyme function. Color the enzyme and its active sites, noting that the shapes of the active sites precisely match those of the substrates. Proceed in a clockwise direction, coloring the arrow, substrates, and the enzyme-substrate complex that is formed when the substrates occupy their specific sites on the enzyme. Observe that the enzyme brings the substrates in close proximity so they can form a bond. Continue clockwise, noting the bond formed between the two substrate molecules. Color the final arrow and the product of the reaction, noting that the unoccupied active sites on the enzyme enable it to catalyze another reaction. In this way, enzymes increase the rates of chemical reactions without being changed by them. Compare this figure with Figure 1.15.

Enzyme kinetics

Enzyme function can be studied by examining the effects of substrate concentration on reaction rate. At a fixed enzyme concentration, reaction rates increase with increasing substrate concentration until they reach a maximum velocity (designated by V_{max}).

Once a reaction has attained its maximum velocity, further increases in substrate concentration no longer accelerate the reaction (Figure 1.17). The reason for this leveling off of reaction velocity is that very high substrate concentrations saturate all of the available binding sites of the enzyme (Figure 1.16).

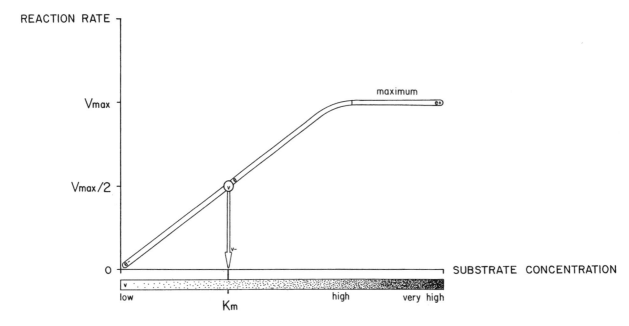

Figure 1.17   Enzyme kinetics. Color the line that shows that the rate of an enzyme-catalyzed reaction increases with increasing substrate concentration until it reaches a maximum value (V_{max}). Color the horizontal band beneath the x-axis that indicates substrate concentration. Note that K_m (the Michaelis constant, a measure of enzyme function) corresponds to the substrate concentration for which the reaction rate is half the maximum velocity, $V_{max}/2$. Compare this figure with Figure 1.16.

Effect of temperature on reaction rates

Rates of biological reactions increase with increasing temperature because higher temperatures cause a greater number of molecules to have sufficient kinetic energy to overcome the activation energy barrier (Figure 1.14). However, since very high temperatures can change the shapes of enzymes (which are proteins) through a process called denaturation, further increases in temperature ultimately inactivate enzymes and cause reaction rates to decline (Figure 1.18).

The Q_{10} effect

The effect of temperature on a chemical reaction can be studied by changing the temperature at which the reaction takes place. The relative extent to which a reaction rate increases when the temperature is raised by 10°C is known as the *Q_{10} effect.* It is calculated by dividing the rate at the higher temperature by the rate at the lower temperature and expressing the ratio as a dimensionless number. For example, the Q_{10} effect would be 2 if a reaction rate doubled in response to a 10°C increment in temperature.

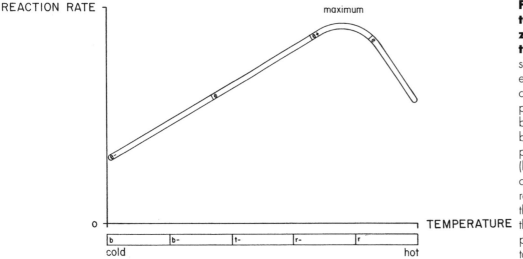

Figure 1.18   Effect of temperature on enzyme-catalyzed reactions. Color the line that shows that the rate of an enzyme-catalyzed reaction increases with increasing temperature until the enzyme begins to become inactivated by structural changes in the protein; beyond this point (labeled maximum), further increases in temperature cause reaction rates to decline. Color the horizontal band beneath the x-axis that indicates the temperature at which the reaction takes place.

chapter **two** metabolism

Exercise increases the rate at which energy is used by the body. It is the function of metabolism to provide this energy. *Metabolism* refers to the entire array of enzyme-catalyzed reactions in which energy sources are stored, mobilized, and utilized. The reactions may occur in specific sequences, so that the product of one reaction is the substrate (raw material) for the next; sequential reactions form a metabolic pathway (Figure 2.1).

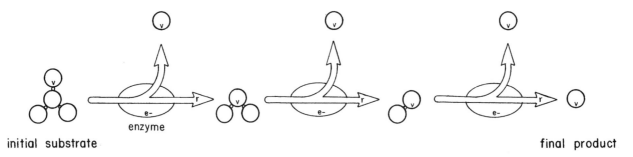

initial substrate   final product

Figure 2.1   Metabolic pathway. Color the figure from left to right and identify the substrates, enzymes, and products associated with each reaction. Note that the initial substrate is converted to a product that is the substrate for the next reaction; the product of the second reaction is the substrate for the third reaction, and so on until the formation of the final product. Thus, a series of reactions forms a metabolic pathway.

Metabolic pathways govern the storage and retrieval of fuels, as well as the breakdown of these fuels with a concomitant transfer of their chemical energy into high-energy phosphate bonds in adenosine triphosphate (ATP). The various energy-requiring functions in the body can use the energy stored in ATP, regardless of the fuel from which the energy was obtained to form the high-energy bond; therefore, ATP can be regarded as the body's energy currency. For example, in working muscle the enzyme ATPase breaks the high-energy bond in ATP, making its energy available for muscle contraction (Figure 2.2).

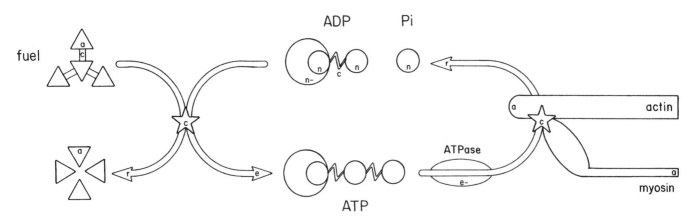

Figure 2.2   Energy transfer from fuel to muscle. Color the catabolic reaction at left in which a more complex molecule of fuel is broken down into its subunits (triangles), the star that symbolizes the energy released by this reaction, and the coupled reaction in which this energy is used to form ATP from ADP and inorganic phosphate (Pi). Color the reaction at right in which ATP is broken down into ADP and Pi, the star that symbolizes the energy that is released by this reaction, and the coupled reaction in which this energy is used for muscle contraction, as indicated by the interaction between the actin and myosin filaments. Thus, it is the high-energy bonds of ATP that supply the energy for muscle contraction. Note that the enzyme ATPase catalyzes the reaction in which ATP is broken down into ADP and Pi; the activity of this enzyme therefore regulates the rate of energy release from ATP breakdown. Compare this figure with Figure 1.13.

Anabolism and catabolism

Anabolism is the term used for metabolic processes that build compounds (e.g., synthesis of proteins from amino acids); anabolism requires an input of energy. *Catabolism* is the term used for metabolic processes that break down compounds (e.g., degradation of glucose to CO_2 and H_2O); catabolism causes the release of energy. Anabolic and catabolic reactions may be coupled so that the energy released from the catabolic reaction is used to drive the anabolic reaction (Figure 2.3).

Energy sources

The major sources of energy in the body are carbohydrates, fats, and proteins. They are provided by food and are therefore classified as *nutrients*. Nutrients must be digested and absorbed into the body in order to be used by cells. The amount of energy that can be extracted from a nutrient by the body is called its energy value and is expressed in units of calories or joules.

Carbohydrates, fats, and proteins can serve as fuels because the energy contained in their carbon-to-hydrogen bonds can be released by enzymes in a controlled, stepwise fashion. Metabolic pathways extract the energy held by the original bonds and use it to make ATP by forming a high-energy bond between ADP and phosphate.

Structure of carbohydrates

In the diet, carbohydrate is found as sugar, starch, and dietary fiber. All types of carbohydrate have chemical formulas in which the ratio of hydrogen (H) to oxygen (O) is 2:1. Carbohydrates are comprised of subunits called *monosaccharides,* which is the form of carbohydrate that is not further digested. The main monosaccharides in the diet are glucose (Figure 2.4), fructose, and galactose.

Disaccharides

Disaccharides are formed when pairs of monosaccharides are linked together by condensation. *Condensation* is the process in which OH is removed from one of the reactants and H is removed from the other at the sites where the two will be linked, thereby releasing a molecule of H_2O (Figure 2.5). The main disaccharides in the diet are sucrose, lactose, and maltose; sucrose (table sugar) is consumed in far greater quantities than the other disaccharides. Sucrose is comprised of glucose plus fructose; lactose is comprised of glucose plus galactose; and maltose is comprised of glucose plus glucose.

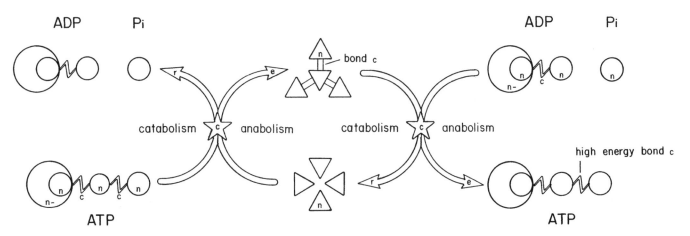

Figure 2.3   Anabolism and catabolism. Color the first catabolic reaction (at left) in which ATP is broken down into ADP plus inorganic phosphate (Pi), the star that symbolizes the energy released by this reaction, and the coupled anabolic reaction in which this energy is used to build the larger, more complex molecule from its subunits (triangles). Color the second catabolic reaction (at right) in which this molecule is broken down into its subunits, the star that symbolizes the energy released by this reaction, and the coupled anabolic reaction in which this energy is used to make ATP by forming a high-energy bond between ADP and Pi. Observe that the energy released by catabolic reactions can be used to drive anabolic reactions that are coupled to them. Note that heat loss is neglected in the hypothetical reactions shown. Compare this figure with Figure 1.11.

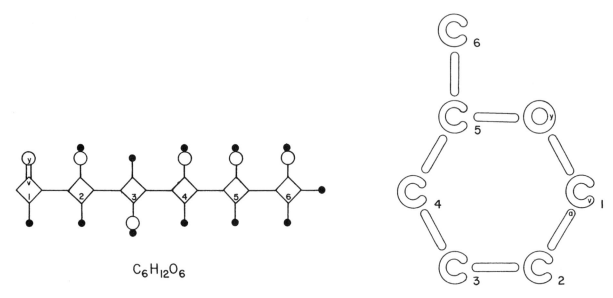

$$C_6 H_{12} O_6$$

Figure 2.4   Structure of glucose. Color the structure at left that depicts glucose as a linear molecule made up of carbon atoms (diamonds); the first carbon at the left (carbon number 1) has a double bond to oxygen (open circle), whereas all other carbons are bonded to hydroxyl (OH) groups and hydrogen atoms (filled circles). Color and compare the structure on the right that depicts glucose as a six-sided ring formed by five carbons and one oxygen; carbon number 6 is outside of the ring (hydrogen atoms and hydroxyl groups are not shown). Note the numbering of the carbons. Glucose is found in nature as a ring structure.

Polysaccharides

Polysaccharides are large, complex molecules that consist of many units of monosaccharides linked together by condensation to form straight or branched chains. Starch is a polysaccharide made by plant cells from units of glucose. Glycogen is a polysaccharide made by animal cells from units of glucose (Figure 2.10). Although both of these polysaccharides can be digested and absorbed, only starch is consumed in the diet in sufficiently large quantities to serve as a major energy source.

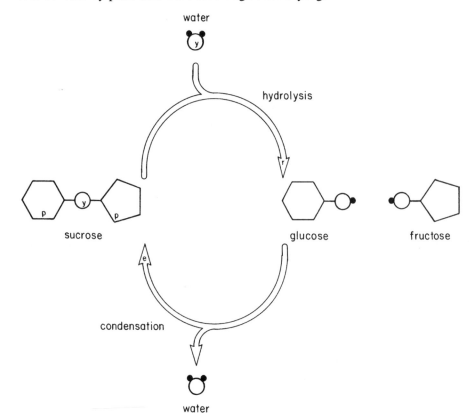

Figure 2.5   Conversions between monosaccharides and disaccharides. Color the disaccharide sucrose and its constituent monosaccharides, glucose and fructose. Although both monosaccharides have six carbons, in glucose five carbons form a six-sided ring with oxygen (Figure 2.4), whereas in fructose four carbons form a five-sided ring with oxygen (details of structures not shown). Observe that sucrose is broken down to glucose plus fructose by hydrolysis, a process in which a molecule of water is added across the bond between them. Note that the water molecule is divided into a hydroxyl group (OH) and a hydrogen atom (H), with the hydroxyl group going to one side of the broken bond and the hydrogen atom joining the oxygen atom on the other side, thereby forming one complete molecule of glucose and one complete molecule of fructose. The reverse process (condensation, arrow at bottom) occurs when glucose and fructose bond to form sucrose in a process in which water is removed at the site where the bond is formed.

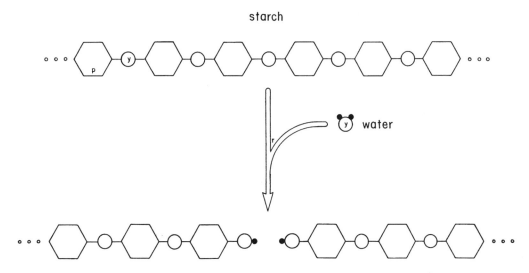

starch

water

Figure 2.6   Digestion of starch. Color the chain of glucose molecules that comprise starch and the shorter chains of glucose molecules that result from hydrolysis; note that the water molecule is divided between the products as shown in Figure 2.5. This reaction, which is catalyzed by enzymes in the mouth (salivary amylase) and small intestine (pancreatic amylase), continues until starch is broken down to maltose (Figure 2.7).

Plants also synthesize a variety of indigestible polysaccharides; these are components of the plant's structure known as *dietary fiber*. Since dietary fiber is not digested and absorbed, it does not serve as an energy source to humans (Figure 3.15); however, its presence in the gastrointestinal tract has been shown to have health-promoting effects.

Digestion and absorption of carbohydrate

In the gastrointestinal (GI) tract the polysaccharide starch is digested to glucose in a series of reactions. Starch is first hydrolyzed to smaller chains of glucose in the mouth and stomach by the enzyme salivary amylase (Figure 2.6); *hydrolysis* is the reverse of the process of condensation since H_2O is added at the site where the bond is to be broken. In the small intestine, pancreatic amylase hydrolyzes starch into units of the disaccharide maltose (Figure 2.7). Maltose is then digested by the enzyme maltase to two units of glucose (Figure 2.5); maltose consumed in the diet is also digested by maltase to two units of glucose.

Lactose and sucrose are hydrolyzed in the intestine by their respective enzymes, lactase and sucrase, into their constituent monosaccharides. Thus, the final digestion products of all dietary carbohydrates are the monosaccharides glucose, fructose, and galactose.

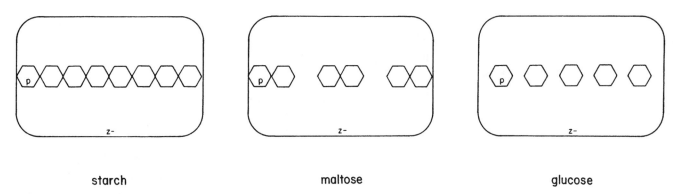

starch   maltose   glucose

Figure 2.7   Stages of starch digestion. Beginning at the left panel, color the original starch molecule (oxygen and hydrogen atoms not shown), then maltose, which is produced by hydrolysis of starch by salivary amylase and pancreatic amylase, and finally glucose (hexagon), which is produced by hydrolysis of maltose by the intestinal enzyme maltase. Note that glucose is the end product of starch digestion.

Glucose, fructose, and galactose in the intestinal lumen of the GI tract enter the mucosal cells which form the lining of the intestine. They pass through and exit the intestinal cells into blood vessels that transport the monosaccharides to the liver (via the portal vein) before they enter the general circulation (Figure 2.8). Although galactose and fructose are absorbed from the diet, they are virtually absent from the general circulation because they are converted to other compounds (mainly glucose) by the liver. For this reason, glucose is the only form of dietary carbohydrate that reaches all cells.

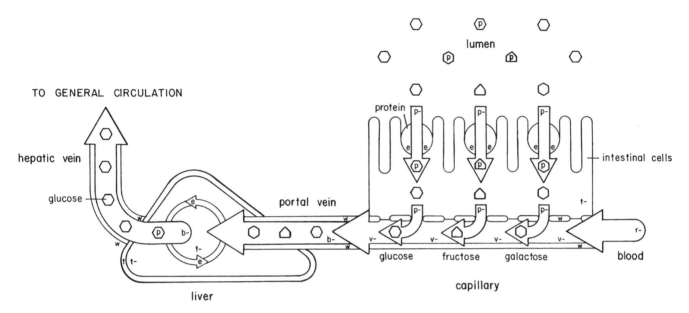

Figure 2.8   Absorption of monosaccharides into the blood. Color and identify the final products of carbohydrate diges-tion—glucose (hexagon), fructose (pentagon), and galactose (rotated hexagon)—which are in the intestinal lumen. Follow the entry of each of these monosaccharides into the intestinal cells by facilitated diffusion and color the corresponding transport proteins. Color the blood supply to the intestinal mucosal cells, the arrows that depict the passage of monosaccharides into the capillary, and their transport to the liver via the portal vein. Observe that fructose and galactose are converted to glucose in the liver. Color the blood leaving the liver via the hepatic vein, noting that glucose is the only form of carbohydrate that enters the general circulation.

Glucose uptake by cells

Cells take up glucose from the blood by *facilitated diffusion,* a process that utilizes transport proteins that span the cell membrane (Figure 2.9). In muscle and adipose tissue, glu-cose uptake is stimulated by the hormone insulin, which causes more glucose transport proteins to migrate to the cell membrane. This mechanism enables muscle and adipose tis-sue to take up more glucose when blood levels of insulin rise after a meal.

Muscle contraction itself increases facilitated diffusion of glucose into muscle, even in the absence of stimulation by in-sulin (Figure 7.23). This mechanism enables working muscle to take up glucose from the blood even though insulin levels fall during exercise.

Once glucose is inside the cell, it receives a phosphate group from ATP to become glucose 6-phosphate (Figure 2.9); this process is called *phosphorylation*. Phosphorylation not only activates glucose for entry into metabolic pathways but it also prevents glucose from leaving the cell.

Glycogen

Glucose is stored in animal cells as the polysaccharide glyco-gen; breakdown of glycogen provides a readily available source of glucose. *Glycogen* is a large molecule made of a chain of glucose that branches frequently, providing many ends where glucose can be added or removed (Figure 2.10). This feature of glycogen's structure permits the processes of glycogen synthesis and glycogen breakdown to proceed rapidly. Skeletal muscle and liver are the main sites of glyco-gen storage in the body.

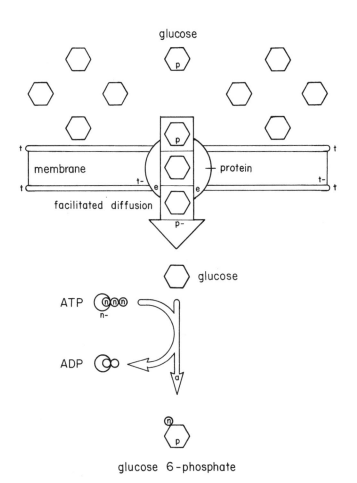

glucose

membrane — protein

facilitated diffusion

glucose

ATP

ADP

glucose 6-phosphate

Figure 2.9   Glucose uptake by cells. Color the glucose molecules in the extracellular space (above the cell membrane), the hatched arrow depicting the entry of glucose into the cell by facilitated diffusion (ignore hatches when coloring), and the transport protein in the cell membrane. A number of different glucose transporters (GLUT), specific to certain tissues, have been identified. For example, GLUT4 is a transport protein found in skeletal muscle (Figure 7.23). Color the phosphorylation of glucose in the cytoplasm, a reaction in which glucose receives a phosphate group on carbon number 6 (Figure 2.4) when ATP is broken down to ADP and Pi. The resulting molecule of glucose 6-phosphate cannot diffuse out of the cell.

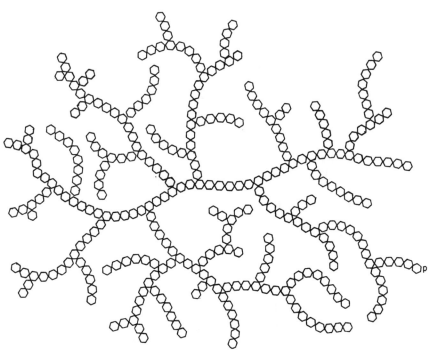

Figure 2.10.   Structure of glycogen. Color the many units of glucose that comprise glycogen (oxygen and hydrogen atoms not shown). Note that the large molecule branches repeatedly; units of glucose can be added to or removed from the ends of its many branches simultaneously.

Glycogen synthesis

Glycogen is a compound that has a variable size. A molecule of glycogen becomes larger when units of glucose are added to it after a meal and smaller when units of glucose are removed from it, as can occur during exercise.

Glucose must be converted to a suitable higher-energy form before it is added to glycogen. In the process of *glycogen* *synthesis* (also called glycogenesis), glucose is first converted to glucose 6-phosphate (Figure 2.9); the phosphate group is moved to carbon number 1 (Figure 2.4) and then replaced by UDP (uridine diphosphate), thereby forming UDP-glucose (Figure 2.11). UDP-glucose is a high-energy compound, and breakage of the bond between UDP and glucose provides the energy needed to add glucose to the end of one of the many branches of an existing glycogen molecule (Figure 2.10).

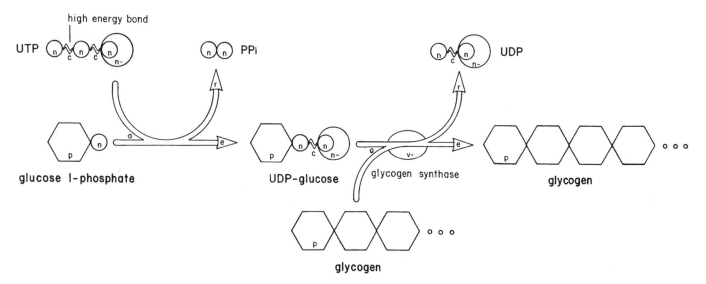

Figure 2.11   Glycogen synthesis. Color the molecules of glucose 1-phosphate (formed from glucose 6-phosphate) and UTP (uridine triphosphate), and the reaction in which UTP loses two phosphates (PPi) and combines with glucose 1-phosphate to form UDP-glucose. Color the subsequent removal of UDP, and the bonding of glucose to another glucose unit at the end of a branch of the glycogen molecule. The addition of glucose to glycogen is catalyzed by the enzyme glycogen synthase; the activity of this enzyme therefore regulates the rate of glycogen synthesis.

The enzyme glycogen synthase catalyzes the addition of glucose to glycogen. Storage of glucose as glycogen can be controlled by increasing or decreasing the activity of this enzyme. After a meal, elevated blood levels of the hormone insulin increase the activity of glycogen synthase, thereby promoting the synthesis of glycogen in liver and muscle.

Glycogenolysis

When the need for glucose increases, such as during exercise or long after a meal, units of glucose are removed from the ends of the many branches of glycogen molecules. This process is called *glycogenolysis* (lysis means splitting).

The enzyme glycogen phosphorylase removes glucose molecules from glycogen by phosphorolysis, the process in which phosphate is added across a bond, thereby breaking the bond (Figure 2.12). This reaction produces units of glucose 1-phosphate, which are rapidly converted to units of glucose 6-phosphate. Glucose 6-phosphate can enter the pathway of glycolysis (see below) or, in the case of the liver but not muscle, can have its phosphate group removed to become free glucose, which can leave the liver cell and enter the blood (Figure 2.13). Thus, liver glycogen, but not muscle glycogen, can serve as a source of blood glucose.

Glycogen phosphorylase activity is stimulated during exercise or in a state of hypoglycemia (low blood glucose concentration). Neural, hormonal, and intracellular signals increase the enzyme's activity and thereby stimulate glycogen breakdown. Stimulation of glycogen phosphorylase activity in muscle provides glucose to be used as a fuel within muscle whereas in liver it supplies glucose to the blood.

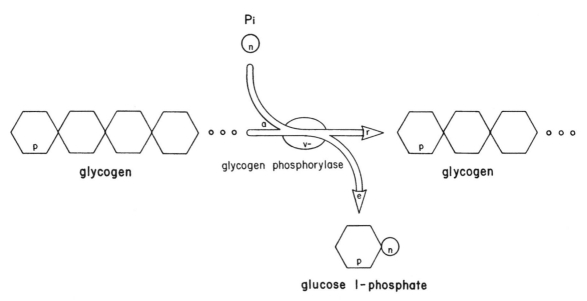

Figure 2.12 Glycogenolysis. Color the end segment of a branch of a glycogen molecule and the arrow depicting the process of phosphorolysis in which phosphate (Pi) is added to carbon number 1 of the glucose unit at the left end of the glycogen molecule, thereby breaking its bond to the next glucose unit. When glucose is removed as glucose 1-phosphate, the glycogen molecule is made smaller by one unit of glucose. This reaction is catalyzed by the enzyme glycogen phosphorylase; the activity of this enzyme therefore regulates the rate of glycogen breakdown.

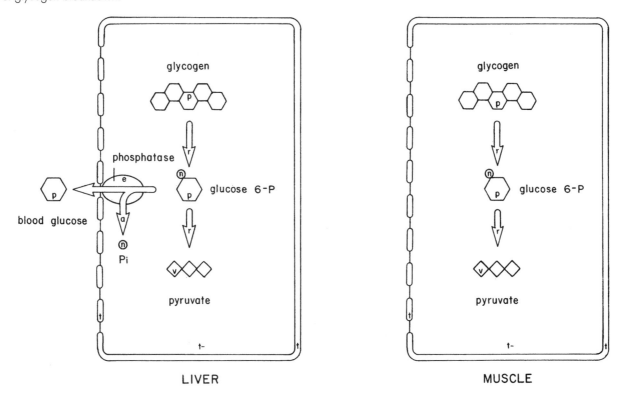

Figure 2.13 Glycogenolysis in liver and muscle. In both panels, color the glycogen molecules at the top, the downward arrows indicating glycogenolysis, and the units of glucose 6-phosphate produced. Color the downward arrows that indicate glycolysis and the molecules of pyruvate formed (hydrogen and oxygen atoms not shown). Color the reaction in liver in which the enzyme glucose 6-phosphatase removes the phosphate group to produce free glucose, which can then leave the cell and enter the blood (left panel). Contrast this with the situation in muscle in which glucose 6-phosphate can only enter glycolysis because muscle does not have the enzyme needed to remove the phosphate group from glucose 6-phosphate (right panel). For this reason, liver glycogen can serve as a source of blood glucose but muscle glycogen cannot.

Glycolysis

Glycolysis is a catabolic pathway that operates in the cytoplasm of all cells. Glycolysis breaks down glucose to two molecules of pyruvic acid in a series of reactions that do not require oxygen (Figure 2.14). Reactions or pathways that can operate in the absence of oxygen are termed *anaerobic;* those

requiring oxygen are termed *aerobic.* Glycolysis is the only energy-yielding (ATP-producing) anaerobic pathway; since glucose is the substrate of glycolysis, it is only fuel that can be metabolized anaerobically. For this reason, anaerobic metabolism is associated with higher rates of glucose utilization and glycogen depletion.

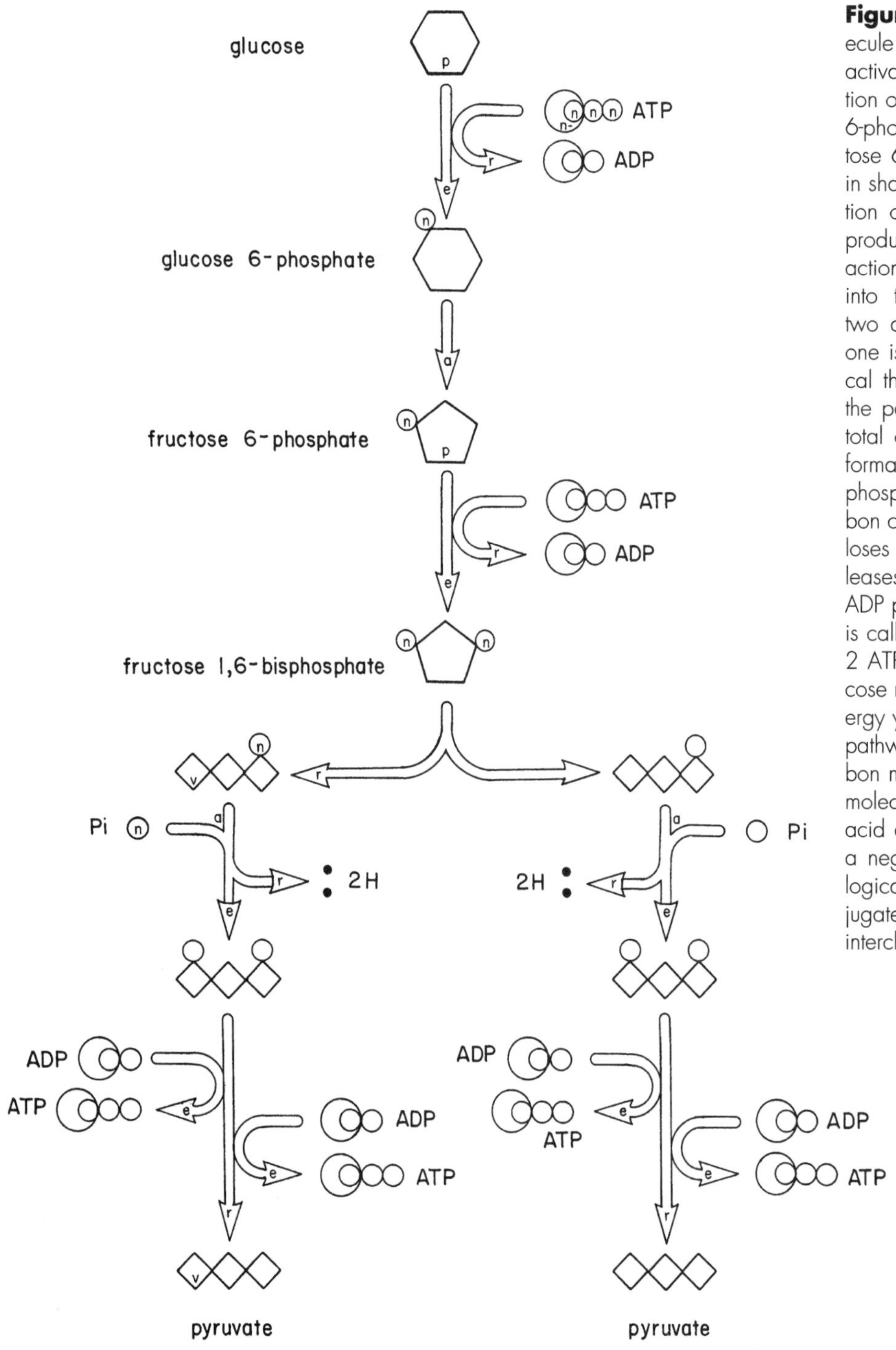

Figure 2.14   Glycolysis. Color the molecule of glucose and the reaction in which it is activated for entry into glycolysis by the addition of phosphate from ATP to become glucose 6-phosphate. Color the reaction in which fructose 6-phosphate is formed, noting its change in shape. Color the reaction in which the addition of a second phosphate group from ATP produces fructose 1,6-bisphosphate and the reaction in which this six-carbon compound splits into two three-carbon compounds (although two different compounds are initially formed, one isomerizes to the other so that two identical three-carbon compounds continue through the pathway). Color the series of reactions (a total of five steps) that ultimately leads to the formation of pyruvate. Note that a second phosphate group is added to each three-carbon compound; each of these compounds then loses a pair of hydrogen atoms (2H) and releases enough energy to form 2 ATP from 2 ADP plus 2 Pi, for a total of 4 ATP; this process is called substrate level phosphorylation. Since 2 ATP are required for activation of each glucose molecule, 2 ATP per glucose is the net energy yield within the pathway. In summary, the pathway of glycolysis breaks down one six-carbon molecule of glucose into two three-carbon molecules of pyruvic acid. Because pyruvic acid dissociates into a hydrogen ion (H+) and a negatively-charged anion at normal physiological pH, the term pyruvate (actually the conjugate base of the acid) can be used interchangeably with pyruvic acid.

Glucose enters glycolysis as glucose 6-phosphate, which may be formed when glucose enters the cell (Figure 2.9) or as a product of glycogenolysis (Figure 2.12). Glucose 6-phosphate, in successive enzyme-catalyzed steps, is changed in shape and receives a second phosphate group from ATP to become fructose 1,6-bisphosphate (Figure 2.14). This compound is cleaved to form two interconvertible three-carbon compounds. Each of these compounds is converted to the three-carbon compound pyruvic acid in a series of reactions in which electrons are removed.

Oxidation and reduction

The process in which electrons are removed is called *oxidation,* and the process in which electrons are added is called *reduction* (Figure 2.15). In the pathways of fuel metabolism, oxidation removes an entire hydrogen atom (one proton plus one electron) because the proton from the hydrogen atom follows the electron that is removed. During oxidation, there-

fore, hydrogen atoms (electrons plus protons) are removed from the substrate of the reaction and are picked up by hydrogen carriers, such as nicotinamide adenine dinucleotide (NAD^+) and flavin adenine dinucleotide (FAD). When NAD^+ receives a pair of hydrogen atoms, it becomes $NADH + H^+$; when FAD receives a pair of hydrogen atoms it becomes $FADH_2$ (Figure 2.16). $NADH + H^+$ and $FADH_2$ are called the reduced forms of NAD^+ and FAD, respectively.

NAD^+ and FAD are examples of *coenzymes,* which are organic compounds that assist enzymes in reactions. Many coenzymes are synthesized from vitamins, which are necessary organic compounds that must be obtained from the diet because they are not synthesized in adequate amounts by the body. NAD^+ is made from the vitamin niacin and FAD is made from the vitamin riboflavin. Deficient intakes of vitamins can lead to decreased production of their respective coenzymes and, therefore, to impaired function of metabolic pathways.

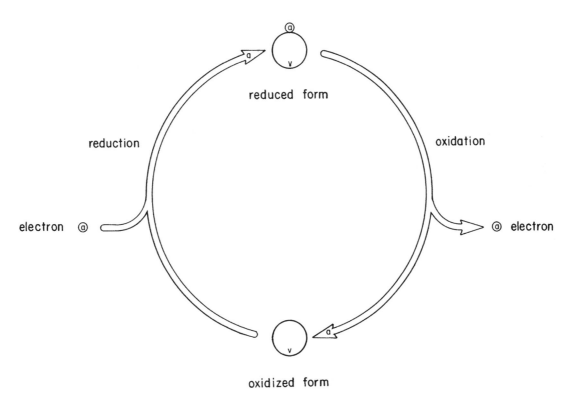

reduced form

reduction

oxidation

electron @

@ electron

oxidized form

Figure 2.15 Oxidation and reduction. Color the reaction (at left) representing the addition of an electron, which is the process of reduction. Note that the product of this reaction is referred to as the reduced form of the original compound. Color the reaction (at right) representing the removal of an electron, which is the process of oxidation. Note that the product of this reaction is referred to as the oxidized form of the compound. Observe that oxidation and reduction are reactions that can be coupled to each other, i.e., electrons that are removed when one compound is oxidized can be used to reduce another compound.

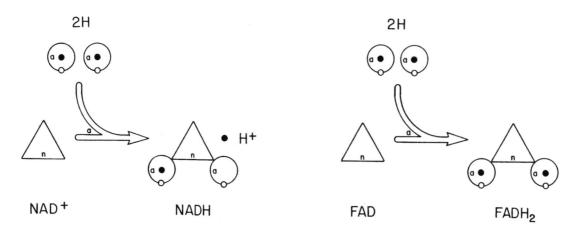

Figure 2.16   Hydrogen carriers. Observe that the coenzymes NAD⁺ (left panel) and FAD (right panel) can each carry two hydrogen atoms (two electrons plus two protons). Color the oxidized forms of the coenzymes (NAD⁺ and FAD), hydrogen atoms (2H), the arrows representing the addition of hydrogen atoms (reduction), and the reduced forms of the coenzymes (NADH + H⁺ and $FADH_2$). Since NAD⁺ has a positive charge, the compound formed by addition of two uncharged hydrogen atoms, NADH + H⁺, is still positively charged. These coenzymes pick up and transport pairs of hydrogen atoms that are released by catabolic pathways, such as glycolysis (Figure 2.17) and the Krebs cycle (Figure 2.18).

Production of NADH + H⁺ in glycolysis

In glycolysis, the oxidation of each of the three-carbon compounds formed from glucose yields a pair of hydrogen atoms that are picked up by NAD⁺, thereby converting it to NADH + H⁺. In total, 2 NADH + 2H⁺ are produced for each molecule of glucose that is converted to two molecules of pyruvic acid (Figure 2.14).

In order for glycolysis to continue, NADH + H⁺ must be recycled to NAD⁺ so that it can pick up more hydrogen atoms that are removed during the operation of the pathway. NAD⁺ can be regenerated either by donating its hydrogen atoms to pyruvic acid (a reaction that takes place in the cytoplasm and does not require oxygen) or by donating its hydrogen atoms to the electron transport chain (a process that takes place in the mitochondria and does require oxygen).

Anaerobic glycolysis

In *anaerobic glycolysis,* NADH + H⁺ is recycled to NAD⁺ by donating its pair of hydrogen atoms to pyruvic acid which then becomes lactic acid (Figure 2.17); this permits glycolysis to continue under anaerobic conditions. The conversion of pyruvate to lactate is catalyzed by the enzyme lactate dehydrogenase (LDH).

Anaerobic glycolysis is a major source of ATP for fast-twitch skeletal muscle fibers that are recruited during high-intensity exercise. Lactate that is produced under these conditions can be metabolized aerobically by cardiac and slow-twitch skeletal muscle fibers or be converted to other compounds such as glucose or amino acids.

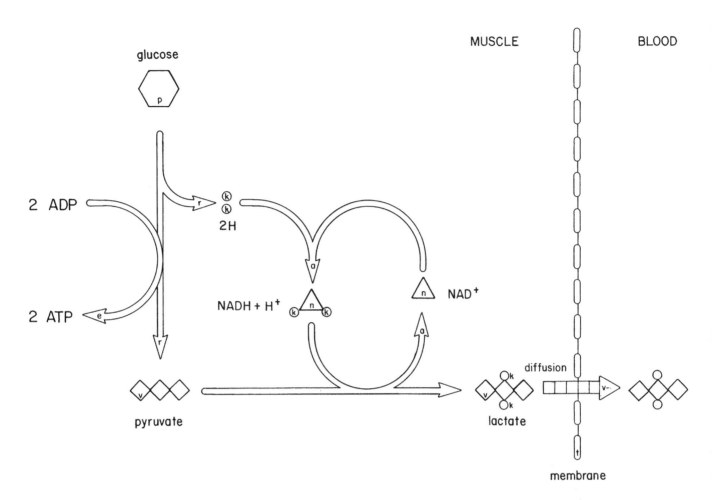

Figure 2.17   Anaerobic glycolysis. Color the arrows depicting the conversion of glucose to pyruvate in the pathway of glycolysis in the cytoplasm. Note that 2ATP and two pairs of hydrogen atoms (open circles) are produced from each molecule of glucose. Observe that each pair of hydrogen atoms (2H) is picked up by NAD^+ to form $NADH + H^+$. Color the reaction in which the transfer of this pair of hydrogen atoms to pyruvate forms lactate, noting that lactate differs from pyruvate by the addition of these two hydrogen atoms. Note also that the terms pyruvate and lactate refer to the conjugate bases of pyruvic acid and lactic acid, respectively. Observe that NAD^+ is regenerated in the process so that it can return to the pathway of glycolysis and pick up another pair of hydrogen atoms. For this reason, the formation of lactic acid enables glycolysis to continue. Anaerobic glycolysis refers to the operation of glycolysis under conditions in which the regeneration of NAD^+ occurs through the production of lactic acid. Color the hatched arrow that shows the diffusion of lactate out of the muscle fiber and into the blood. The removal of lactate from the cell also promotes glycolysis by preventing the buildup of pyruvate (end product) that would otherwise inhibit the pathway by the law of mass action.

Krebs cycle

Carbohydrates, fats, and proteins can all be converted to compounds that can enter the *Krebs cycle* (also known as the citric acid cycle or the tricarboxylic acid cycle). The Krebs cycle (Figure 2.18), which takes place in the mitochondria, is considered to be an aerobic pathway because its operation requires a continuous supply of oxygen.

Acetyl CoA is the major substrate entering the Krebs cycle; other substrates can enter at later steps in the pathway. Acetyl CoA consists of a two-carbon acetyl group bound to coenzyme A (which is derived from the vitamin pantothenic acid).

Pyruvic acid is converted to acetyl CoA in the mitochondria by the removal of CO_2 and the addition of coenzyme A. Acetyl CoA can also be formed from the breakdown of fatty acids (Figure 2.35) and amino acids (Figure 2.40). When acetyl CoA enters the Krebs cycle, the acetyl group attaches to oxaloacetic acid, which is a four-carbon compound, and forms citric acid, a six-carbon compound. Citric acid undergoes a series of oxidations during which two carbons are released as CO_2, and oxaloacetic acid is regenerated upon completion of each cycle of the pathway.

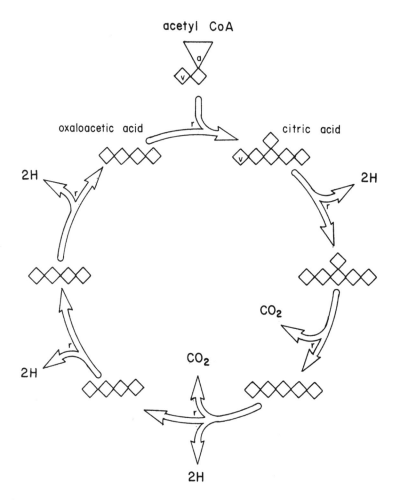

acetyl CoA

oxaloacetic acid

citric acid

2H

2H

CO_2

CO_2

2H

2H

Figure 2.18   Krebs cycle. Color the molecule of acetyl CoA and the reaction in which its two-carbon acetyl group combines with a four-carbon molecule of oxaloacetic acid to form a six-carbon molecule of citric acid (note that coenzyme A is removed). Color the compounds in the cycle and count the number of carbons in each. Note that the cycle has been simplified by omitting four steps (e.g., isomerizations) in which no hydrogen atoms (oxidation) or CO_2 molecules are removed. Observe that four pairs of hydrogen atoms are removed and that two molecules of CO_2 are released with each turn of the cycle; completion of the cycle is marked by regeneration of oxaloacetic acid.

In the Krebs cycle, oxidation occurs at four different steps in the pathway where pairs of hydrogen atoms are picked up by the coenzymes NAD^+ and FAD so that they become $NADH + H^+$ and $FADH_2$, respectively (Figure 2.19). The hydrogen atoms are carried as $NADH + H^+$ and $FADH_2$ to the electron transport chain where the energy in the electrons is captured to make high-energy bonds in ATP.

Electron transport chain

A series of compounds that can alternately function as electron donors and electron acceptors are organized on the inner membrane of the mitochondria (Figure 2.20); they comprise the *electron transport chain*. These compounds are mainly proteins with attached metal-containing ring structures that reflect only some wavelengths of light and so have color; hence these compounds are called *cytochromes*. The components of the electron transport chain are ordered so that the

compound with the strongest tendency to give up electrons is at the beginning of the sequence and the compound with the strongest tendency to accept electrons is at the end; the initial donor of electrons is $NADH + H^+$ and the final acceptor is O_2.

Chemiosmotic-coupling mechanism

The electrons lose much of their energy as they are passed down the electron transport chain. Part of this energy is used ultimately to form ATP from ADP and phosphate; the remaining energy is dissipated as heat. The proposed mechanism for this coupling of electron transport with ATP synthesis (i.e., oxidative phosphorylation) is called the *chemiosmotic-coupling mechanism* and operates as follows (Figure 2.21).

Hydrogen atoms carried as $NADH + H^+$ and $FADH_2$ are brought to the electron transport chain, where each hydrogen atom separates into its proton and electron. Because the inner

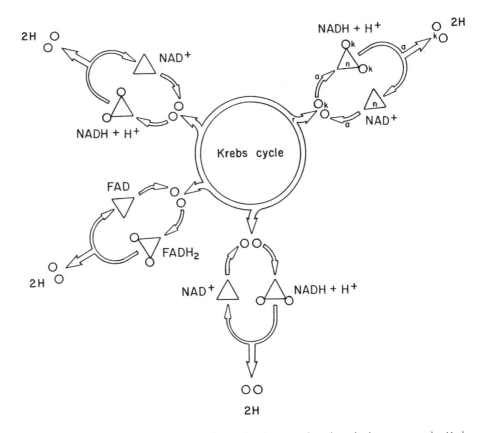

Figure 2.19   Hydrogen carriers in the Krebs cycle. Color the central circle, which represents the Krebs cycle, and its arrows, noting that the positions of the arrows correspond to the positions of similar arrows in Figure 2.18. Color the reactions in which three pairs of hydrogen atoms are picked up by NAD$^+$ and one pair of hydrogen atoms is picked up by FAD. These coenzymes transport the hydrogen atoms to the electron transport chain as NADH + H$^+$ and FADH$_2$, respectively. NAD$^+$ and FAD, which are regenerated by transferring the hydrogen atoms to the electron transport chain, can then pick up more pairs of hydrogen atoms released by the Krebs cycle. Note that for each turn of the Krebs cycle, two molecules of CO$_2$ are released, four pairs of hydrogen atoms are produced, and oxaloacetric acid is regenerated.

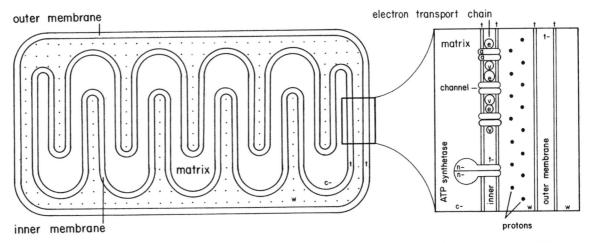

Figure 2.20   Structure of a mitochondrion. Color the inner and outer mitochondrial membranes, and the gel-like matrix surrounded by the inner membrane (left panel). Identify and color the two membranes, the matrix, and the electron transport chain in the magnification at right. Observe that the electron transport chain, which resides within the inner membrane, contains channels through which protons are actively transported from the matrix to the space between the membranes, and that this mechanism produces a high concentration of protons in the space between the inner and outer membranes. Identify the enzyme ATP synthetase, noting that it spans the inner mitochondrial membrane.

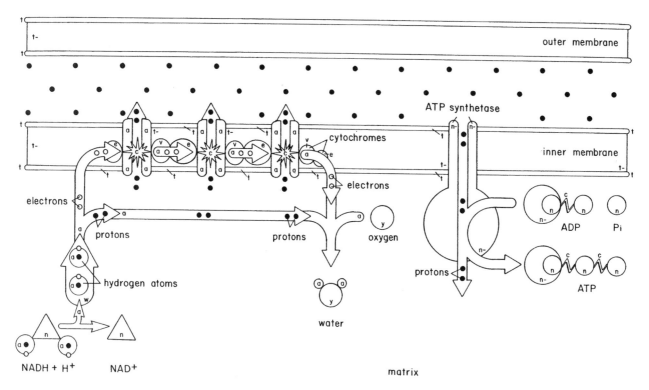

Figure 2.21   Electron transport chain. Color the membranes of the mitochondrion and note the location of the matrix, where the Krebs cycle takes place. Begin at the lower left, coloring the hydrogen atoms that are brought to the electron transport chain as part of NADH + H$^+$. Color the coenzyme molecules, the pair of hydrogen atoms that are removed, and the arrows indicating their separation into their constituent protons (filled circles) and electrons (open circles). Note that the protons initially remain on the matrix side of the membrane. Color the arrows that show the passage of electrons along the electron transport chain (from left to right in this illustration), coloring the cytochromes and the flashes that indicate the release of energy from the electrons; note that each flash causes two protons to be actively transported across the inner mitochondrial membrane. Observe that this process establishes a high density of protons in the space between the inner and outer mitochondrial membranes. Color the arrows that indicate the reuniting of electrons and protons in the matrix to form the hydrogen atoms that combine with oxygen to form water. Color the oxygen and water molecules and note that these reactions cannot proceed in the absence of oxygen because oxygen serves as the final electron acceptor. At the right, color the enzyme ATP synthetase and observe the channel through which protons pass in going down their electrochemical gradient to reenter the matrix. Observe that the energy released by the passage of one pair of protons is sufficient to synthesize one molecule of ATP from one molecule of ADP plus one molecule of Pi. Color the molecules of ATP, ADP, and Pi, noting the high-energy bonds. Observe that each pair of hydrogen atoms carried as NADH + H$^+$ yields three molecules of ATP. Each pair of hydrogen atoms carried as FADH$_2$ yields only two molecules of ATP because the electrons from these hydrogen atoms enter the electron transport chain at a point where they only transport four protons across the inner mitochondrial membrane. Compare this figure with Figure 2.20.

mitochondrial membrane is permeable to electrons but not to protons, only the electrons enter the membrane; the protons remain in the mitochondrial matrix. The electrons are passed along the chain of cytochromes, with a release of energy at each transfer. At three sites in the chain, the energy that is released is used to transport two protons (H$^+$) across the inner mitochondrial membrane into the space between the inner and outer mitochondrial membranes. The resultant accumulation of protons between the two membranes produces both a chemical gradient (due to the difference in the concentration of particles on the two sides of the membrane) and an electrical gradient (due to the difference in the density of positive charges) across the inner membrane. The resulting electrochemical gradient provides the driving force that causes protons to reenter the matrix through a channel within the enzyme ATP synthetase. The energy released as each pair of protons passes through the channel is used to make ATP from ADP and phosphate.

After passing through the electron transport chain, the electrons reunite with protons in the matrix to form hydrogen atoms, which then combine with oxygen to form H$_2$O. Thus, the function of oxygen in aerobic metabolism is to accept hydrogen at the end of the electron transport chain.

Dependence of the Krebs cycle on oxygen

The operation of the electron transport chain requires a continuous supply of oxygen. Because the activity of the Krebs cycle is tightly coupled to that of the electron transport chain, the cycle does not operate under anaerobic conditions. This coupling is due to the fact that NADH + H^+ and $FADH_2$ produced by the Krebs cycle can only be recycled to NAD^+ and FAD, respectively, through the action of the electron transport chain. Therefore, in the absence of oxygen the electron transport chain is not active, NAD^+ and FAD are not regenerated, and the Krebs cycle does not operate.

Aerobic glycolysis

In *aerobic glycolysis*, NADH + H^+ is recycled to NAD^+ by donating its pair of hydrogen atoms to the electron transport chain; this process requires oxygen. *Hydrogen shuttle systems* transport pairs of hydrogen atoms from the cytoplasm into the mitochondria because NADH + H^+ cannot cross the mitochondrial membranes. The two major hydrogen shuttle systems are the malate-aspartate shuttle and the α-glycerol phosphate shuttle (Figure 2.22); the first predominates in cardiac muscle and the second predominates in skeletal muscle.

NADH + H^+ in the cytoplasm transfers its pair of hydrogen atoms to another hydrogen carrier that accepts them inside the mitochondrion. The intramitochondrial hydrogen acceptor is NAD^+ for the malate-aspartate shuttle and the hydrogen acceptor is FAD for the α-glycerol phosphate shuttle. Because electrons of the hydrogen atoms carried as NADH + H^+ and $FADH_2$ enter the electron transport chain at different points (Figure 2.21), use of the malate-aspartate shuttle results in production of 3 ATP per pair of hydrogen atoms whereas use of the α-glycerol phosphate shuttle results in production of 2 ATP per pair of hydrogen atoms. This difference in hydrogen carriers explains why the complete oxidation of one molecule of glucose yields 36 ATP in skeletal muscle but 38 ATP in cardiac muscle.

Anaerobic production of ATP

The reason that anaerobic glycolysis can provide energy as ATP in the absence of oxygen, and therefore independently of the electron transport chain, is that the high-energy bond in ATP can be made within the glycolytic pathway. Through the process known as substrate level phosphorylation, a phosphate group that is removed from the substrate is transferred to ADP to form ATP. Each of the two three-carbon units derived from glucose goes through two such reactions, thereby producing 4 ATP per molecule of glucose. However, because 2 ATP are used to activate each molecule of glucose (Figure 2.14), there is a net yield of only 2 ATP per molecule of glucose in anaerobic glycolysis.

Energy yield of anaerobic and aerobic metabolism

Under anaerobic conditions NADH + H^+ produced in glycolysis donates its hydrogen atoms to pyruvic acid, thereby forming lactic acid. Under aerobic conditions, NADH + H^+ donates its hydrogen atoms to the electron transport chain, where the energy in their electrons is extracted to form ATP. For this reason, glycolysis produces more ATP under aerobic conditions than anaerobic conditions (6 vs. 2 ATP per glucose in skeletal muscle, Figure 2.22). Aerobic conditions also permit the conversion of pyruvic acid to acetyl CoA , which can then be oxidized by the Krebs cycle and electron transport chain to yield an additional amount of ATP.

In sum, aerobic metabolism of one molecule glucose produces six molecules of CO_2 and shows a net yield of 36 ATP in skeletal muscle (Figure 2.23). In contrast, anaerobic metabolism of one molecule of glucose produces two molecules of lactic acid and shows a net yield of 2 ATP. The tally for aerobic metabolism of glucose in skeletal muscle includes 2 ATP produced anaerobically in glycolysis, 4 ATP produced from aerobic processing of 2 NADH +2 H^+ formed during glycolysis, 6 ATP derived from the conversion of pyruvic acid to acetyl CoA (2 NADH + 2H^+), and 18 ATP from 6 NADH + 6H^+, 4 ATP from 2 $FADH_2$, and 2 GTP (energy equivalent to 2 ATP) generated in the Krebs cycle (Figure 2.23).

Gluconeogenesis

Plasma levels of glucose must be kept sufficiently high (nominally $\geq$ 60 mg/dL) for normal function of the central nervous system. Since exercise increases the removal of glucose from the blood by muscle, plasma glucose must be replenished to maintain normal levels. The liver supplies glucose to the blood by breaking down its glycogen stores (glycogenolysis) and by synthesizing new glucose from noncarbohydrate compounds in the energy-requiring pathway of *gluconeogenesis*.

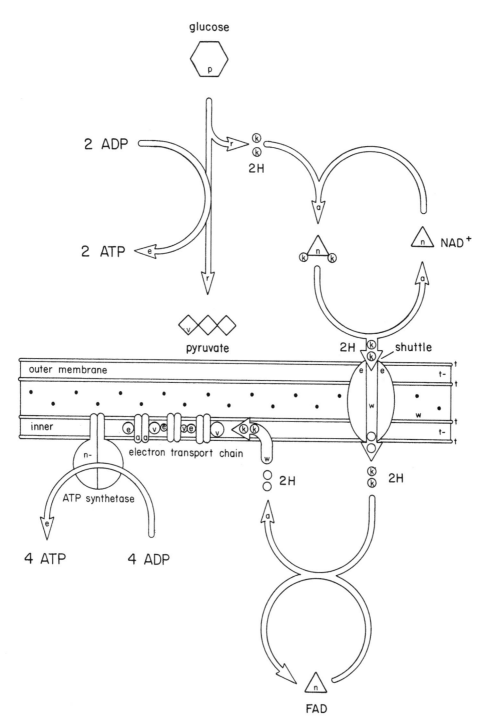

Figure 2.22   Aerobic glycolysis. Color the arrows depicting the conversion of glucose to pyruvate in the pathway of glycolysis in the cytoplasm. Note that 2 ATP and two pairs of hydrogen atoms (open circles) are produced for each molecule of glucose (Figure 2.14). Color the reaction in which a pair of hydrogen atoms (2H) is picked by NAD^+ and transferred to a hydrogen shuttle that transports them across both mitochondrial membranes and into the matrix; note that NAD^+ is regenerated in the process. Color the reaction in which the hydrogen atoms from the shuttle are picked up by FAD and transferred to the electron transport chain, noting that FAD is regenerated in the process. Color the membranes, the electron transport chain, and the molecule of ATP synthetase, noting that 4 ATP can be produced aerobically from the two pairs of hydrogen atoms that are removed during glycolysis. Thus, aerobic glycolysis yields a total of 6 ATP per molecule of glucose whereas anaerobic glycolysis yields a total of 2 ATP per molecule of glucose (Figure 2.17). In cardiac muscle, the hydrogen atoms from the shuttle system are picked up in the matrix by NAD^+, rather than FAD; the electrons from these hydrogen atoms enter the electron transport chain at a point where they can produce 6 ATP aerobically from the two pairs of hydrogen atoms that are removed during glycolysis. For this reason, aerobic glycolysis yields a total of 8 ATP per molecule of glucose in cardiac muscle but 6 ATP per molecule of glucose in skeletal muscle.

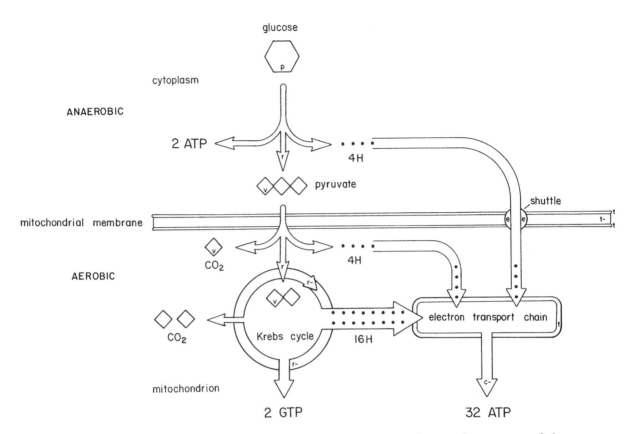

Figure 2.23   Anaerobic and aerobic production of ATP. Color the arrows depicting the conversion of glucose to pyruvate in the pathway of glycolysis, noting that 2 ATP (net yield) are produced anaerobically in the cytoplasm. Observe that four hydrogen atoms (4H, filled circles) are removed during glycolysis. Color the reaction in which each of the two molecules of pyruvate is broken down to CO_2 plus a two-carbon acetyl group in acetyl CoA which enters the Krebs cycle, noting that another 4H are removed per molecule of glucose in the process. Observe that 16 H are removed per molecule of glucose in the Krebs cycle. Count the hydrogen atoms, noting that a total of 24 hydrogen atoms are brought to the electron transport chain per molecule of glucose. The energy in their electrons is used to produce 32 ATP aerobically per molecule of glucose; another 2 ATP per molecule of glucose are obtained from 2 GTP (a high-energy compound) produced in the Krebs cycle. Thus, the net yield is 36 ATP per molecule of glucose aerobically, compared with 2 ATP per molecule of glucose anaerobically. This difference in ATP production explains why anaerobic metabolism is associated with higher rates of glucose utilization and glycogen depletion than aerobic metabolism.

The raw materials for gluconeogenesis include pyruvic acid, lactic acid, amino acids (all except leucine) and glycerol (Figure 2.24). Pyruvic acid produced in glycolysis is released by muscle and other tissues into the blood. Lactic acid that is formed by anaerobic glycolysis is also released into the blood (Figure 2.17) and can be reconverted to pyruvic acid in the liver and used as a substrate for gluconeogenesis. Amino acids whose NH_2 groups (Figure 2.37) have been removed are also used for gluconeogenesis, as is glycerol released into the blood from triglyceride breakdown in adipose tissue (Figure 2.30).

During strenuous exercise, production of lactic acid is increased; lactic acid leaves muscle and enters the general circulation (since lactic acid dissociates into lactate plus H^+, the terms lactic acid and lactate are often used interchangeably). The liver converts lactate to glucose through the pathway of gluconeogenesis and releases this newly formed glucose into the blood. This energy-costing conversion of lactate to glucose is part of the *Cori cycle* (Figure 2.25).

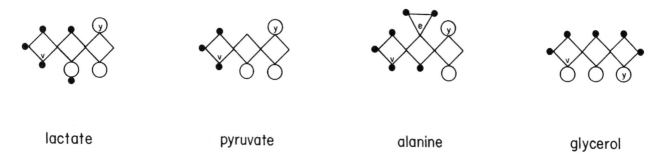

lactate   pyruvate   alanine   glycerol

Figure 2.24   Substrates for gluconeogenesis. Color and identify the carbon (diamonds), oxygen (open circles), and hydrogen (filled circles) atoms in each of the three-carbon substrates for gluconeogenesis. Note that alanine contains a nitrogen atom (triangle). The liver can synthesize glucose from each of these compounds.

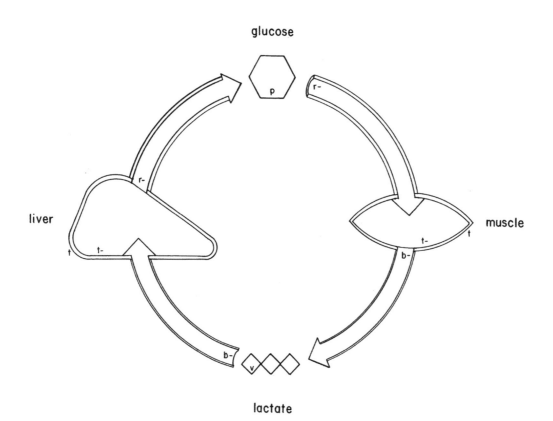

Figure 2.25   Cori cycle. Color the glucose molecule and continue clockwise, coloring the arterial blood that transports glucose to muscle and the subsequent release of lactate into venous blood. Color the molecule of lactate, the arrow indicating its transport to the liver, and its conversion to glucose by the pathway of gluconeogenesis in the liver. This cycling of lactate and glucose between muscle and liver is known as the Cori cycle. The Cori cycle provides glucose, the only substrate for anaerobic glycolysis. Because glycolysis is an exergonic process which releases energy, gluconeogenesis must be an endergonic process which requires an input of energy (Figure 1.10).

Pathway of gluconeogenesis

In a general sense, gluconeogenesis is the reverse of glycolysis (Figure 2.26) and uses many of the same enzymes as glycolysis. However, three of the reactions of glycolysis are not reversible; for these three steps the enzymes of gluconeogenesis catalyze reverse reactions. These enzymes are active only in liver (the major site of gluconeogenesis) and kidney (a minor site of gluconeogenesis).

Both glycogenolysis and gluconeogenesis lead to the production of glucose 6-phosphate, a form of glucose that does not leave the cell. The enzyme glucose 6-phosphatase in liver removes the phosphate group, yielding glucose that can leave the cell and enter the blood (Figure 2.13).

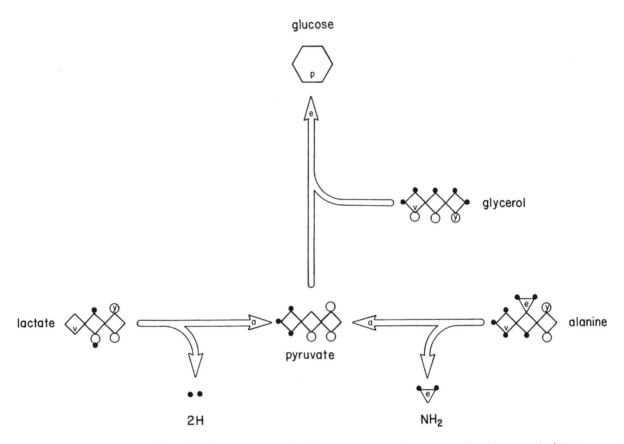

Figure 2.26 Gluconeogenesis. Color the reaction in which lactate is converted to pyruvate by the removal of 2H (arrow at left) and the reaction in which alanine is converted to pyruvate by the removal of an amino group (NH$_2$, arrow at right). Color the reaction in which pyruvate is converted to glucose in the pathway of gluconeogenesis (upward arrow), noting that glycerol can enter the pathway at an intermediate step. Observe that two three-carbon compounds are required to synthesize one six-carbon molecule of glucose. Compare this figure with Figure 2.24.

Summary of carbohydrate metabolism

Glucose, whether it is taken up by the cell from the blood or derived from glycogen within the cell, is first metabolized by the pathway of glycolysis to pyruvic acid. Pyruvate can be converted anaerobically to lactate which can leave the cell and be metabolized by other cells to yield energy or be converted to other forms, such as glucose or amino acids (Fig. 2.27). Pyruvate can also be converted aerobically to acetyl CoA and then metabolized to CO$_2$ and H$_2$O by the Krebs cycle and the electron transport chain. Aerobic metabolism provides a much greater ATP yield per molecule of glucose than does anaerobic metabolism (Figure 2.23).

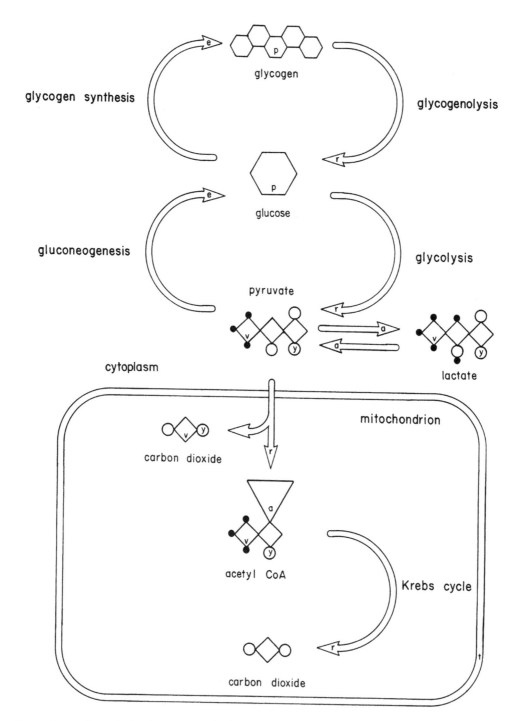

Figure 2.27 Overview of carbohydrate metabolism. Begin at the top by coloring the glycogen molecule and continue down the right side by coloring the arrow that indicates glycogenolysis, the glucose molecule produced by this pathway, the arrow indicating glycolysis and the molecule of pyruvate that is produced. Color the molecule of lactate and the arrows that show that it is reversibly synthesized from pyruvate. Continue up the left side, coloring the arrows for gluconeogenesis and glycogen synthesis. Observe that anabolic pathways are indicated by upward arrows, whereas catabolic pathways are indicated by downward arrows. Color the downward arrow from pyruvate showing its entry into the mitochondrion and its irreversible conversion to acetyl CoA and carbon dioxide. Color acetyl CoA and its breakdown to carbon dioxide in the Krebs cycle. Note from the two-way arrows that pyruvate and lactate can be used to make glucose. Also note from the one-way arrow that acetyl CoA cannot be used to make glucose.

Metabolism of fat

Fat is a major source of energy in the resting state and during prolonged low-intensity exercise. Fat is obtained mainly from the diet but can also be synthesized in the body from carbohydrate. Unlike carbohydrate and protein, fat is not soluble in water.

The primary subunit of fat is the fatty acid (Figure 2.28), which consists of a chain of carbons terminating in a car-

boxyl group (COOH). The major form of fat found in the diet is triglyceride (also known as triacylglycerol), which is comprised of three fatty acids bound in ester linkage (Figure 2.29) to the alcohol glycerol (Figure 2.30). The term lipid includes fat as well as other compounds that are not water-soluble, such as cholesterol.

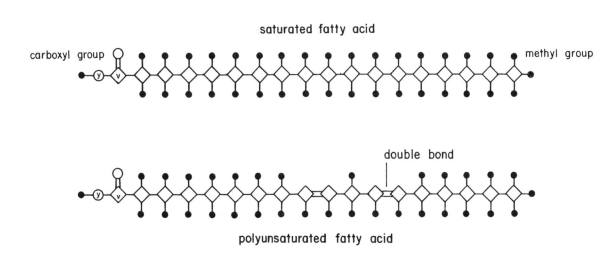

Figure 2.28 **Structure of fatty acids.** Color the carbon (diamonds) and oxygen (open circles) atoms and identify the hydrogen atoms (filled circles) in the saturated fatty acid (top panel). Note the carboxyl group (COOH) at the left end of the chain and the methyl group (CH$_3$) at the right end. Repeat this process for the polyunsaturated fatty acid (bottom panel). Compare the two molecules, noting that saturated fatty acids have no carbon-to-carbon double bonds, whereas polyunsaturated fatty acids have two or more carbon-to-carbon double bonds. Both saturated and polyunsaturated fatty acids are found in the diet and in the body.

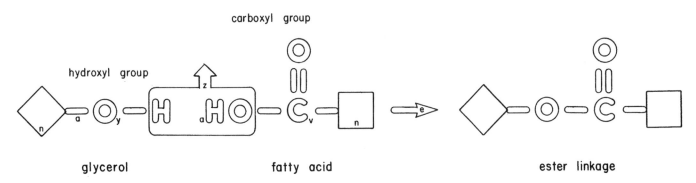

Figure 2.29 **Esterification.** Color the portion of the glycerol molecule shown, noting its hydroxyl group (OH). Color the portion of the fatty acid shown, noting its carboxyl group (COOH). Color the region depicting the water that is removed in the process of condensation. Color the arrow that indicates the process of esterification and the ester linkage that is formed between glycerol and the fatty acid. Since each glycerol molecule has three hydroxyl groups, it can form ester linkages with three fatty acids. A glycerol molecule attached to three fatty acids is called a triglyceride.

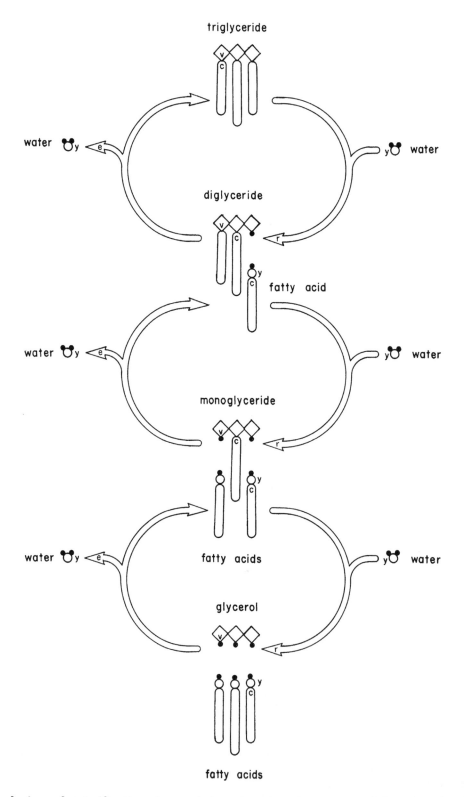

Figure 2.30   Lipolysis and esterification. Begin with the triglyceride at the top, proceed down the right side and color each of the three steps at which a fatty acid is removed by the addition of a molecule of water (hydrolysis) at the ester linkage, until free glycerol is produced. Note that the names of the compounds correspond to the number of fatty acids. Removal of fatty acids from triglyceride is the process of lipolysis. Now proceed up the left side for each of three steps of condensation in which a fatty acid is added to glycerol and a molecule of water is removed; this is the process of esterification which can produce triglyceride from glycerol plus three fatty acids. Compare this figure with Figure 2.29.

Digestion and absorption of fat

Dietary fat is emulsified by bile in the small intestine; emulsification divides fat into small droplets that present more surface area to digestive enzymes than did the original larger droplet, and causes fat to mix with water thereby forming a suspension. Pancreatic lipase is the major enzyme of triglyceride digestion; it is secreted by the pancreas into the small intestine where the enzyme removes fatty acids by hydrolysis (Figure 2.30).

Digested fat forms tiny particles with bile called *micelles*. Micelles diffuse to the mucosal cells that form the inner surface of the intestine; the digested fat and most of the bile enter the intestinal mucosal cells. Intestinal cells incorporate dietary fat into large particles comprised of fat and protein (lipoprotein particles) called *chylomicrons*. Chylomicrons are released into the lymphatic system, which slowly empties into the general circulation so that absorbed fat enters the blood several hours after the fat is consumed (Figure 2.31).

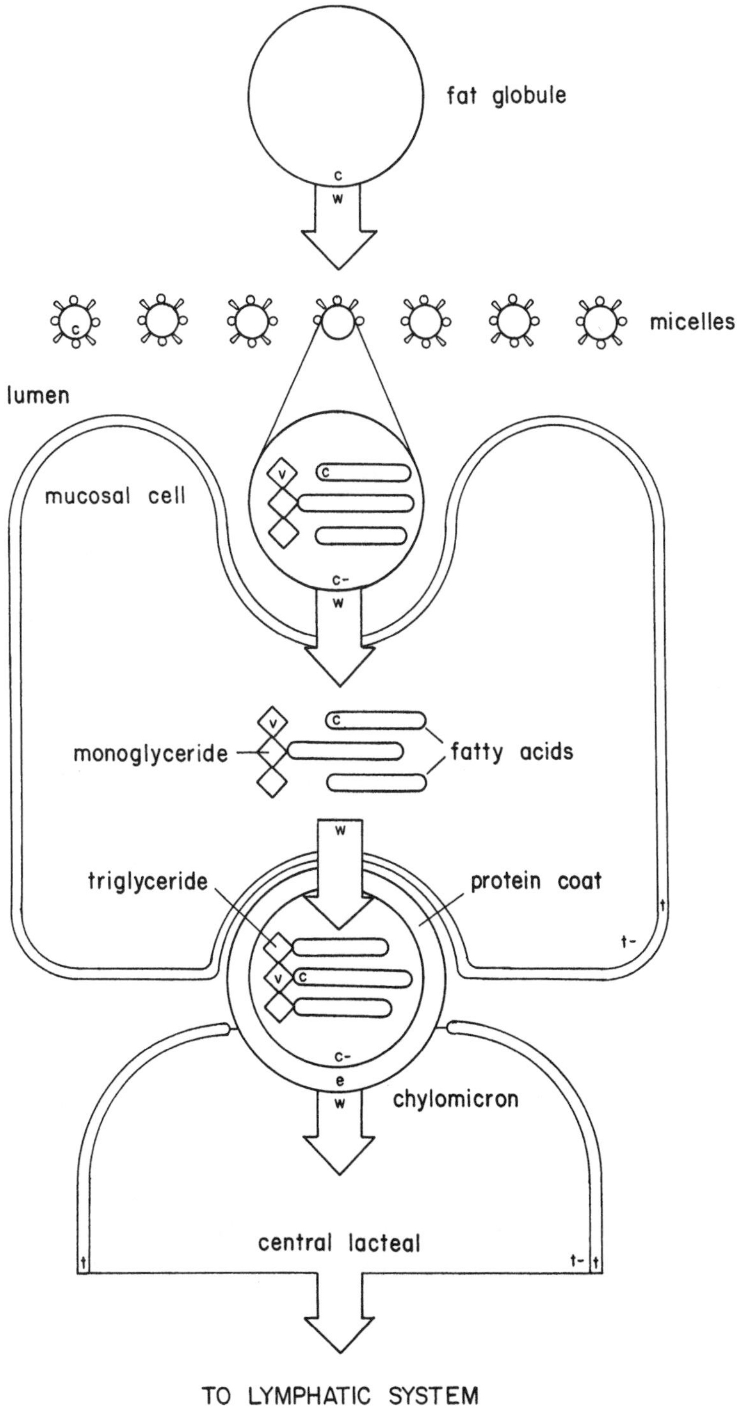

fat globule

micelles

lumen

mucosal cell

monoglyceride — | — fatty acids

triglyceride   protein coat

chylomicron

central lacteal

TO LYMPHATIC SYSTEM

Figure 2.31   Absorption of fat. Color the globule of dietary fat in the intestinal lumen and its emulsification and digestion which result in the formation of micelles. Observe that the magnified micelle contains a monoglyceride and two fatty acids. Observe that the contents of the micelle enter the intestinal mucosal cell where they are packaged as a chylomicron. A chylomicron is a kind of lipoprotein particle that contains triglyceride in the center, surrounded by cholesterol and phospholipids, and is coated with specific proteins. Color the chylomicron, noting that it leaves the mucosal cell by exocytosis, and enters the lymphatic circulation via an open-ended duct called a central lacteal. Chylomicrons eventually enter the blood at the site where the lymphatic vessels empty into the general circulation.

Storage of triglyceride

After a meal most of the dietary fat, which is carried by chylomicrons, is taken up by fat depots known as adipose tissue (Figure 11.3). The enzyme in adipose tissue responsible for fat uptake, *lipoprotein lipase,* is released into the blood in response to the high plasma insulin levels that occur after a meal. Lipoprotein lipase attaches to the chylomicron where it hydrolyzes the triglyceride into glycerol plus three fatty acids (Figure 2.32). The fatty acids enter the adipocyte (fat cell) where three fatty acids bond with one molecule of glycerol that was produced by adipose tissue from glucose, thereby forming a new triglyceride by the process of esterification (Figure 2.29). The triglyceride molecule that is produced is added to the large lipid droplet that occupies most of the volume of the adipocyte (Figure 11.2).

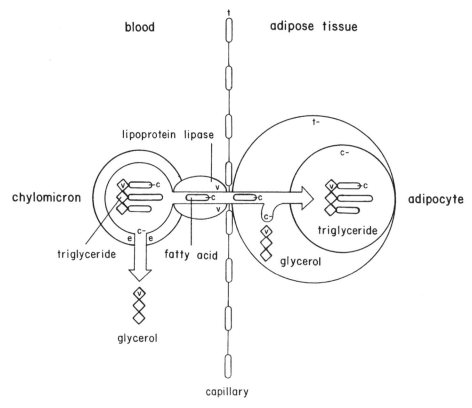

Figure 2.32   Storage of dietary fat in adipose tissue. Color the triglyceride molecule within the chylomicron in the blood. Color the enzyme lipoprotein lipase that is secreted by adipose tissue into the capillary, where it hydrolyzes the triglyceride contained in chylomicrons and very low density lipoprotein (VLDL) particles (Figure 2.34) into three fatty acids plus glycerol. Color the capillary membrane, noting that fatty acids cross the membrane to enter the adipocyte (fat cell) while glycerol remains in the blood and will be taken up by the liver. Color the adipocyte, the glycerol that it synthesizes from glucose, the triglyceride molecule, and the fat droplet in which it is stored. Note that triglyceride is formed by combining this glycerol with incoming fatty acids.

Muscle also produces lipoprotein lipase (Figure 2.33); this enzyme permits muscle to take up fatty acids carried by chylomicrons and very low density lipoprotein particles (VLDL, Figure 2.34). Muscle tissue stores a much smaller amount of triglyceride than does adipose tissue. The mechanisms that regulate the storage and mobilization of triglyceride within muscle differ in some respects from those in adipose tissue. For example, during exercise lipoprotein lipase in muscle, but not adipose tissue, removes fatty acids from triglycerides in the blood for transport into the cell (Figure 2.33). In this way, circulating triglyceride is directed to muscle for use as a fuel, instead of to adipose tissue for storage.

Synthesis of fat

Although fat in the body is largely derived from fat in the diet, it also may be synthesized from carbohydrate when there is excess energy intake, particularly with high-sucrose diets. Synthesis of fatty acids takes place mainly in the liver in humans, but under some conditions it also occurs in adipose tissue. The fatty acids that are synthesized are esterified with glycerol to form triglycerides (Figure 2.30); these triglycerides are exported from the liver to other tissues in VLDL particles (Figure 2.34).

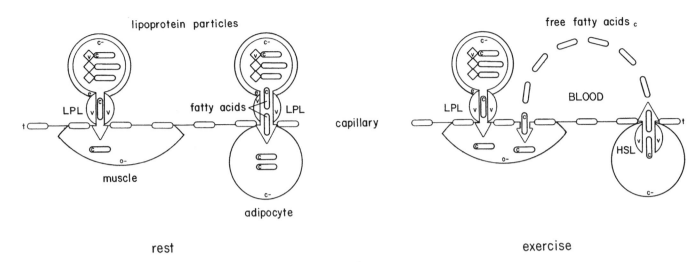

Figure 2.33   Triglyceride flux in muscle and adipose tissue. Begin with the left panel, which depicts conditions at rest. Color the lipoprotein particles in the blood, their triglyceride molecules, and the enzyme lipoprotein lipase (LPL) that is released into the capillary by muscle cells and fat cells (adipocytes). Color the fatty acids released by triglyceride breakdown, noting that, at rest after a meal, fatty acids are taken up by both muscle cells and adipocytes. Color the lipoprotein particle, its triglyceride molecule, and the enzyme in the right panel, which depicts conditions during exercise. Observe that muscle releases LPL and takes up fatty acids from lipoprotein particles. Observe that the adipocyte does not take up fatty acids during exercise, but instead breaks down its stored triglyceride to fatty acids and glycerol through the action of another enzyme, hormone-sensitve lipase (HSL). Observe also that the free fatty acids released from the adipocyte are taken up by the muscle cell. Thus, muscle receives fatty acids from two extracellular sources during exercise. Compare this figure with Figure 2.32.

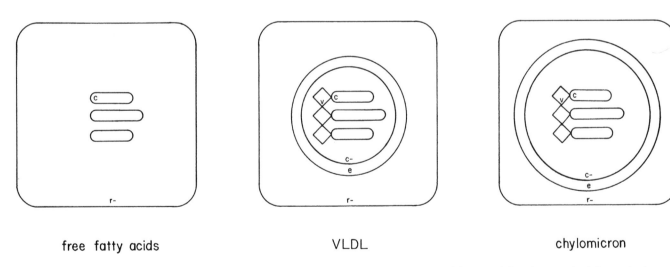

Figure 2.34   Forms of fat in the blood. Color the three unattached molecules of fatty acid (free fatty acids, left panel), the very low density lipoprotein particle (VLDL) which carries fat as triglyceride (middle panel), and the larger lipoprotein particle, the chlyomicron, which also carries fat as triglyceride (right panel). Free fatty acids are derived from the lipolysis of triglyceride that is stored in adipose tissue (Figure 2.33). The triglyceride contained in the chylomicron is derived from absorbed dietary fat, whereas the triglyceride in the VLDL particle is mainly fat synthesized in the liver from carbohydrate.

Circulating lipids

Fats are found in the blood both as triglycerides and as free fatty acids (i.e., fatty acids that are not incorporated into triglyceride). Circulating triglyceride is packaged in lipoprotein particles such as chylomicrons and VLDL (Figure 2.34); their triglyceride is hydrolyzed by lipoprotein lipase and the fatty acids that are released are taken up by cells (Figures 2.32 and 2.33). Free fatty acids (FFA) in the blood result from the breakdown of triglycerides stored in adipose tissue; free fatty acids are also taken up by cells.

In addition to the circulating lipids that provide fuel to tissues, other forms of lipids are found in the circulation, including low density lipoprotein (LDL) and high density lipoprotein (HDL) particles. LDL particles transport cholesterol to cells and HDL particles transfer cholesterol and enzymes among lipoprotein particles and facilitate the transport of cholesterol from the blood to the liver.

Lipolysis

Triglyceride in adipose tissue is hydrolyzed by the process of *lipolysis* into three fatty acids plus glycerol, which are released into the blood (Figure 2.30). The enzyme hormone-sensitive lipase (HSL) initiates lipolysis. Increased activity of the sympathetic nervous system during exercise stimulates hormone-sensitive lipase, thereby stimulating lipolysis (Figure 2.33). During strenuous exercise, blood levels of lactate may rise enough to inhibit lipolysis and thereby decrease fatty acid output from adipose tissue. This inhibition of lipolysis by lactate could be due to the conversion of lactate to glycerol by adipose tissue and subsequent re-esterification of fatty acids with glycerol to form triglyceride.

A consequence of increased lipolysis in adipose tissue is that plasma levels of free fatty acids may rise markedly during prolonged exercise; usage of fat by muscle during exercise is related to the concentration of free fatty acids in the blood. The triglyceride stores within muscle are also subject to lipolysis, yielding fatty acids plus glycerol.

Adipose tissue does not reuse the glycerol produced by lipolysis, so glycerol leaves the adipocyte and enters the blood. For this reason, blood levels of glycerol are used to measure the rate of lipolysis in adipose tissue. Liver takes up glycerol and converts it to glucose in the pathway of gluconeogenesis (Figure 2.26) or uses it to esterify fatty acids to form triglyceride (Figure 2.30).

Oxidation of fat

Fatty acids that are taken up by tissues and used for fuel are broken down first into two-carbon acetyl units attached to coenzyme A, thereby forming acetyl CoA. A fatty acid that

consists of sixteen carbons will produce eight units of acetyl CoA. The process through which this breakdown occurs is called *β-oxidation* (beta-oxidation, Figure 2.35).

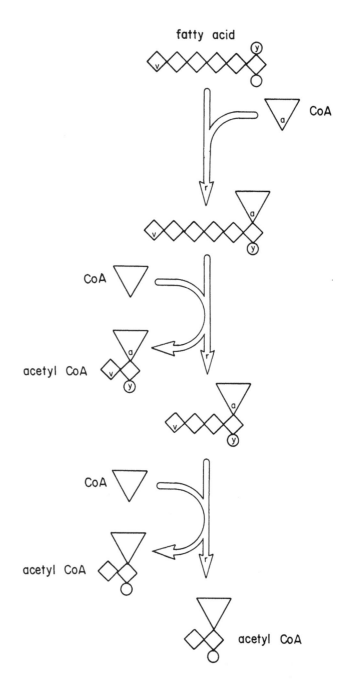

Figure 2.35 β-oxidation. Color and count the carbon atoms (diamonds) in the fatty acid at the top, noting the addition of CoA at the beginning of the pathway. Color the reactions in which the fatty acid loses units of acetyl CoA. At each step, count the carbon atoms that are removed and those that remain. Note that by the end of the pathway, three acetyl CoA have been produced from the original six-carbon fatty acid through the process of β-oxidation, which is an aerobic pathway that occurs in the mitochondria.

β-oxidation is an aerobic pathway that yields energy stored as ATP. Hydrogen atoms in fatty acids are removed by this pathway and transferred to the coenzymes NAD$^+$ and FAD, which carry them to the electron transport chain (Figure 2.21) where their energy is used to form high-energy bonds in ATP. Acetyl CoA produced by β-oxidation of fatty acids is then metabolized in the Krebs cycle (Figure 2.18), to yield an additional amount of ATP (Figure 2.36).

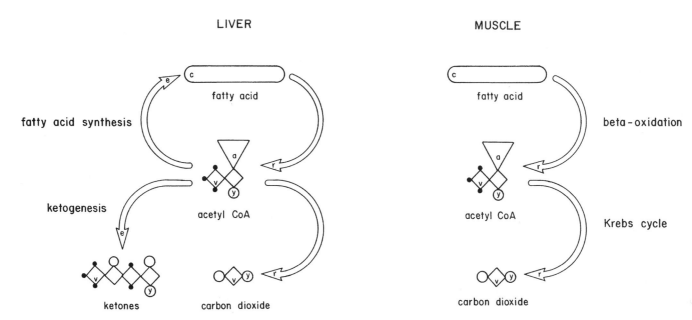

Figure 2.36   Metabolism of fatty acids. For both liver and muscle, color the fatty acid molecule at the top and continue down the right side, coloring the arrows that indicate β-oxidation and the molecules of acetyl CoA that are produced. Continue downward, coloring the arrows that represent the Krebs cycle and the molecules of carbon dioxide that are produced. For the left panel, color the other two arrows from acetyl CoA, which show that the liver can synthesize fatty acids and ketones (also called ketone bodies or ketoacids) from acetyl CoA. Color the ketone molecule, noting its number of carbons and the carboxyl group (COOH) at one end. Compare the metabolism of fatty acids in liver and muscle, considering that muscle uses fatty acids as a fuel whereas liver exports fuels in various forms to other tissues.

Ketogenesis

When free fatty acid levels in plasma are elevated (as in exercise, starvation, or uncontrolled diabetes mellitus), the liver converts fatty acids to a more water-soluble fuel, known as ketoacids or ketones; this process is called *ketogenesis* (Figure 2.36). These four-carbon compounds (β-hydroxybutyrate and acetoacetate) are released into the blood and taken up by muscle and other tissues where they are broken down to units of acetyl CoA and metabolized in the Krebs cycle.

Although plasma levels of ketoacids observed during exercise do not normally lower the pH of the blood, the combination of strenuous exercise and diabetes can increase plasma ketoacid levels markedly, causing metabolic acidosis (Figure 6.18). Individuals with diabetes must therefore monitor their blood levels of ketoacids when engaging in strenuous exercise and reduce their activity or take other action (e.g., injection of insulin) if levels of ketoacids are too high.

Metabolism of fat during exercise

Quantitatively, fat represents a much greater potential source of energy than does carbohydrate. Not only does each gram of fat provide more than twice the energy as the same amount of carbohydrate (Figure 3.15) but, unlike carbohydrate, there is a virtually inexhaustible supply of fat in adipose tissue in the well-fed individual.

During light exercise fat can provide most of the energy used by muscle. The fraction of the energy provided by fat varies with exercise intensity and duration as well as the state of training. For example, high-intensity exercise promotes carbohydrate metabolism, whereas long-duration exercise promotes fat metabolism (Figure 3.22).

Metabolism of protein

Protein is a quantitatively less important fuel than either carbohydrate or fat during exercise. Protein generally accounts for less than 2% of the fuel metabolized during exercise of less than an hour's duration; during prolonged exercise protein can account for as much as 10% of the total energy usage.

Digestion and absorption of protein

Dietary protein is digested in the gastrointestinal tract into *amino acids* (Figure 2.37). There are twenty different amino acids that are important in the human diet. They are linked together in linear sequences to form all the proteins found in living things, including our bodies and the plant and animal-derived foods that we eat.

All amino acids share certain characteristics; each has an amino group (NH_2) and a carboxyl group (COOH) attached to a central, or alpha, carbon (Figure 2.37). Each different type of amino acid has a specific side chain (linear or ring structure) that is attached to the alpha carbon. It is the side chain (or R group) that makes one amino acid different from another, and gives the amino acid its identity. For example, branched-chain amino acids have R groups that are not simple, straight chains of carbons (Figure 2.38).

Metabolism of amino acids

Amino acids that are absorbed from digested proteins in food may be used to synthesize new proteins, to form a variety of nonprotein compounds (such as neurotransmitters), or to provide energy. New proteins are synthesized by forming peptide bonds between amino acids; the sequence of amino acids in each protein is directed by the cell's DNA. Amino acids are also utilized for a number of other anabolic purposes besides protein synthesis. For example, portions of amino acids are used in the synthesis of the heme in hemoglobin, of purines and pyrimidines that make up nucleic acids, and of neurotransmitters like norepinephrine and serotonin.

Proteins within cells are constantly being degraded by hydrolysis of their peptide bonds (Figure 2.39) to their constituent amino acids, thereby providing an endogenous source of amino acids. The short life span of most proteins enables cells to readily adapt to changes in their environment by changing their proteins (e.g., making new enzymes and transport proteins). The increased rate of protein breakdown during exercise also enhances the supply of amino acids that are available for use as fuel.

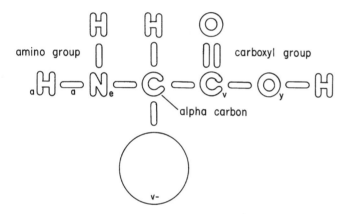

Figure 2.37   Structure of amino acids. Color the alpha carbon and the four groups that bond to it: amino group (NH_2), hydrogen atom (H), carboxyl group (COOH), and the group that differs according to the identity of each amino acid (R group, shown as a large circle). In the case of the amino acid glycine, for example, the R group is a hydrogen atom, while in the amino acid leucine, the R group is a branched chain of carbons.

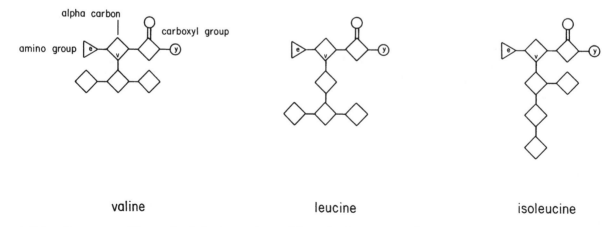

valine   leucine   isoleucine

Figure 2.38   Structure of branched-chain amino acids. Color the structures of each branched-chain amino acid; identify the alpha carbon, the carboxyl group (COOH), and the amino group (NH_2). Compare the R groups, noting that they each consist of a branched chain of carbons. Skeletal muscle preferentially utilizes branched-chain amino acids, over other amino acids, as a fuel. Compare this figure with Figure 2.37.

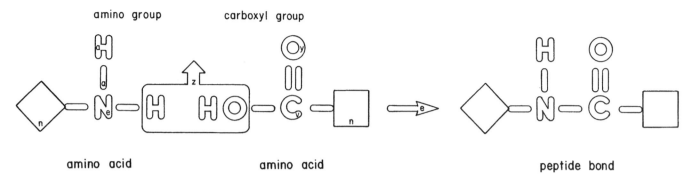

amino group   carboxyl group

amino acid   amino acid   peptide bond

Figure 2.39   Peptide bond. Color the atoms that make up the portions of the individual amino acids on the left side of the arrow; note that the amino group (NH$_2$) of one amino acid is aligned with the carboxyl group (COOH) of the other amino acid. Color the region that represents the water that is removed as these groups are joined by condensation. Color the arrow that indicates the formation of the peptide bond and the dipeptide that results. Because each amino acid contains both an amino group and a carboxyl group (Figure 2.37), each amino acid can bind to two other amino acids, one on each side, and long chains (peptides) can be formed. Note also that peptide bonds can be broken by the process of hydrolysis, the reverse reaction of condensation, in which a molecule of water is added to each peptide bond. Compare this figure with Figure 2.29.

Gluconeogenesis from amino acids

Amino acids that are absorbed from the diet or that are released from the breakdown of tissue proteins may be converted to glucose through the pathway of gluconeogenesis (Figure 2.26). Before amino acids can be converted to glucose or oxidized as fuel, they must lose their NH$_2$ groups (Figure 2.37). Removal of NH$_2$ groups from amino acids occurs mainly in the liver; an exception is the removal of amino groups from branched-chain amino acids (Figure 2.38), which takes place in muscle.

The portion of the amino acid that remains after the amino group has been removed is called its *carbon skeleton* or α-ketoacid (Figure 2.40). It is the carbon skeleton that is converted to glucose in gluconeogenesis or that is oxidized to forms that can enter the Krebs cycle to release energy.

Some carbon skeletons can enter the Krebs cycle directly. For example, the carbon skeleton of the amino acid aspartate is oxaloacetate, which is an intermediate compound in the Krebs cycle (Figure 2.18). Other carbon skeletons must be changed extensively before they can enter the Krebs cycle.

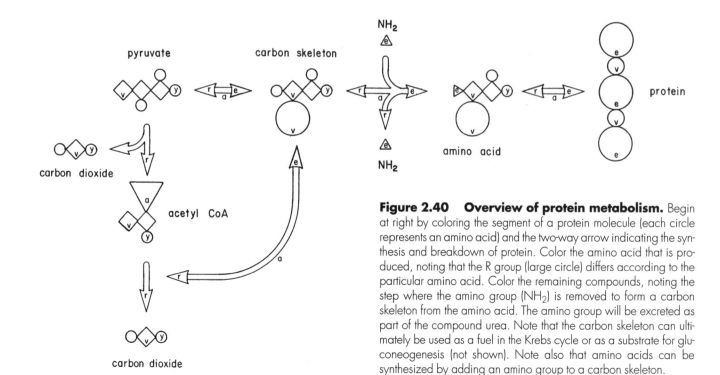

pyruvate   carbon skeleton   NH$_2$ protein

carbon dioxide

acetyl CoA

amino acid

NH$_2$

carbon dioxide

Figure 2.40   Overview of protein metabolism. Begin at right by coloring the segment of a protein molecule (each circle represents an amino acid) and the two-way arrow indicating the synthesis and breakdown of protein. Color the amino acid that is produced, noting that the R group (large circle) differs according to the particular amino acid. Color the remaining compounds, noting the step where the amino group (NH$_2$) is removed to form a carbon skeleton from the amino acid. The amino group will be excreted as part of the compound urea. Note that the carbon skeleton can ultimately be used as a fuel in the Krebs cycle or as a substrate for gluconeogenesis (not shown). Note also that amino acids can be synthesized by adding an amino group to a carbon skeleton.

Fate of the amino group

The amino group of an amino acid may be reused to make a new amino acid by combining with a carbon skeleton that has been synthesized in the cell; for example, pyruvic acid combines with an amino group to form the amino acid alanine. The synthesis of alanine from pyruvic acid that is produced by muscle glycolysis is a major way in which muscle rids itself of the NH₂ that is produced when amino acids are used as fuel. Alanine is released by muscle into the blood and is taken up by the liver, where the amino group is removed to reform pyruvate, which is then used to make glucose by gluconeogenesis. This cycle is known as the *alanine shuttle* (Figure 2.41).

The amino group can be excreted from the body as part of the compound, urea. The *urea cycle* is an energy-requiring pathway that operates in the liver to produce urea, which is then released into the blood (Figure 2.41). Because urea is not taken up by tissues, the amount of urea that is excreted in urine can be used as a measure of amino acid breakdown.

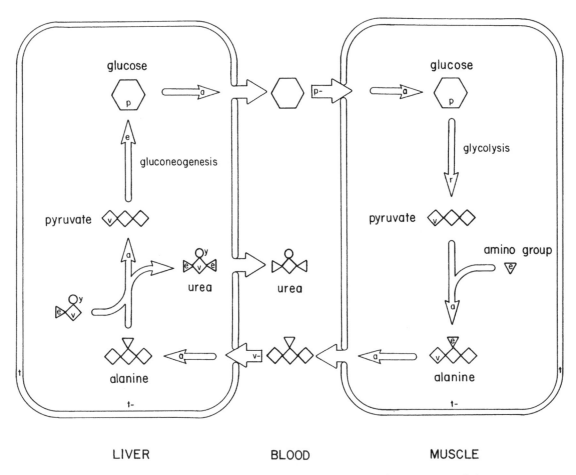

LIVER   BLOOD   MUSCLE

Figure 2.41   Alanine shuttle. Begin in the right panel, color the arrow depicting the conversion of glucose to pyruvate in glycolysis and the reaction in which pyruvate is converted to alanine by the addition of an amino group (triangle). Amino groups are released during the breakdown of amino acids for fuel; their direct release into the blood would cause a metabolic derangement (high blood ammonia levels) and so attachment of the amino group to pyruvate to form alanine provides a safe way to transport amino groups in the blood. Color the export of alanine to the blood, its uptake by liver (left panel), and the subsequent removal of the amino group to produce pyruvate from alanine. The amino group is used by the liver to form urea, which then enters the blood. The kidney clears the blood of urea and excretes it in the urine. Color the arrow depicting gluconeogenesis, the glucose formed from pyruvate, and the release of glucose into the blood. The alanine shuttle, like the Cori cycle (Figure 2.25) represents a relationship between liver and muscle metabolism that involves the breakdown of glucose by muscle and the resynthesis of glucose by the liver.

Effect of exercise on protein metabolism

Protein metabolism is influenced by exercise in two respects: (1) protein catabolism is increased, releasing amino acids that can be used as fuel; and (2) protein anabolism is increased, adding protein to muscle. The former effect predominates during exercise of high intensity and/or long duration, whereas the latter effect predominates during recovery. Therefore, although exercise promotes degradation of muscle protein and amino acid catabolism, regular exercise does not result in muscle atrophy in the well-fed individual because protein synthesis is increased during the postexercise period. In addition, muscle protein content can be enhanced by appropriate training techniques coupled with appropriate nutritional support.

Summary

Carbohydrates, fats, and proteins are metabolized to release energy that is used to form high-energy bonds in ATP. All fuels ultimately can be oxidized to CO_2 and H_2O in the aerobic pathways of the Krebs cycle and electron transport chain, thereby extracting all available energy. Glucose is the only fuel that can be metabolized anaerobically to yield energy to be stored in ATP.

Fuels may be stored or mobilized from storage as needed: glucose is stored as glycogen, fatty acids are stored as triglyceride, and amino acids are stored as protein. There is also considerable interconversion among carbohydrates, fats, and proteins (Figure 2.42). Metabolic pathways provide a steady supply of energy within each cell, drawing both on the

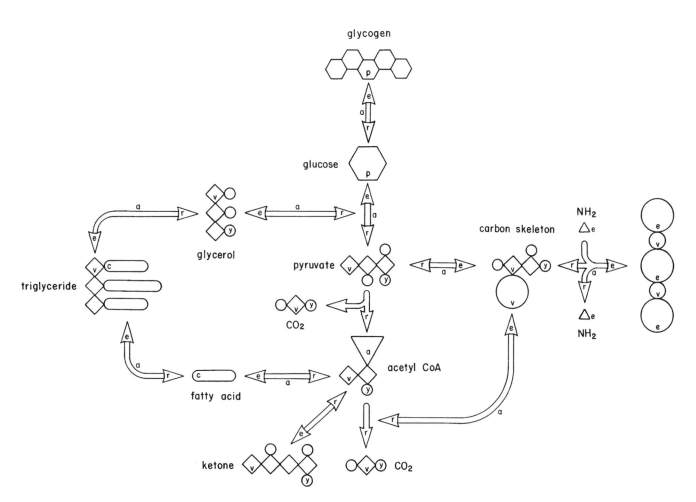

Figure 2.42 Overview of metabolism. Color the glycogen molecule (at top) and continue downward until you reach carbon dioxide, observing whether each pathway is anabolic or catabolic. Color the triglyceride molecule (at left), its breakdown to glycerol and fatty acids by lipolysis and the paths that glycerol and fatty acids follow. Color the protein molecule (at right) and the arrow indicating its breakdown into individual amino acids (not shown) and loss of the amino group to form carbon skeletons. Observe where carbohydrate, fat, and protein enter metabolic pathways, which pathways are reversible and which are not, and how the fuels can be interconverted. Observe that a path can be traced from glucose to fatty acids, but not from fatty acids to glucose. Compare this figure with Figures 2.27, 2.36, and 2.40.

cell's own fuel stores and on fuels transported in the blood from other tissues. Despite the high fuel consumption of muscle during exercise, blood glucose levels are maintained through the provision of glucose by metabolic pathways in the liver. The regulation of metabolic pathways is a function of the endocrine system (Chapter 7).

chapter **three**
energy systems

Energy for skeletal muscle contraction is obtained from the breakdown of adenosine triphosphate (ATP) into adenosine diphosphate (ADP) and inorganic phosphate (Pi). The ATP used during exercise is supplied by three different energy systems: (1) the ATP-PCr (phosphagen) system; (2) the glycolytic (glycogen-lactic acid) system; and (3) the oxidative (aerobic) system (Figure 3.1). The ATP-PCr and glycolytic systems are referred to as *anaerobic* sources of ATP because their operation does not require the presence of oxygen; the oxidative system is referred to as an *aerobic* source of ATP because its operation requires a continuous supply of oxygen.

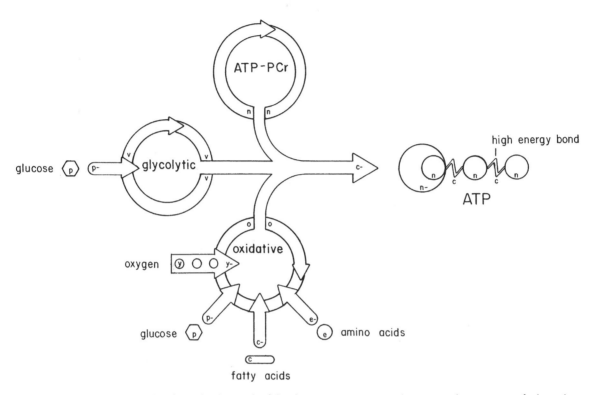

Figure 3.1   Energy systems. Identify and color each of the three energy systems, the arrows that represent fuels and oxygen, and the molecule of ATP, noting its high-energy bonds. The ATP-PCr system is an immediate source of energy because it represents energy stored in the high-energy bonds of ATP and PCr; note that the release of this stored energy does not require fuels or oxygen. The ATP-PCr system is not considered to be a metabolic pathway because it consists of a single reaction, rather than a sequence of reactions (Figure 2.1). The glycolytic system is a short-term source of energy; note that the only fuel the glycolytic system consumes is glucose and that its operation does not require a supply of oxygen (Figure 2.17). The oxidative system, which includes the aerobic pathways of the Krebs cycle (Figure 2.18) and the electron transport chain (Figure 2.21), is a long-term source of energy. Observe that the oxidative system can convert glucose, fatty acids, and amino acids to forms that can enter the Krebs cycle. Also observe that the operation of the oxidative system requires a continuous supply of oxygen (to serve as the final electron acceptor in the electron transport chain).

Because the systems differ both in terms of the rate and duration with which they can supply ATP, the relative contributions of each system to the overall production of ATP vary with the intensity and duration of exercise.

ATP-PCr system

The *ATP-PCr system* stores its energy in the form of high-energy phosphate bonds in ATP and phosphocreatine (PCr, a high-energy compound found in skeletal muscle). The energy released from the breakdown of ATP into ADP and phosphate is used for muscle contraction (Figure 2.2). ATP is then resynthesized from ADP and phosphate utilizing energy stored in the high-energy bonds in PCr or ADP. The energy released from the breakdown of phosphocreatine (also called creatine phosphate) into creatine and phosphate is used to regenerate ATP (Figure 3.2). This reaction enables PCr breakdown to replenish the supply of ATP; this helps maintain high levels of ATP in working muscle at the expense of declining levels of PCr. The energy released from the breakdown of ADP into AMP (adenosine monophosphate) and phosphate is also used to regenerate ATP; this reaction uses two molecules of ADP to produce one molecule of ATP plus one molecule of AMP (Figure 3.3).

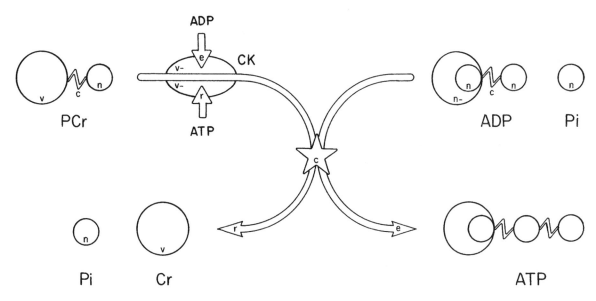

Figure 3.2 Use of PCr to regenerate ATP. Color the PCr molecule, noting its high-energy bond, the catabolic reaction (arrow at left) in which PCr is broken down into Cr and inorganic phosphate (Pi), and the star symbolizing the energy released by this reaction. Color the anabolic reaction (arrow at right) in which this energy is used to form ATP from ADP and Pi. Color the molecules of ATP, ADP, and Pi, noting the high-energy bonds in ATP and ADP. Observe that the breakdown of PCr is catalyzed by the enzyme creatine kinase (CK) and that CK activity is stimulated by high levels of ADP (small downward arrow) but inhibited by high levels of ATP (small upward arrow). This modulation of creatine kinase activity by the prevailing levels of ADP and ATP enables the rate of PCr breakdown to be high during intense exercise (when ATP levels are low and ADP levels are high) and low at rest (when ATP levels are high and ADP levels are low). This mechanism helps maintain high levels of ATP in exercising muscle at the expense of declining levels of PCr. Compare this figure with Figure 1.13.

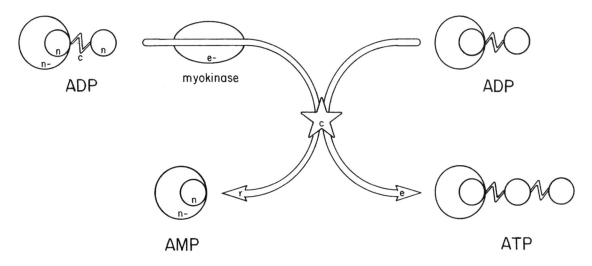

Figure 3.3 Use of ADP to regenerate ATP. Color the molecules of ADP, noting their high-energy bonds. Color the catabolic reaction (arrow at left) in which ADP is broken down into AMP and Pi, and the star symbolizing the energy released by this reaction. Color the anabolic reaction (arrow at right) in which this energy is used to form ATP from ADP and Pi. Color the molecule of ATP, noting its high-energy bonds. Thus, two molecules of ADP can be used to form one molecule of ATP and one molecule of AMP; high levels of AMP therefore indicate a high rate of ATP utilization. This reaction in muscle is catalyzed by the enzyme myokinase. Compare this figure with Figure 1.12.

Muscle monitors its depletion of ATP by the ADP/ATP ratio and by the level of AMP in the cell. The ADP/ATP ratio increases when ATP is broken down to ADP and phosphate, and the level of AMP increases when two ADP are used to make ATP and AMP. Thus, increases in the ADP/ATP ratio and/or increases in the level of AMP signal the need to synthesize more ATP.

In muscle, the rate of PCr breakdown is regulated by the enzyme creatine kinase (CK) (Figure 3.2) and the rate of ADP breakdown is regulated by the enzyme myokinase. Creatine kinase activity is stimulated by increases in the ADP/ATP ratio and by low levels of ATP, which are conditions that indicate the high rate of ATP usage that occurs during intense exercise. Conversely, CK activity is inhibited by decreases in the ADP/ATP ratio and by high levels of ATP, which are conditions that indicate the low rate of ATP usage that occurs at rest. This modulation of CK activity by the prevailing levels of ATP and ADP provides a means by which the rate of PCr breakdown can parallel the rate of ATP utilization; this causes the activity of the ATP-PCr system to be high during intense exercise and low at rest.

Glycolysis

Glycolysis is a catabolic pathway in which one six-carbon molecule of glucose is broken down into two three-carbon molecules of pyruvic acid in the cytoplasm (Figure 2.14). The pairs of hydrogen atoms that are removed during the steps of glycolysis are picked up by NAD^+ and carried as $NADH + H^+$.

Two versions of glycolysis have been defined to indicate the mechanism by which $NADH + H^+$ unloads its hydrogen atoms to become NAD^+ again: (1) anaerobic (a fast process that does not require the presence of oxygen); and (2) aerobic (a slower process that requires a continuous supply of oxygen). In anaerobic glycolysis, $NADH + H^+$ donates its pair of hydrogen atoms to pyruvic acid, which then becomes lactic acid (Figure 2.17). In aerobic glycolysis, $NADH + H^+$ donates its pair of hydrogen atoms to the electron transport chain in the mitochondria (Figure 2.22). Thus, lactic acid is the product of anaerobic glycolysis whereas pyruvic acid is the main product of aerobic glycolysis. Pyruvate formed in aerobic glycolysis is subsequently oxidized to carbon dioxide and water in the aerobic pathways of the Krebs cycle and the electron transport chain.

Glycolytic system

The *glycolytic system* refers to the pathway of anaerobic glycolysis in which two molecules of ATP are formed when one molecule of glucose is broken down to two molecules of lactic acid. Glucose is the only fuel that can be consumed anaerobically because anaerobic glycolysis is the only ATP-

yielding metabolic pathway that does not require the presence of oxygen.

In contrast, the pathways of aerobic glycolysis, the Krebs cycle, and the electron transport chain, which are components of the oxidative system, yield a net gain of 36 molecules of ATP for each molecule of glucose that is completely oxidized to CO_2 and H_2O in skeletal muscle. Stated another way, the anaerobic pathways of the glycolytic system yield two ATP per glucose whereas the aerobic pathways of the oxidative system yield 36 ATP per glucose in skeletal muscle (and 38 ATP in cardiac muscle) (Figure 2.23). This difference in ATP production explains why the glycolytic system consumes more glucose than the oxidative system to produce the same amount of ATP. It also explains why increased activity of the glycolytic system, as occurs during high-intensity exercise, is accompanied by higher rates of glucose utilization, glycogen depletion, and lactate production.

The activity of the glycolytic system depends on: (1) the activity of its rate-limiting enzyme [phosphofructokinase (PFK)]; and (2) the amount of glucose available to serve as a substrate for the pathway.

PFK activity is stimulated by increases in the ADP/ATP ratio and by high levels of AMP, conditions that indicate a high rate of ATP utilization. Conversely, PFK activity is inhibited by high levels of ATP and PCr, conditions that indicate a low rate of ATP utilization (Figure 3.4). This modulation of PFK activity by the prevailing levels of ATP and its breakdown products provides a means by which the rate of ATP production by glycolysis can keep pace with the rate of ATP utilization by working muscle.

Effect of glycogen breakdown on glycolysis

Since glucose is the major substrate for glycolysis, the activity of the glycolytic system also depends on the amount of glucose available to enter the pathway. Muscle glycogen, a stored form of glucose, is an important source of glucose in exercising muscle; glycogen is broken down to units of glucose (actually glucose 1-phosphate) by glycogenolysis (Figure 2.12).

Because the rate-limiting enzyme in glycogenolysis is glycogen phosphorylase (Figure 3.4), factors that stimulate the activity of this enzyme increase the supply of glucose for glycolysis. In skeletal muscle, these factors include: (1) calcium ions that are released into the sarcoplasmic reticulum during muscle contraction; (2) epinephrine, a hormone that is released by the adrenal gland during exercise; and (3) increases in the ADP/ATP ratio or high levels of AMP, conditions that result from a high rate of ATP breakdown.

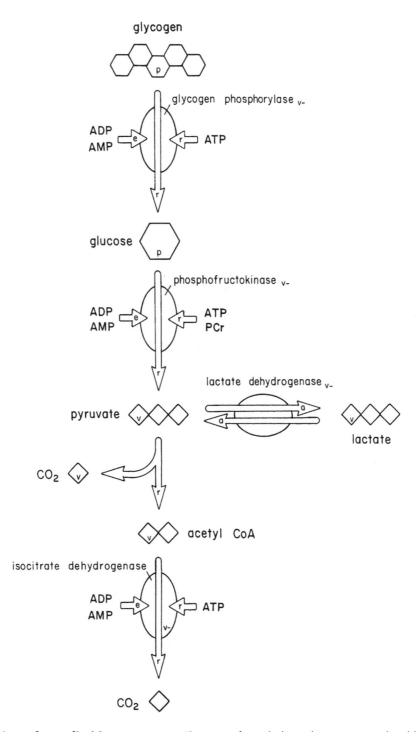

Figure 3.4   Modulation of rate-limiting enzymes. The rates of metabolic pathways are regulated by modulators, which are substances that increase or decrease the activity of the rate-limiting enzyme, i.e., the one that exhibits the lowest maximum velocity (V_{max}, Figure 1.17) in the pathway. Color the glycogen molecule at the top, and then continue down, coloring the arrows, the rate-limiting enzymes, and the products of the pathways; note that the product of one pathway is the substrate for the pathway just beneath it. Color the modulators of the rate-limiting enzymes in each pathway, noting that catabolic pathways are stimulated (green horizontal arrows) by high levels of ADP and AMP and inhibited (red horizontal arrows) by high levels of ATP. Identify the pathways of glycogenolysis (Figure 2.12), glycolysis (Figure 2.14), and the Krebs cycle (Figure 2.18). Cytochrome oxidase, the rate-limiting enzyme of the electron transport chain, is not shown. Observe that the modulation of rate-limiting enzymes by the prevailing levels of ATP and ADP is a mechanism whereby the activity of energy-yielding pathways can be regulated in accordance with the rate of ATP utilization.

Lactic acid formation

As noted above, pyruvic acid formed during glycolysis has two possible fates in muscle: (1) it can be converted to lactic acid, another three-carbon compound, in a reaction that does not require oxygen, i.e., anaerobically; or (2) it can be completely oxidized to carbon dioxide and water in a series of reactions that do require oxygen, i.e., aerobically. Lactic acid is formed when two hydrogen atoms (carried as NADH + H$^+$) are taken up by pyruvic acid; this reaction takes place in the cytoplasm and is catalyzed by the enzyme lactate dehydrogenase (Figure 3. 5). Thus, factors that increase the concentration of pyruvic acid and/or hydrogen atoms in the cytoplasm or that increase the activity of lactate dehydrogenase promote the formation of lactic acid.

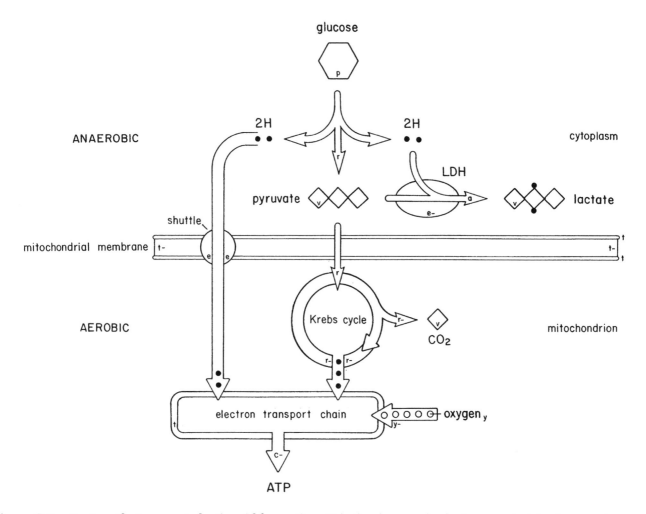

Figure 3.5   Factors that promote lactic acid formation. Color the glucose molecule, the arrow depicting its conversion to pyruvate in glycoloysis, and the pyruvate molecule; note that this is an anaerobic pathway that takes place in the cytoplasm. Color the mitochondrial membrane, the next downward arrow, and the icons for the Krebs cycle and electron transport chain. Color the CO_2 molecule produced by the Krebs cycle, identify the hydrogen atoms (filled circles) that are transported from the Krebs cycle to the electron transport chain, and color the arrow depicting the oxygen supply to the electron transport chain; note that these pathways are aerobic and take place in the mitochondria. Identify the hydrogen atoms (filled circles) that are released during glycolysis; observe that a pair of hydrogen atoms (2H) can be picked up by pyruvate to form lactate and that this reaction is catalyzed by the enzyme lactate dehydrogenase (LDH). Color the enzyme and the lactate molecule, noting that it differs from the pyruvate molecule by the addition of two hydrogen atoms. Follow a pair of hydrogen atoms (2H) removed in glycolysis as they are transported by a hydrogen shuttle system across the mitochondrial membrane to enter the electron transport chain, where the energy in their electrons can be extracted to form ATP. Observe that the rate at which lactic acid is formed is determined by the concentrations of pyruvate and hydrogen atoms (carried as NADH + H$^+$) in the cytoplasm and by the activity of the enzyme lactate dehydrogenase (LDH). Thus, lactic acid is formed when the rate of production of pyruvate and hydrogen atoms by glycolysis exceeds their rate of removal by the Krebs cycle and electron transport chain, respectively. These considerations explain why low mitochondrial enzyme activity, low mitochondrial oxygen supply, and high LDH activity are factors that promote the formation of lactic acid. Compare this figure with Figure 2.23.

In light of the above considerations, lactic acid is formed when the rate of production of pyruvate and hydrogen atoms by glycolysis exceeds their rate of removal by the Krebs cycle and electron transport chain, respectively. Reduced activity of the electron transport chain leads to a decrease in the rate at which pyruvate is oxidized to CO_2 by the Krebs cycle; this could increase the concentration of pyruvate in the cytoplasm and thereby accelerate the formation of lactic acid. Reduced activity of the electron transport chain also leads to a decrease in the rate at which hydrogen atoms are removed from the cytoplasm by the hydrogen shuttle system, which transports them to the electron transport chain. This could increase the concentration of hydrogen atoms (carried as $NADH + H^+$) in the cytoplasm and thereby accelerate the formation of lactic acid (Figure 3.5).

Lactic acid accumulation could therefore be due to low mitochondrial enzyme activity, as found in fast-twitch skeletal muscle fibers, or to an insufficient oxygen supply. For this reason, muscle hypoxia (low O_2 levels) is a condition that has been implicated in the buildup of lactic acid during exercise. However, given that the O_2 levels in exercising muscles do not normally fall low enough to impair mitochondrial function, and that well-oxygenated muscle fibers produce lactic acid (even at rest), the role played by muscle hypoxia in the production of lactic acid during exercise remains unclear.

Isozymes of lactate dehydrogenase

The conversion of pyruvic acid to lactic acid is a reversible reaction that is catalyzed by the enzyme lactate dehydrogenase (LDH). The two basic subunits of LDH are the muscle type (M), found predominantly in fast-twitch skeletal muscle fibers, and the heart type (H), found predominantly in cardiac muscle and slow-twitch skeletal muscle fibers. Type M has a high affinity for pyruvate and promotes the conversion of pyruvate to lactate while type H has a lower affinity for pyru-

vate and promotes the opposite conversion, from lactate to pyruvate (Figure 3.4). Because LDH is made up of different combinations of these basic subunits, different forms, called *isozymes,* of LDH exist.

Based on their contractile properties, skeletal muscle fibers can be characterized as slow-twitch fibers or fast-twitch fibers (Table 4.1). The LDH isozyme found in slow-twitch skeletal muscle fibers and in cardiac muscle fibers favors the conversion from lactate to pyruvate, whereas the LDH isozyme found in fast-twitch skeletal muscle fibers favors the opposite conversion, from pyruvate to lactate. Thus, increased activity of fast-twitch fibers is another factor that promotes the formation of lactic acid (Figure 3.5). These differences in LDH help explain why high-intensity exercises, which employ fast-twitch fibers (Figure 4.27), cause blood levels of lactate to rise, whereas low-intensity exercises, which do not employ fast-twitch fibers, do not cause blood levels of lactate to rise (Figure 3.12).

Oxidative system

The *oxidative system* collectively refers to the pathways of the Krebs cycle and the electron transport chain, as well as all other oxidative pathways that donate hydrogen atoms to the electron transport chain (e.g., aerobic glycolysis, β-oxidation and amino acid catabolism). The oxidative system, which breaks down fuels into CO_2 and H_2O, is also known as the aerobic system because its operation requires a continuous supply of O_2 to serve as the final electron acceptor in the electron transport chain. In contrast to the glycolytic system, which can only use glucose as a fuel, the oxidative system can extract energy from carbohydrate (glucose), fat (fatty acids), and protein (amino acids) and store it in the form of high-energy bonds in ATP (Figure 3.6).

Figure 3.6 Oxidative system. The oxidative system, also known as the aerobic system, collectively refers to the reactions of the Krebs cycle and the electron transport chain, as well as all other oxidative pathways that donate hydrogen atoms to the electron transport chain. Color the icon for the oxidative system, the fuels, and their arrows, noting that the oxidative system can convert carbohydrate (glucose), fat (fatty acids), and protein (carbon skeletons of amino acids) to forms that can be used to make high-energy bonds in ATP. Color the arrows that indicate the oxygen consumed and carbon dioxide produced, noting that the operation of the oxidative system requires a continuous supply of oxygen to break down fuels to CO_2 and H_2O. The relative amounts of O_2 consumed and CO_2 produced by the oxidative system are determined by the specific chemical reaction in which the fuel is completely oxidized to CO_2 and H_2O. Compare this figure with Figure. 3.1.

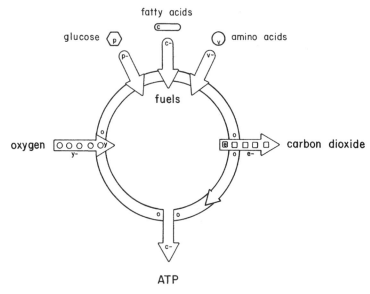

chapter **three**

The rate-limiting enzyme of the Krebs cycle is isocitrate de-hydrogenase, and the rate-limiting enzyme of the electron transport chain is cytochrome oxidase. The activity of these enzymes is stimulated by an increase in the ADP/ATP ratio, a condition that indicates a high rate of ATP utilization, and is inhibited by high levels of ATP, a condition that indicates a low rate of ATP utilization (Figure 3.4). The modulation of rate-limiting enzymes by the prevailing levels of ATP and ADP enables the activity of the oxidative system to keep pace with the rate at which working muscles utilize ATP. Thus, the activity of the oxidative system, and therefore the rate at which oxygen is consumed, is tightly coupled to the rate at which work is performed. As a result, oxygen consumption is proportional to work rate (Figure 3.11).

Functional differences among energy systems

The maximal rate of ATP production is highest in the ATP-PCr system (~4 mol ATP/min), lower in the glycolytic system (~2.5 mol ATP/min), and lowest in the oxidative system (~1 mol ATP/min). In contrast, the duration of maximal ATP production is shortest in the ATP-PCr system (~10 s), longer in the glycolytic system (~1.5 min), and longest in the oxida-tive system (indefinite, given a continuous supply of fuels and oxygen) (Figure 3.7).

Figure 3.7 Maximal rates and du-rations of ATP production. Color the rectangles that depict the maximal energy re-leased by the ATP-PCr system (top panel), gly-colytic system (middle panel), and oxidative system (bottom panel). The height of each rec-tangle indicates the maximal rate of ATP pro-duction, expressed in units of mol ATP/min, and the width of each rectangle indicates the duration of maximal ATP production, ex-pressed in units of seconds (top panel), min-utes (middle panel), and hours (bottom panel). These differences in the maximal rates and du-rations of ATP production are responsible for the following functional differences among the energy systems: (1) The ATP-PCr system is well-suited for activities that require high-inten-sity, short-duration power surges; (2) the gly-colytic system is well-suited for activities that require sustained power; and (3) the oxidative system is well-suited for continuous submaxi-mal activities that require endurance.

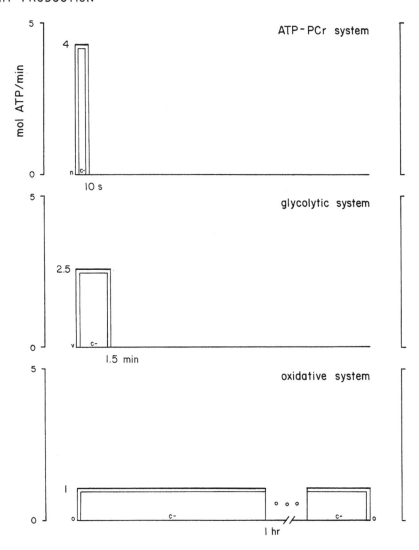

ATP PRODUCTION

These differences in the maximal rates and durations of ATP production are responsible for the following functional differences among the energy systems: (1) The ATP-PCr system is well-suited for activities that require high-intensity, short-duration power surges, such as the 100-meter dash or weight lifting; (2) the glycolytic system is a major source of ATP for activities that require sustained power, such as the 400-meter dash; and (3) the oxidative system is well-adapted for continuous submaximal activities that require endurance, such as cross-country skiing and marathon running.

These different properties of the energy systems explain why the relative contributions of each system to the overall production of ATP vary with the intensity and duration of exercise.

Anaerobic and aerobic components of ATP production

The ATP consumed during any given physical activity can be partitioned into an anaerobic component due to the operation of the ATP-PCr and glycolytic systems and an aerobic component due to the operation of the oxidative system. This analysis reveals that high-intensity, short-duration exercises rely heavily on anaerobic sources of ATP, whereas, at the opposite extreme, low-intensity, long-duration exercises rely heavily on aerobic sources of ATP (Figure 3.8).

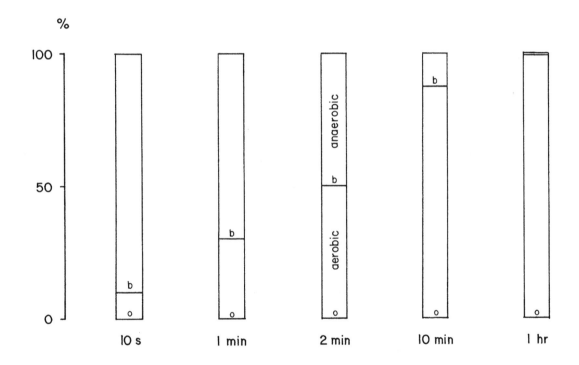

DURATION OF MAXIMAL EXERCISE

Figure 3.8   ATP supply during maximal exercises of different durations. Color the bars from left to right, noting that their heights represent the total amount of energy expended (normalized as 100%) during maximal exercises of different durations. Observe that each bar is partitioned into a lower aerobic component (representing the operation of the oxidative system) and an upper anaerobic component (representing the combined operation of the ATP-PCr and glycolytic systems) so that the relative contributions of aerobic and anaerobic sources of ATP can be visualized from the relative heights of each of its components. Observe that longer durations of maximal exercise are associated with progressively smaller anaerobic components coupled with correspondingly larger aerobic components. Observe also that the energy for a maximal exercise of 10 s duration is derived primarily from anaerobic sources (left bar), of 2 min duration is derived equally from aerobic and anaerobic sources (middle bar), and of 1 hr duration is derived almost entirely from aerobic sources (right bar). For this reason, the oxidative system is the primary energy source for physical activities that require endurance. Compare this figure with Figure 3.7.

Oxygen consumption during exercise

The rate at which oxygen is consumed by the body ($\dot{V}O_2$, in L/min) can be regarded as a measure of the aerobic production of ATP and thus, the ability to perform continuous exercise.

A common practice in engineering is to analyze the response of a system to a change in its stimulus in terms of an initial *transient* phase (during which the response varies with time) and a subsequent *steady-state* phase (during which the response does not change with time). In accord with this procedure, the oxygen consumption observed during a period of continuous submaximal exercise can be characterized by: (1) an initial transient period during which $\dot{V}O_2$ rises gradually from its resting steady-state level to a new, higher steady-state level; (2) a subsequent steady-state period in which $\dot{V}O_2$ remains constant at the higher level; and (3) a transient recovery period following the cessation of exercise during which $\dot{V}O_2$ gradually returns to the resting level (Figure 3.9).

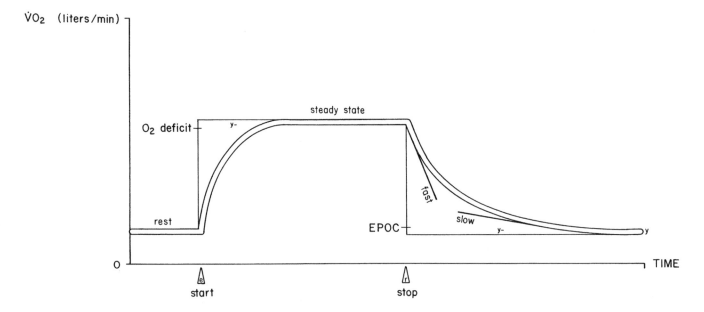

Figure 3.9   Oxygen uptake during exercise. Color the line that depicts oxygen uptake ($\dot{V}O_2$, in liters/min) plotted against time and identify the times at which a fixed intensity of submaximal exercise begins and ends. Note that oxygen uptake gradually increases from its resting level to a higher steady-state level following the onset of exercise and gradually returns to its resting level during the recovery period following the cessation of exercise. Observe that steady-state refers to a condition of dynamic equilibrium in which $\dot{V}O_2$ does not change with time. Because $\dot{V}O_2$ is expressed in units of LO_2/min and time is expressed in units of min, the area contained in a $\dot{V}O_2$-time diagram represents a volume of oxygen, i.e., LO_2/min $\cdot$ min = LO_2. Identify and color the areas labeled O_2 deficit and EPOC (excess postexercise oxygen consumption); note that the EPOC is larger than the O_2 deficit. The O_2 deficit represents the oxygen needed to replenish that portion of the ATP that is derived from anaerobic sources (the ATP-PCr and glycolytic systems) during the initial transient period of exercise. Note that the recovery period is characterized by a fast component (which includes the oxygen used to replenish the high-energy bonds of the ATP-PCr system and to reload depleted oxygen stores) and a slow component. Other factors that contribute to EPOC include: (1) higher body temperature; (2) increased activity of the heart and respiratory muscles; (3) elevated levels of hormones that increase metabolic rate; and (4) endergonic reactions in which the lactate formed during exercise is converted to glucose or amino acids (Figure 3.10). Mild exercise during the recovery period accelerates the rate of lactate removal, presumably by increasing the blood flow to tissues that remove lactate from the blood (Figure 3.14). However, heavy exercise during the recovery period can lead to the formation of lactic acid and thereby retard the rate at which blood lactate levels return to baseline.

The fact that $\dot{V}O_2$ does not increase instantaneously to its higher steady-state level indicates that anaerobic energy sources (the ATP-PCr and glycolytic systems) contribute a portion of the ATP that is used during the initial transient period. Another portion of the ATP is derived from aerobic energy sources (the oxidative system) that operate using oxygen extracted from existing O_2 stores in muscle and blood. For this reason, O_2 stores can become depleted during the initial phase of exercise, as evidenced by the lower O_2 levels in venous blood (Figure 6.14).

However, once the steady-state level has been reached, the fact that $\dot{V}O_2$ remains constant indicates that the ATP requirements of exercise can be met entirely by aerobic energy sources. This aerobic supply of ATP is made possible through the combined operation of the cardiorespiratory system, which delivers fuels and O_2 to exercising muscles, and the oxidative system, which produces ATP through metabolic pathways that require O_2 (Figure 3.6).

Oxygen deficit

The *oxygen deficit* refers to the difference between the amount of oxygen actually consumed during the initial transient period of exercise and that consumed during a steady-state period of equal time. The magnitude of the oxygen deficit can be visualized from the area between the actual response in which $\dot{V}O_2$ gradually rises to its steady-state level and a hypothetical response in which $\dot{V}O_2$ instantly reaches its steady-state level (Figure 3.9). The oxygen deficit varies with exercise intensity; high-intensity exercises incur a larger O_2 deficit than low-intensity exercises because they utilize more anaerobically derived ATP.

The magnitude of the oxygen deficit also varies with the fitness of the individual performing the exercise. Trained persons incur a smaller O_2 deficit than untrained persons, because they are able to reach steady state in a shorter period of time. This difference in performance is due to training-induced improvements in the ability of the cardiopulmonary system to deliver fuels and O_2 to exercising muscles, as well as improvements in the capacity of trained muscles to oxidize fuels for energy.

Excess postexercise oxygen consumption (EPOC)

Oxygen consumption remains elevated during the recovery period that follows the cessation of exercise (Figure 3.9). The magnitude and duration of this phase of the $\dot{V}O_2$ response depends on the intensity and duration of the preceding exercise. The amount of oxygen consumed above the resting level during the recovery period has traditionally been called the *oxygen debt* and has more recently been called the *excess postexercise oxygen consumption* (EPOC); this latter notation is more accurate insofar as the oxygen debt is not due entirely to the extra oxygen needed to restore the preexercise levels of energy sources, oxygen stores, and blood lactate. Like the O_2 deficit, the magnitude of the EPOC can be visualized from the area between the actual $\dot{V}O_2$ response in which $\dot{V}O_2$ gradually declines to the resting level and a hypothetical response in which the $\dot{V}O_2$ response instantly returns to the resting level when exercise stops (Figure 3.9).

The EPOC can be partitioned into a fast component (lasting 2–3 min) and a slow component (lasting longer than 30 min) (Figure 3.9). Factors that contribute to the fast component include the oxygen used to: (1) metabolize fuel to replenish the high-energy bonds of the ATP-PCr system; and (2) reload the depleted O_2 stores in muscle and blood. Other factors that contribute to the elevated oxygen consumption during the re-

covery period include the effects of: (1) higher body temperature, which increases metabolic rate and therefore O_2 consumption; (2) increased activity and therefore higher O_2 consumption of the heart and respiratory muscles; (3) elevated levels of hormones that increase metabolic activity, such as catecholamines and thyroid hormone; and (4) endergonic (energy absorbing) metabolic pathways in which ~30% of the lactate formed during exercise is converted either to glucose (~20%) or amino acids (~10%). The remainder of the lactate (~70%) is converted to pyruvate which, in turn, is completely oxidized to CO_2 and H_2O in the oxidative system (Figure 3.10). Thus, the major portion of the lactate formed during exercise substitutes for pyruvate that would otherwise have to be supplied by glucose or glycogen. This lactate, which is consumed as a fuel in exergonic (energy releasing) metabolic pathways, does not result in extra O_2 consumption and therefore does not contribute to the EPOC.

Effect of exercise intensity on oxygen consumption

The effect of exercise intensity on oxygen consumption can be analyzed by plotting measured values of $\dot{V}O_2$ (in liters/min) against work rate (in watts, a measure of exercise intensity). Analysis of $\dot{V}O_2$-work rate data obtained during a graded exercise test (in which work rate is progressively incremented) yields a graph that can be characterized by a steep, essentially linear portion in which $\dot{V}O_2$ is dependent on work rate, and a flat, nearly horizontal portion in which $\dot{V}O_2$ is independent of work rate (Figure 3.11).

The linear portion corresponds to the range of exercise intensities over which a given increment in work rate (ΔWR) is matched by a proportional increment in oxygen consumption ($\Delta \dot{V}O_2$). The horizontal portion corresponds to the range of exercise intensities over which a given increment in work rate no longer elicits higher oxygen consumption, indicating that the oxidative system is operating at its maximal capacity. The maximal level of O_2 uptake attained under these conditions is designated as $\dot{V}O_2max$ (Figure 3.11).

Factors that influence $\dot{V}O_2max$

Individual values of $\dot{V}O_2max$ depend on the fitness of the person performing the exercise and on the type of exercise performed. As for fitness, highly trained endurance athletes exhibit substantially higher values of $\dot{V}O_2max$ (Figure 9.22) and can sustain substantially higher maximal work rates than untrained persons. For this reason, $\dot{V}O_2max$ can be regarded as a quantitative measure of *aerobic capacity*. As for type of exercise, continuous exercises that employ a larger muscle mass yield higher $\dot{V}O_2max$ values than do exercises that employ a smaller muscle mass.

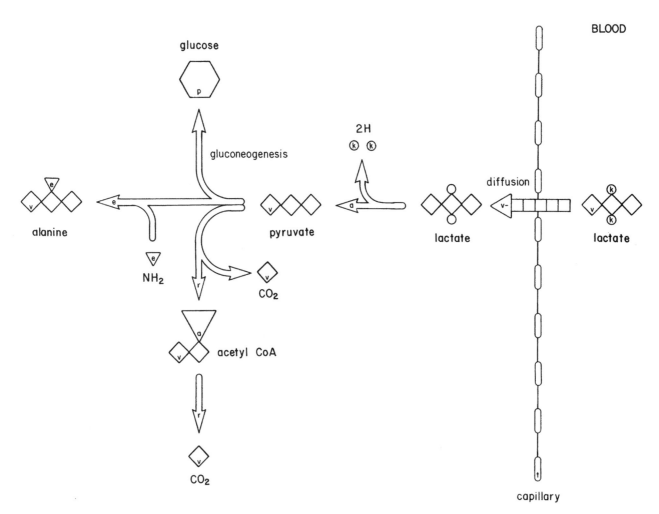

Figure 3.10 **Fates of lactate.** Color the lactate molecule in the blood, the hatched arrow that depicts its diffusion through the capillary wall (ignore hatches when coloring), and the lactate molecule that has entered the cell. Color the arrow depicting the reaction in which a pair of hydrogen atoms (2H, open circles) is removed from the lactate molecule, the hydrogen atoms, and the resulting pyruvate molecule; note that lactate differs from pyruvate by two hydrogen atoms. Color the arrows and the products of the reactions. Observe that pyruvate can be used to form glucose in the anabolic pathway of gluconeogenesis (Figure 2.26) or it can be used to form the amino acid alanine in the alanine shuttle (Figure 2.41); note that alanine differs from pyruvate by an amino group (NH_2). Observe that pyruvate can also be broken down to CO_2 and H_2O in the catabolic pathways of the oxidative system (Figure 2.27), where its energy can be extracted to form high-energy bonds in ATP. Most of the lactate formed during exercise is converted to CO_2 and H_2O by the oxidative system (~70%); the remainder is converted to glucose (~20%) or alanine (~10%).

These considerations explain why individual $\dot{V}O_2$max values exhibited by trained cross-country skiers (who utilize both upper and lower extremities) are higher than either those of trained cyclists (who primarily utilize the lower extremities) or those of untrained cross-country skiers. They also explain why $\dot{V}O_2$max values obtained on a cycle ergometer (a lower-extremity exercise) are higher than those obtained on an arm ergometer (an upper-extremity exercise). Values of maximum oxygen consumption obtained during treadmill exercise have been found to be ~10% higher than those observed during cycle ergometry and ~15% higher than those observed during arm ergometry. For this reason, it is common practice to designate treadmill values as $\dot{V}O_2$max and ergometer val-

ues as $\dot{V}O_2$peak. These findings indicate that caution should be exercised when comparing $\dot{V}O_2$max values obtained under different exercise conditions.

Effect of exercise intensity on blood lactate levels

Blood levels of lactate remain essentially constant from rest to moderate exercise, but rise markedly from moderate to strenuous exercise (Figure 3.12).

Studies in which subjects are infused with glucose that contains radioactive carbon atoms have shown that lactic acid is

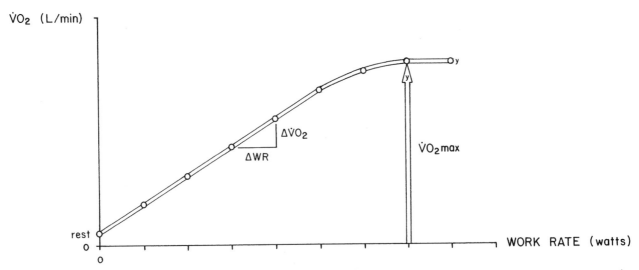

Figure 3.11 **Effect of exercise intensity of oxygen consumption.** Color the line that plots oxygen consumption ($\dot{V}O_2$, in L/min) against work rate (WR, in watts, a measure of power output). Identify the data points (small circles) that indicate $\dot{V}O_2$ values measured at different work rates during a graded exercise test; note that rest corresponds to a work rate of zero (y-intercept). Observe that the relationship between $\dot{V}O_2$ and work rate is characterized by a steep, essentially linear portion in which a given increment in work rate (ΔWR) is matched by a proportional increment in $\dot{V}O_2$ ($\Delta\dot{V}O_2$). Observe that the relationship between $\dot{V}O_2$ and work rate is also characterized by a flat portion in which $\dot{V}O_2$ is constant, independent of work rate. The maximum value of $\dot{V}O_2$ is designated as $\dot{V}O_2$max, a quantitative measure of aerobic capacity. $\dot{V}O_2$max values can range from ~3 L/min in healthy sedentary individuals to ~ 5 L/min in marathon runners. Values of $\dot{V}O_2$max and thus, the capacity to perform continuous submaximal exercises, can be increased by endurance training (Figure 9.22). In practice, commonly used criteria to determine $\dot{V}O_2$max during a graded exercise stress test include: (1) a leveling off of $\dot{V}O_2$ ($\Delta\dot{V}O_2 < 150$ mL/min) in the face of a higher work rate; (2) blood levels of lactate > 8 mmol/L; and (3) values of respiratory exchange ratio ($R = \dot{V}CO_2/\dot{V}O_2$) exceeding 1.15 (Figure 3.24).

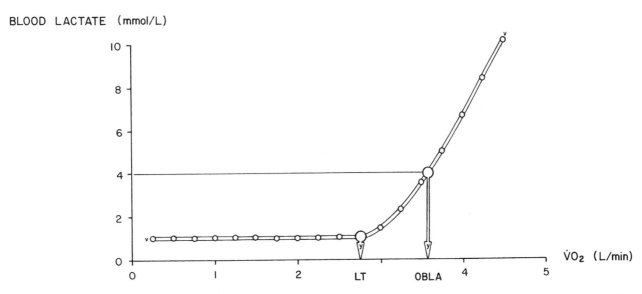

Figure 3.12 **Effect of exercise intensity on blood lactate levels.** Color the line that depicts blood levels of lactate (in mmol/L) plotted against oxygen consumption ($\dot{V}O_2$, in L/min), a measure of exercise intensity. Identify the data points (small circles) that represent the blood lactate concentration measured at different exercise intensities. Note that blood levels of lactate remain low over the range from rest to moderate exercise and increase markedly over the range from moderate to strenuous exercise. Identify the lactate threshold (LT, the point at which blood levels of lactate rise above the resting level) and the onset of blood lactate accumulation (OBLA, the point at which blood lactate levels rise to some predetermined level, in this case 4 mmol/L). Given that resting values of blood lactate are nominally 1 mmol/L, OBLA represents a fourfold increase in blood lactate. The functional significance of the lactate threshold is that it corresponds to the highest intensity of continuous exercise that can be performed in the absence of a buildup in blood lactate.

formed continuously at all levels of exercise and that fivefold increases in lactic acid production can occur without a concomitant buildup in blood lactate levels. These findings support the view that the low blood levels of lactate observed over the range from rest to moderate exercise result from a dynamic equilibrium in which the rate of lactate production is matched by an equal rate of lactate removal (Figure 3.13).

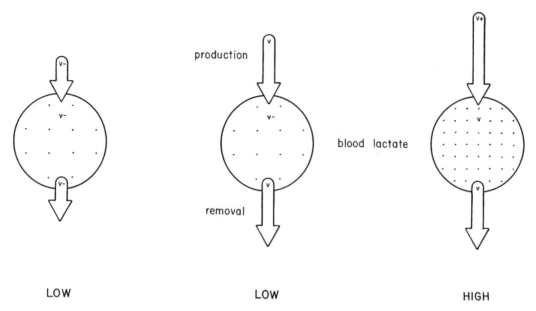

Figure 3.13   Determinants of blood lactate levels. Color the panels from left to right, noting that the length of the top arrow indicates the rate of lactate production, the length of the bottom arrow indicates the concomitant rate of lactate removal, and the density of dots in each circle represents the blood lactate concentration associated with each condition. Note that the rate of lactate production is low in the left panel, intermediate in the middle panel, and high in the right panel. Observe that these rates of lactate production are matched by equal rates of lactate removal in the left and middle panel; blood levels of lactate are therefore low in these conditions. Also observe that the rate of lactate production exceeds the rate of lactate removal in the right panel; blood levels of lactate are therefore high in this condition. These examples demonstrate that the concentration of lactate in the blood is not an accurate measure of lactate production.

During exercise, lactate formed in fast-twitch muscle fibers can diffuse out of the muscle and enter the blood or it can shuttle directly to adjacent slow-twitch muscle fibers where the lactate can be consumed as a fuel. For this reason, some of the lactate formed in working muscle is consumed within the same muscle and never enters the blood. At the same time, lactate is removed from the blood by other tissues that either consume lactate as a fuel (lactate may be the preferred fuel of cardiac muscle and slow-twitch skeletal muscle fibers), or convert it to other compounds, such as glucose or amino acids. Thus, an observed increase in blood lactate concentration could be due to an increase in the rate of lactate production and/or a decrease in the rate of lactate removal (Figure 3.14). A relevant outcome of these considerations is that the concentration of lactate in the blood is not an accurate measure of lactate production.

Factors that could increase the rate of lactic acid production include: (1) increased activity of lactate dehydrogenase (due to increased activity of fast-twitch muscle fibers, Figure 4.27); (2) increased concentration of pyruvate in the cytoplasm (due to a failure of the Krebs cycle to keep pace with glycolytic production of pyruvate, Figure 3.5); or (3) increased concentration of hydrogen atoms carried as $NADH + H^+$ (due to a failure of the hydrogen shuttle system to keep pace with glycolytic production of hydrogen atoms, Figure 3.5). A factor that could decrease the rate of lactate removal is reduced blood flow to tissues that either consume lactate as a fuel, such as cardiac and skeletal muscle, or convert lactate to glucose, such as the liver (Figure 3.14).

Lactate threshold (LT)

Two parameters that are used to identify the point at which lactate begins to accumulate in the blood are the *lactate threshold* (LT) and the *onset of blood lactate accumulation* (OBLA) (Figure 3.12). The lactate threshold (also referred to as the anaerobic threshold or the lactate breakpoint) is defined as the highest exercise intensity that can be sustained without an increase in blood lactate above the resting level. OBLA is defined as the exercise intensity for which blood levels of lactate rise to some predetermined amount, usually 2.0 or 4.0 mmol/L.

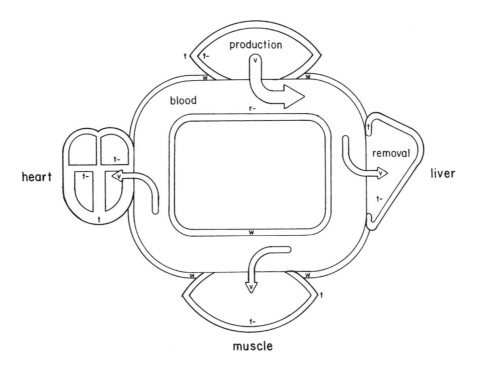

Figure 3.14 Lactate production and removal. Begin at the top and work clockwise as you color the organs, the arrows that depict the production and removal of lactate, and the blood. Note that liver, skeletal muscle, cardiac muscle, and kidney (not shown) can remove lactate from the blood. Note also that skeletal muscle is not only a major site of lactate production but also a major site of lactate removal. The liver can convert lactate to glucose (Cori cycle, Figure 2.25) or amino acids, or oxidize lactate to CO_2 and H_2O (Krebs cycle, Figure 2.18). Skeletal and cardiac muscle can convert lactate to amino acids or oxidize lactate to CO_2 and H_2O, but cannot convert lactate to glucose because the pathway of gluconeogenesis (Figure 2.26) does not operate in muscle.

Given that lactic acid causes fatigue in skeletal muscle, the functional significance of the lactate threshold is that it is an index of the highest level of exercise intensity that can be sustained indefinitely. For this reason, a higher lactate threshold is associated with the capacity to sustain a higher intensity of continuous exercise. By normalizing exercise intensity as a percent of $\dot{V}O_2$max, both LT and OBLA can be expressed in units of %$\dot{V}O_2$max. The lactate threshold occurs at 55% to 65% $\dot{V}O_2$max in untrained individuals and at 65% to 75% $\dot{V}O_2$max in endurance trained individuals. This difference in performance is due to training-induced improvements in the delivery of fuels and oxygen to exercising muscles, coupled with improvements in the oxidative capacity of trained muscles.

Physiological fuel value of nutrients

The oxidative system can extract energy from carbohydrates, fats, and proteins and store this energy in the form of high-energy bonds in ATP; for this reason, these three types of nutrients can serve as fuels for continuous exercise (Figure 3.6). The *physiological fuel value* of each nutrient, defined as the amount of usable energy per gram of nutrient, is determined by three factors: (1) its heat of combustion, a measure of the total amount of energy stored in its molecular bonds; (2) its

% digestibility, a measure of the degree to which the nutrient is absorbed into the body; and (3) its urinary nitrogen loss, which represents the unusable energy contained in the NH_2 groups that are ultimately excreted as urea.

Table 3.1, itemizing the approximate physiological fuel value of nutrients, shows that carbohydrate provides 4 kcal/g, fat provides 9 kcal/g, and protein provides 4 kcal/g. In addition,

Table 3.1	Physiological fuel value of nutrients		
	Carbohydrate	Fat	Protein
Heat of combustion (kcal/g)	4.1	9.4	5.6
Digestibility	98%	95%	92%
Unavailable NH_2 (kcal/g)			1.3
Physiological fuel value (kcal/g)	4.0	9.0	4.0

ethanol provides 7 kcal/g and dietary fiber provides 0 kcal/g (because it is not digestible by humans) (Figure 3.15). These results demonstrate that: (1) one gram of carbohydrate contains the same number of usable calories as one gram of protein; and (2) one gram of fat contains more than twice as many usable calories as one gram of carbohydrate or one gram of protein. For this reason, fat is said to be calorically dense than carbohydrate or protein.

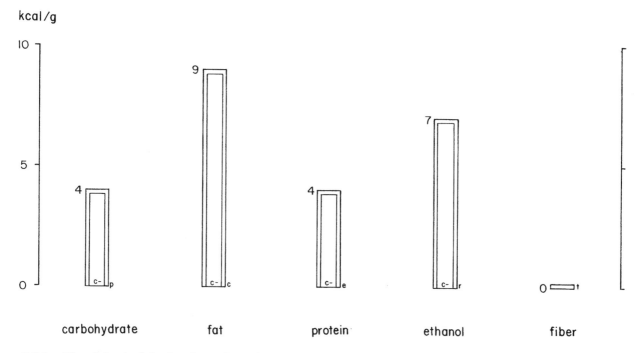

Figure 3.15 **Physiological fuel value of nutrients.** Color the bar graph from left to right, noting that the energy content of each nutrient (in kcal/g) can be visualized from the height of the bar. Observe that 1 g of carbohydrate contains the same number of usable calories as 1 g of protein and that 1 g of fat contains more than twice as many usable calories as 1 g of carbohydrate or 1 g of protein. Thus, fat is more calorically dense than carbohydrate or protein.

Energy content of nutrients

The number of calories in a specified amount of a nutrient can be calculated by multiplying the number of grams of the nutrient by its corresponding physiological fuel value. For example, 10 g of carbohydrate yields 40 kcal (10 g · 4 kcal/g = 40 kcal), whereas 10 g of fat yields 90 kcal (10 g · 9 kcal/g = 90 kcal).

Similarly, the total number of calories in a mixture of nutrients can be calculated by adding the number of calories in each of its constituents. For example, a glass of milk containing 12 g of carbohydrate, 10 g of fat, and 8 g of protein provides 170 kcal, i.e., the sum of its carbohydrate (48 kcal), fat (90 kcal), and protein (32 kcal) calories.

Direct calorimetry

Direct calorimetry is a method of determining energy expenditure by measuring the rate at which heat is produced by the body.

The method employs a calorimeter, which is an insulated, airtight chamber. The heat produced by the body warms the water that is pumped through pipes embedded in the walls of the calorimeter and warms the air that is pumped through the chamber of the calorimeter. Direct calorimetry is based on the premise that the amount of heat produced by the body is equal to the heat picked up by the water plus the heat picked up by the air; these latter values are derived from measured temperature differences between the incoming and outgoing water and air (Figure 3.16).

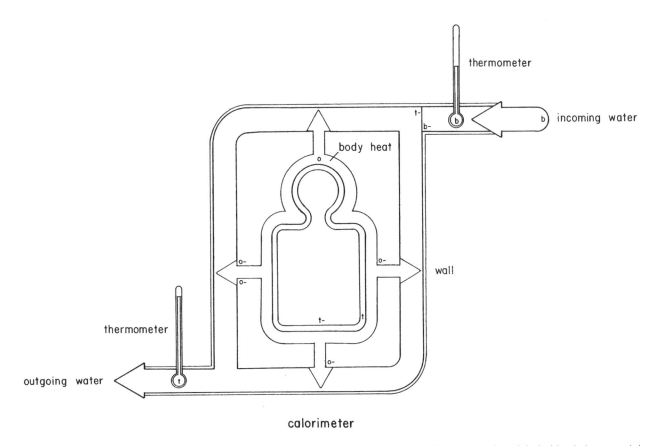

Figure 3.16   Direct calorimetry. Color the icon for the person in the calorimeter, the aura (outline) labeled body heat, and the interior of the calorimeter; observe that body heat is transferred to water that flows through the walls. Color the arrow labeled incoming water and follow the water around the walls of the calorimeter until you reach the arrowhead labeled outgoing water. Color the thermometers that detect the temperatures of the incoming and outgoing water; note that the outgoing water is warmer than the incoming water because it absorbed body heat. Given that the thermal properties of water are known (1 cal raises the temperature of 1 g of water by 1° C), the rate at which the body produces heat (in kcal/min) can be determined from measurements of the rate at which water flows through the calorimeter in conjunction with measurements of the temperature of the incoming and outgoing water. Differences in temperature between the incoming and outgoing air, which also picks up body heat, are not shown in this simplified diagram. Direct calorimetry is an accurate method of measuring heat production at rest, but is not well-suited for the assessment of energy expenditure in many athletic, recreational, and occupational activities. For example, it is not an accurate method of assessing energy expenditure during cycle ergometry because the friction between the belt and flywheel generates heat (Figure 3.28).

Although direct calorimetry is an accurate method of measuring heat production, its applicability to the study of exercise is limited because the calorimeter is unwieldy, expensive to build and maintain, and not well-suited for the assessment of energy expenditure in many athletic, recreational, and occupational activities.

Thermal equivalent for oxygen

The *thermal equivalent for oxygen* refers to the amount of energy (in kcal) that is released when 1 liter of oxygen is consumed in the complete oxidation of a given fuel to CO_2 and H_2O. In particular, ~4.7 kcal of energy are released when 1 liter of oxygen is consumed in the burning of fat and ~5.0 kcal of energy are released when 1 liter of oxygen is consumed in the burning of carbohydrate (Figure 3.17). It follows that an intermediate amount of energy (more than 4.7 kcal but less than 5.0 kcal) is released when 1 liter of oxygen is consumed in the burning of a mixture of carbohydrate and fat.

These findings explain why the amount of heat produced by the body can be inferred from the amount of oxygen consumed and the chemical composition of the fuel. They also provide the theoretical basis for *indirect calorimetry,* which is a method of estimating energy expenditure from measurements of oxygen consumption coupled with measurements of fuel utilization.

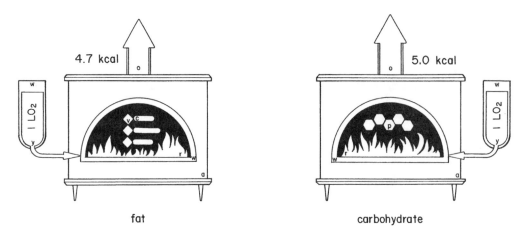

Figure 3.17 **Thermal equivalent for oxygen.** Color the fuels, fire, oxygen supply, and arrow indicating heat production in each panel. Note that 4.7 kcal of energy are released when 1 liter of O_2 is consumed in the burning of fat (triglyceride) and that 5.0 kcal of energy are released when 1 liter of O_2 is consumed in the burning of carbohydrate (glucose). These findings explain why the amount of heat produced by the body can be derived from measurements of oxygen consumption coupled with measurements of fuel utilization, the basis for the method of indirect calorimetry.

Indirect calorimetry

A widely used method of indirect calorimetry is *open-circuit spirometry,* in which expired air is collected (Figure 3.18) and analyzed to determine the amounts of oxygen consumed and carbon dioxide produced over a given time period. The method is based on the assumptions that: (1) the O_2 consumed by the body is given by the difference between the amount of O_2 in inspired and expired air; and (2) the CO_2 produced by the body is given by the difference between the amount of CO_2 in expired and inspired air. This enables O_2 consumption and CO_2 production to be calculated from measurements of the volume of expired air (V_E, in liters) and the fractional concentrations of oxygen (F_EO_2, in %) and carbon dioxide (F_ECO_2, in %) in expired air (Figure 3.19).

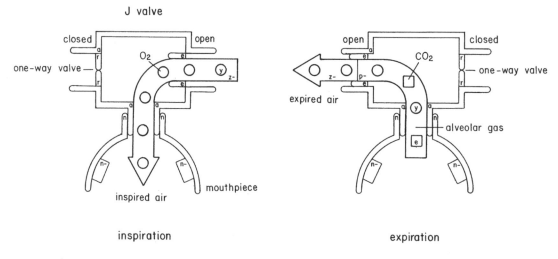

Figure 3.18 **J valve.** A J valve is a device that causes inspiration to occur through an inspiratory port and expiration to occur through an expiratory port; this permits expired air to be collected and analyzed. Identify the one-way valves and the mouthpiece, noting that the one-way valve at the right is open during inspiration (left panel) and that the other one-way valve is open during expiration (right panel). Color the arrows labeled inspired air and expired air and the molecules of O_2 (circles) and CO_2 (squares) contained within them. Observe that inspired air is atmospheric air (containing 20.9% O_2 and 0% CO_2, Table 6.1) and that expired air is made up of a mixture of two components: an initial component of inspired air (that ventilated the region of the lung where no gas exchange takes place) and a secondary component of alveolar gas (that ventilated the region of the lung where gas exchange takes place) (Figure 6.20). Count the molecules of O_2 and CO_2 in inspired and expired air, noting that expired air contains less O_2 and more CO_2 than inspired air. These considerations explain why differences between the O_2 and CO_2 contents of inspired and expired air can be used to determine the amount of O_2 consumed and the amount of CO_2 produced over any given period of time.

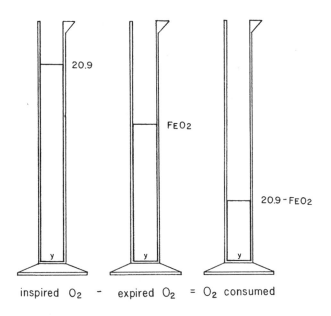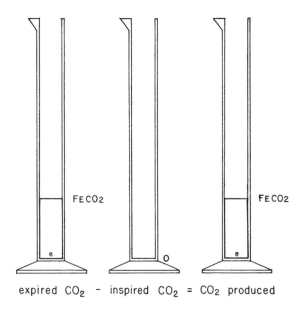

inspired O_2 − expired O_2 = O_2 consumed   expired CO_2 − inspired CO_2 = CO_2 produced

Figure 3.19   Principles of open-circuit spirometry. Color the gas contained in each cylinder from left to right in each panel. Observe that the degree to which a cylinder is filled represents the fractional concentration of the gas as a percent. Note that the fractional concentration of O_2 is 20.9% in inspired air and is F_EO_2 in expired air, and that the fractional concentration of CO_2 is 0% in inspired air and is F_ECO_2 in expired air. Observe that the O_2 consumed is given by the difference between the inspired and expired O_2 (left panel) and that the CO_2 produced during the same time period is given by the difference between the expired and inspired CO_2 (right panel). Because the volume of any particular constituent of a gas mixture is given by the product of its fractional concentration and the total volume of the mixture, the volume of O_2 consumed (VO_2) over a given period of time is $(20.9 - F_EO_2)$% of the volume of air expired during the same time period (V_E), i.e., $VO_2 = (20.9 - F_EO_2) \cdot V_E/100$. Similarly, the amount of CO_2 produced in the time period is $(F_ECO_2) \cdot V_E/100$. These considerations show that O_2 consumption and CO_2 production can be derived from measurements of expired volume (V_E, obtained using a Douglas bag or derived from devices that measure expiratory airflow) in conjunction with measurements of the fractional concentrations of O_2 and CO_2 in expired air (F_EO_2 and F_ECO_2, respectively, obtained from gas analyzers).

Respiratory quotient (RQ)

The *respiratory quotient* (RQ) is a metabolic parameter that is used as a measure of fuel utilization; it is calculated by dividing the number of carbon dioxide molecules that are produced by the number of oxygen molecules that are consumed during the complete oxidation of any given fuel to CO_2 and H_2O. Under resting steady-state conditions, RQ can be derived from the simultaneous measurements of CO_2 production ($\dot{V}CO_2$) and O_2 consumption ($\dot{V}O_2$) obtained from an analysis of expired air, i.e.,

$$RQ = \dot{V}CO_2/\dot{V}O_2$$

RQ for carbohydrate

The RQ value for a particular fuel can be determined by balancing the specific chemical equation in which the fuel is completely oxidized to CO_2 and H_2O. For example, the com-

plete oxidation of one molecule of glucose ($C_6H_{12}O_6$) consumes 6 molecules of O_2 and produces 6 molecules of CO_2 and 6 molecules of H_2O (Figure 2.27), i.e.,

$$C_6H_{12}O_6 + 6\,O_2 \rightarrow 6\,CO_2 + 6\,H_2O$$

It follows from this equation that the RQ for glucose is $6CO_2/6O_2 = 1$. Given that carbohydrates are digested into monosaccharides and the C:H:O ratio of monosaccharides is 1:2:1 (Figure 2.4), the complete oxidation of glucose to CO_2 and H_2O requires that only one O_2 molecule be added for each carbon atom of the glucose molecule to balance the equation. For this reason, the RQ for carbohydrate is 1 (Figure 3.20).

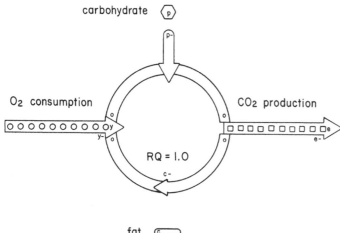

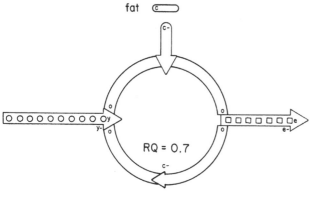

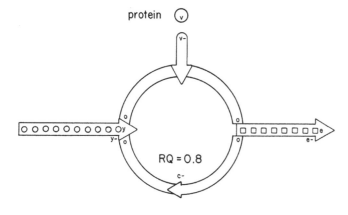

Figure 3.20   Respiratory quotient. Color the icon for the oxidative system, the fuel and its arrow, and the arrows labeled O_2 consumption and CO_2 production in each panel. Count the O_2 molecules (circles) and CO_2 molecules (squares) associated with the complete oxidation of each fuel to CO_2 and H_2O. Observe that the consumption of 10 molecules of O_2 yields 10 molecules of CO_2 during the oxidation of carbohydrate (top panel), 7 molecules of CO_2 during the oxidation of fat (middle panel), and 8 molecules of CO_2 during the oxidation of protein (bottom panel). Thus, the RQ for carbohydrate is 1.0, the RQ for fat is 0.7, and the RQ for protein is 0.8. These differences in RQ reflect corresponding differences in the chemical compositions of carbohydrate, fat, and protein. These considerations explain why RQ can serve as a quantitative measure of fuel utilization.

molecules are consumed than CO_2 molecules are produced whenever a fatty acid is completely oxidized to CO_2 and H_2O. As a result, the RQ for fat is less than 1.

As an example, the complete oxidation of one molecule of palmitic acid ($C_{16}H_{32}O_2$) consumes 23 O_2 molecules to produce 16 molecules of CO_2 and 16 molecules of H_2O, i.e.,

$$C_{16}H_{32}O_2 + 23\,O_2 \rightarrow 16\,CO_2 + 16\,H_2O$$

It follows from this equation that the RQ for fat is 16 CO_2/23 $O_2 \approx 0.7$ (Figure 3.20).

RQ for protein

The chemical composition of protein differs from those of carbohydrate and fat. Proteins are broken down into individual amino acids and the NH_2 groups are removed from the amino acids, leaving the carbon skeletons (Figure 2.40). The NH_2 groups are ultimately excreted from the body in the form of urea; the remaining carbon skeletons are eventually oxidized to CO_2 and H_2O in the Krebs cycle and electron transport chain.

A comparison of the CO_2 production and O_2 consumption associated with the complete oxidation of protein reveals that the RQ for protein is ~0.8 (Figure 3.20). Because protein normally accounts for less than 2% of the substrates used during exercise of less than 1 hour duration, carbohydrate and fat are the major sources of fuel under most conditions and therefore are the major determinants of RQ. However, protein breakdown can be an appreciable source of energy during periods of stress, as can occur during prolonged intense exercise or during starvation.

RQ for fat

The chemical composition of fat differs from that of carbohydrate in that fatty acids contain fewer oxygen atoms in relation to hydrogen atoms than does glucose—there is only one O_2 per fatty acid molecule, regardless of the number of its carbons (Figure 2.28). The balancing of the equation in which fatty acids are oxidized to CO_2 and H_2O therefore requires that one O_2 molecule be added for each carbon atom and that additional oxygen atoms be added to make H_2O from the pairs of hydrogen atoms that are not accompanied by an oxygen. The outcome of these considerations is that a greater number of O_2

Nonprotein RQ

The *nonprotein RQ* is defined as the $\dot{V}CO_2/\dot{V}O_2$ value associated with the complete oxidation of a mixture of carbohydrate and/or fat but not protein. Since each value of nonprotein RQ corresponds to a unique combination of carbohydrate and fat, nonprotein RQ can be used to partition the total number of calories obtained from a mixture of carbohydrate and fat into one component due to carbohydrate metabolism and another component due to fat metabolism. Stated another way, nonprotein RQ can be used to quantify the actual percentages of carbohydrate and fat calories obtained from a mixture of carbohydrate and fat.

As an example, a nonprotein RQ of 0.7 corresponds to a fuel mixture made up of 100% fat and 0% carbohydrate, whereas, at the opposite extreme, a nonprotein RQ of 1.0 corresponds to a fuel mixture made up of 0% fat and 100% carbohydrate. As another example, a nonprotein RQ of 0.85 (the midpoint between 0.7 and 1.0) corresponds to a fuel mixture in which 50% of the calories are derived from fat and the remaining 50% of the calories are derived from carbohydrate (Figure 3.21).

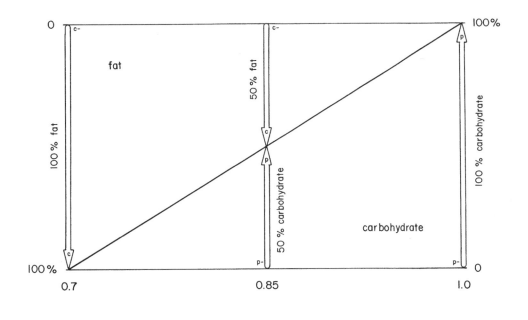

nonprotein RQ

Figure 3.21 Use of nonprotein RQ to determine fuel utilization. Color the rectangle, noting that the area above the diagonal line represents fat calories and the area below the diagonal line represents carbohydrate calories. Note also that the height of the rectangle represents the total number of calories (100%) associated with any given mixture of carbohydrate and fat. This analysis enables a vertical line (corresponding to any given nonprotein RQ) to partition the energy content of a mixture of carbohydrate and fat into two components: one due to carbohydrate and one due to fat. Observe that the sum of the carbohydrate calories (lower component) and fat calories (upper component) always equals 100%. Note that a nonprotein RQ of 0.7 indicates that 100% of the calories are derived from fat, whereas, at the opposite extreme, a nonprotein RQ of 1.0 indicates that 100% of the calories are derived from carbohydrate. Also note that a nonprotein RQ of 0.85 corresponds to a fuel mixture in which 50% of the calories come from carbohydrate and 50% of the calories come from fat. Thus, nonprotein RQ can be used to determine the relative contributions of carbohydrate and fat to the total energy expenditure. The energy contents of nutrients (in kcal) can be converted to grams of nutrients using their physiological fuel values (Table 3.1).

Effect of protein breakdown on urinary nitrogen

Because NH_2 groups released during protein breakdown are excreted in the form of urea, protein breakdown can be estimated from measurements of urinary nitrogen; each gram of urinary nitrogen is associated with a CO_2 production of ~4.8 liters coupled with an O_2 consumption of ~6.0 liters that can be attributed to the catabolism of protein (note that the RQ associated with these values is 4.8/6.0 = 0.8, the RQ for protein). Values of nonprotein RQ can then be obtained by subtracting the CO_2 production and O_2 consumption due to protein breakdown from the total CO_2 production and O_2 consumption.

Effect of exercise intensity and duration on fuel utilization

The actual amounts of carbohydrate and fat that are metabolized during any particular physical activity depend on: (1) the intensity and duration of the exercise (Figure 3.22); (2) the composition of the diet (high-carbohydrate diets promote carbohydrate utilization); and (3) the state of training of the person performing the exercise (endurance training increases fat utilization and decreases carbohydrate utilization at any given level of submaximal exercise) (Figure 9.28).

An increase in exercise intensity causes a relative increase in carbohydrate breakdown coupled with a corresponding decrease in fat breakdown (Figure 3.22, left panel). On the other hand, an increase in exercise duration causes a relative decrease in carbohydrate breakdown coupled with a corresponding increase in fat breakdown (Figure 3.22, right panel). Thus, high-intensity exercises promote carbohydrate catabolism, whereas long-duration exercises promote fat catabolism.

Factors that cause carbohydrate utilization to increase at higher-intensity exercise include: (1) increased recruitment of fast-twitch fibers (Figure 4.27), which derive energy from the pathway of anaerobic glycolysis (in which glucose is consumed at high rates); (2) higher blood levels of epinephrine, which promotes glycogen breakdown in liver and muscle and thereby increases the amount of glucose available to enter glycolysis; and (3) high blood levels of lactate, which inhibit triglyceride breakdown and thereby decrease the availability of fatty acids to serve as substrates.

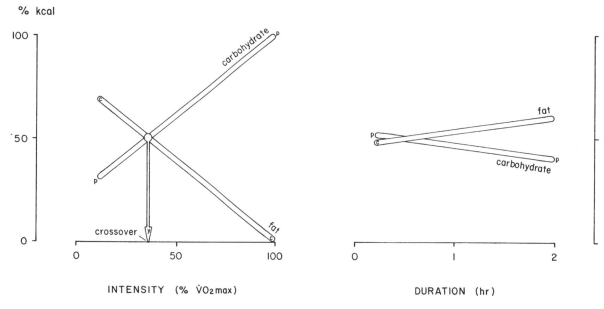

Figure 3.22   Effect of exercise intensity and duration on fuel utilization. Color the lines that depict the relative contributions of carbohydrate and fat to the total energy expenditure plotted against exercise intensity (expressed as % $\dot{V}O_2$max, left panel) and exercise duration (in hr, right panel). Note that the calories derived from carbohydrate (line labeled carbohydrate) plus the calories derived from fat (line labeled fat) equal 100% in all conditions shown. It follows that an increase in either component is accompanied by a corresponding decrease in the other component. Observe that an increase in exercise intensity (left panel) causes an increase in carbohydrate utilization (line with positive slope) coupled with a corresponding decrease in fat utilization (line with negative slope). Note also that fat normally contributes more calories than carbohydrate at rest (left endpoints of lines) and that carbohydrate contributes all of the calories at maximal exercise (right endpoints of lines); the crossover point is the exercise intensity at which 50% of the energy comes from carbohydrate and 50% of the energy comes from fat. Observe also that an increase in the duration of a fixed intensity exercise (right panel) causes an increase in fat utilization (line with positive slope) coupled with a corresponding decrease in carbohydrate utilization (line with negative slope). These findings demonstrate that high-intensity exercise promotes carbohydrate utilization, whereas long-duration exercise promotes fat utilization. Modified from G. Brooks et al. *J Appl Physiol* 76:2253, 1994.

Respiratory exchange ratio (R)

The *respiratory exchange ratio* (R, or RER), is another metabolic parameter defined as the ratio of $\dot{V}CO_2$ to $\dot{V}O_2$ (the same equation as that used to calculate RQ), i.e.,

$$R = \dot{V}CO_2/\dot{V}O_2$$

R is the same as RQ whenever the values of $\dot{V}CO_2$ and $\dot{V}O_2$ obtained from an analysis of expired air can be attributed entirely to the oxidation of fuels by aerobic pathways in the mitochondria. However, R differs from RQ when there is nonmetabolic production of CO_2 (see below) or when there is a change in the storage of O_2 or CO_2. Some exercise-related conditions in which R differs from RQ include: (1) lactic acid production, as occurs during anaerobic glycolysis (Figure 2.17); (2) hyperventilation, as occurs during very intense exercise (Figure 6.44); and (3) recovery from exhaustive exercise.

Because of its low pK (pH at which equal amounts of the dissociated and non-dissociated forms of the acid exist), lactic acid almost completely dissociates into hydrogen ions and lactate ions. The hydrogen ions are buffered predominantly by the bicarbonate system. The formation of lactic acid therefore produces hydrogen ions (H^+) which diffuse out of muscle cells and enter the blood where they combine with bicarbonate ions (HCO_3^-) already present in blood; this process produces *nonmetabolic CO_2* according to the following reaction (Figure 3.23), i.e.,

$$H^+ + HCO_3^- \rightleftarrows H_2CO_3 \rightleftarrows CO_2 + H_2O$$

A consequence of this nonmetabolic production of CO_2 is that the rate of CO_2 elimination in expired air exceeds the rate of CO_2 production by aerobic metabolism (Figure 3.24). As a result, R is larger than RQ. These results explain why

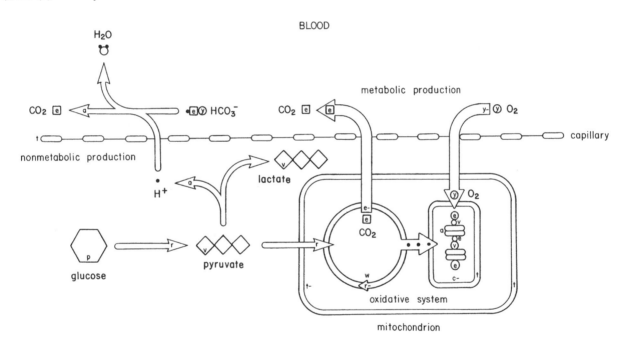

Figure 3.23 Metabolic and nonmetabolic production of CO₂. Color the glucose molecule and the arrow that depicts its breakdown to pyruvate in the pathway of glycolysis in the cytoplasm. Color the mitochondrial membrane, the icons for the Krebs cycle and electron transport chain (collectively labeled oxidative system), and the arrow that depicts the entry of pyruvate into the mitochondrion, where it is ultimately oxidized to CO_2 and H_2O. Color the O_2 molecules (circles), the capillary wall, and the arrow that indicates the diffusion of O_2 from the blood into the mitochondrion . Color the CO_2 molecules (squares) that are produced in the mitochondrion and the arrow that indicates the diffusion of CO_2 from the mitochondrion into the blood. This CO_2 is called metabolic CO_2 and its relationship to O_2 consumption is determined by the RQ of the fuel consumed in the oxidative system (Figure 3.20). Return to the pyruvate molecule in the cytoplasm and color the reaction in which pyruvic acid is converted to lactic acid; identify the hydrogen ion (H^+) that is released when lactic acid dissociates into H^+ and lactate. Color the arrow that shows the diffusion of H^+ into the blood and its combination with a bicarbonate ion (HCO_3^-) already present in blood. Color the bicarbonate ion, and the CO_2 and H_2O molecules that are produced by the reaction between H^+ and HCO_3^-. The CO_2 produced by the reaction between H^+ and HCO_3^- is called nonmetabolic CO_2. Observe that the total amount of CO_2 produced under these conditions is given by the sum of the metabolic CO_2 (due to the oxidation of fuels in the mitochondrion) and the nonmetabolic CO_2 (due to the buffering of H^+ by HCO_3^-). These considerations explain why the formation of lactic acid gives rise to an increase in CO_2 production coupled with a decrease in the blood level of bicarbonate. Compare this figure with Figure 3.5.

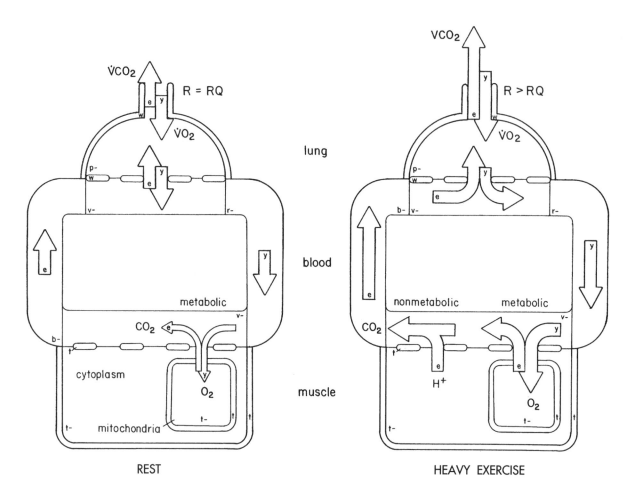

Figure 3.24   Effect of lactic acid formation on respiratory exchange ratio. Begin by coloring the left panel, which illustrates conditions at rest. Color the arrow labeled $\dot{V}O_2$ and follow the clockwise path in which O_2 is transported from the atmosphere into the mitochondria of the cell, coloring the structures as you go. Color the arrow labeled CO_2 in the mitochondria, and follow the clockwise path in which CO_2 is transported to the atmosphere, where it is ultimately expired (arrow labeled $\dot{V}CO_2$). Observe that the O_2 consumption and CO_2 production measured at the mouth are due entirely to the oxidation of fuels in the mitochondria. R is therefore the same as RQ under these conditions. Color the arrow labeled $\dot{V}O_2$ in the right panel, which illustrates conditions during heavy exercise. Follow the clockwise path in which O_2 is transported from the atmosphere into the mitochondria, noting that the flow of O_2 is greater (larger arrow) during heavy exercise than at rest. Color the arrow which indicates that the metabolic production of CO_2 is also greater (larger arrow) during heavy exercise than at rest. Color the arrow that depicts the nonmetabolic production of CO_2 (due to the buffering of H^+ by HCO_3^-) [Figure 3.23]. Note that the total CO_2 production (long vertical arrow in blood) is given by the sum of the metabolic CO_2 (arrow from mitochondria) and the nonmetabolic CO_2 (arrow from cytoplasm). Observe that the expired CO_2 (arrow labeled $\dot{V}CO_2$) exceeds the metabolic CO_2; R therefore exceed RQ under these conditions. Note also that the $\dot{V}CO_2$ arrow is longer than the $\dot{V}O_2$ arrow, indicating that the formation of lactic acid can cause R to exceed 1; thus, the observation of R > 1 during strenuous exercise can be regarded as evidence of nonmetabolic CO_2 production. Compare this figure with Figure 3.23.

the formation of lactic acid leads to an increase in R coupled with a decrease in the blood levels of HCO_3^- (Figure 3.25).

During hyperventilation, the rate of CO_2 elimination in expired air exceeds the rate of CO_2 production by metabolism (Fig. 6.23), and R is larger than RQ. Conversely, during recovery from exhaustive exercise, CO_2 is retained to replace the depleted HCO_3^- levels in blood. Under these conditions, the rate of CO_2 elimination in expired air is less than the rate of CO_2 production by metabolism, and R is smaller than RQ.

Components of energy expenditure

The major components of the *total daily energy expenditure* (TDEE) include: (1) the resting metabolic rate (RMR); (2) the thermic effect of feeding (TEF); and (3) the thermic effect of exercise (TEE) (Figure 3.26).

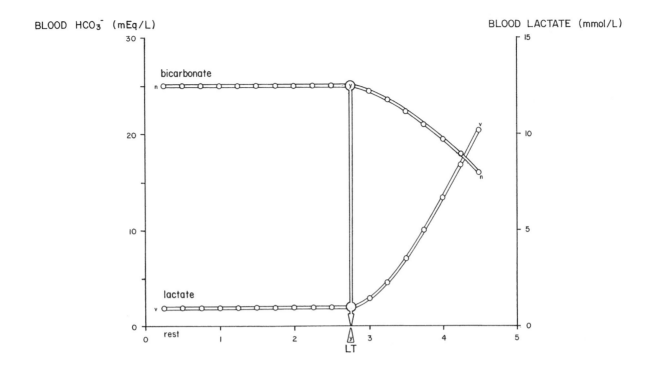

BLOOD HCO₃⁻ (mEq/L)

BLOOD LACTATE (mmol/L)

OXYGEN CONSUMPTION (L/min)

Figure 3.25   Effect of lactic acid formation on blood levels of bicarbonate. Color the lines that depict blood levels of bicarbonate (in mEq/L) and lactate (in mmol/L, redrawn from Figure 3.12) plotted against oxygen consumption ($\dot{V}O_2$, in L/min), a measure of exercise intensity. Identify the data points (small circles) that represent the blood levels of bicarbonate and lactate observed at different exercise intensities. Observe that blood levels of bicarbonate remain at the normal level (~ 25 mEq/L) over the range from rest to moderate exercise and fall over the range from moderate to strenuous exercise. Note also that the exercise intensity at which they begin to fall coincides with the lactate threshold (LT). These findings demonstrate that lactic acid production causes blood levels of bicarbonate to fall; this condition is referred to as metabolic acidosis (Figure 6.18). Modified from E. Hultman et al. *Exer Sport Rev* 8:41, 1986.

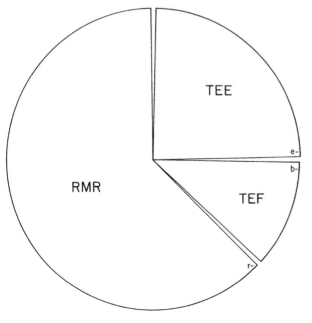

Figure 3.26   Components of total daily energy expenditure. Identify and color each of the components of the total daily energy expenditure (TDEE) and note the relative contributions from resting metabolic rate (RMR), thermic effect of exercise (TEE), and thermic effect of feeding (TEF). TEE is a highly variable component, ranging from 15% TDEE in sedentary persons to more than 30% TDEE in active persons.

71

Resting metabolic rate (RMR)

The *basal metabolic rate* (BMR) is the minimum level of energy expenditure needed to maintain the vital functions of the body. It is determined by measuring O_2 consumption under somewhat restricted conditions—during bed rest (in the morning) following a 12 to 18 hour fast prior to the test. The *resting metabolic rate* (RMR) is determined by measuring O_2 consumption under less stringent conditions—2 to 4 hours after a light meal with no exercise for 30 minutes prior to the test. These differences in procedure explain why RMR values are ~10% higher than BMR values.

The BMR in a given individual varies with body surface area; larger persons have higher BMR values than smaller persons. Body surface area is estimated from a nomogram based on height and weight (Figure 3.27). Values of BMR, normalized as kcal/hr per m^2, decrease by 2% and 3% per decade after age 20 in women and men, respectively. The BMR of women is 5% to 10% lower than that of men of the same size; this difference reflects differences in body fat, which is less metabolically active than lean body mass.

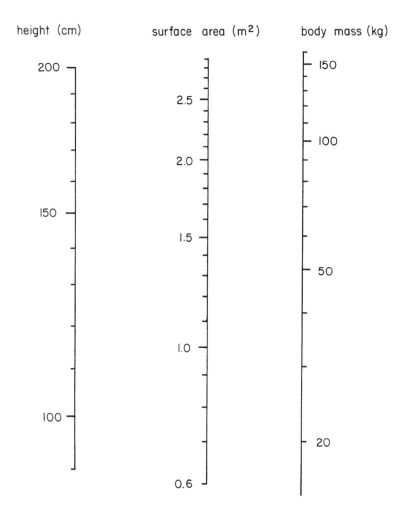

Figure 3.27 Nomogram for body surface area. This figure shows a nomogram that can be used to estimate body surface area (in m^2, middle axis) from body height (in cm, left axis), and body mass (in kg, right axis). Plot your height on the left axis, your body mass on the right axis, and connect the two plotted points with a straight line. The point at which this line intersects the middle axis is the calculated value of your body surface area.

gray blue canary green black navy orange pink red tan violet white yellow azure [+] and [–] mean use heavy and light pressure, respectively

Thermic effect of feeding (TEF)

The *thermic effect of feeding* (TEF) refers to the energy used in the digestion, absorption, and assimilation of ingested nutrients; this component accounts for ~65% of TEF. TEF also includes the increase in metabolism caused by the effects of ingesting food on the activity of the sympathetic nervous system; this component accounts for the remaining ~35% of TEF. Although the TEF of individual nutrients varies (TEF of protein > carbohydrate > fat) it is a common practice to estimate TEF as 10% of an individual's total energy intake.

Thermic effect of exercise (TEE)

The *thermic effect of exercise* (TEE) refers to the energy used in the performance of physical activities. TEE is a highly variable component of TDEE, ranging from 15% TDEE in sedentary persons to more than 30% TDEE in active persons (Figure 3.26).

Efficiency of exercise

The *efficiency of exercise* is defined as the ratio of the work output to the energy input above resting level (estimated by indirect calorimetry) (Figure 1.9).

Physical activities for which work output can readily be obtained include cycle ergometry, stair climbing, and exercise on an inclined treadmill. External work (in joules) during cycle ergometry can be estimated from the product of the external force applied to the flywheel by the friction belt (F), the velocity of the flywheel at the point of contact with the friction belt (v, determined by the diameter of the flywheel and the pedaling frequency), and cycling duration (T), i.e., work = F · v · T (Figure 3.28). External work (in joules) during stair climbing can be estimated from the product of body weight [the product of body mass (m, in kg) and the acceleration of gravity ($g = 9.8 \text{ m/s}^2$)] and vertical height (h, in m), i.e. work = m · g · h (Figure 1.4). Similarly, external work (in

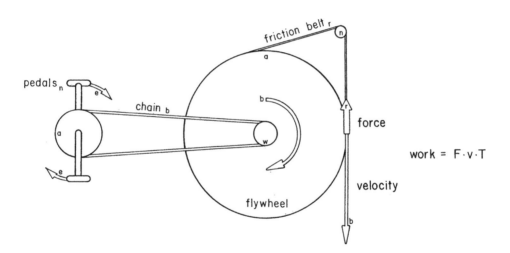

Figure 3.28   External work during cycle ergometry. Color the pedals, chain, flywheel, and friction belt. Observe that tightening the friction belt increases the force against which the flywheel must spin. Color the arrows labeled force and velocity, noting that force is determined by the friction belt adjustment and that velocity is determined by the flywheel diameter and the pedaling frequency. Physical principles dictate that power, or work rate (in watts), is given by the product of force (in N) and velocity (in m/s) and that work (in joules) is given by the product of power (in watts) and time (in seconds). Thus, the external work performed on a cycle ergometer under steady-state conditions can be calculated from the product of force (F), velocity (v) and time (T), i.e., work = F · v · T.

joules) during exercise on an inclined treadmill can be estimated from the product of body weight (w = mg) and vertical height [determined by treadmill belt speed (V), angle of inclination (θ), and exercise duration (T)], i.e., work = mg · T · $V\sin\theta$ (Figure 3.29).

However, physical activities for which work output cannot be readily obtained include horizontal walking and running, cross-country skiing, and swimming. As an illustrative

example, energy expenditure during horizontal walking (Figure 3.30) is due to the movement of the body's center of gravity in the vertical, horizontal, and lateral directions. For this reason, external work during walking cannot be determined from such factors as body weight, walking speed, or walking distance. Thus, the usefulness of efficiency as a measure of physical performance is sometimes limited by the lack of accurate methods for quantifying external work.

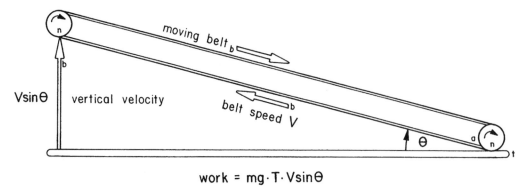

$$\text{work} = mg \cdot T \cdot V\sin\Theta$$

Figure 3.29   External work during inclined treadmill exercise. Color the treadmill and identify the angle at which the treadmill is inclined (θ). Note that treadmill belt speed (designated as V) can be expressed as the vector sum of a horizontal velocity (given by $V\cos\theta$) and a vertical velocity (given by $V\sin\theta$). Because the horizontal component of work (used to move the body in the horizontal direction) can usually be neglected in comparison to the vertical work (used to move the body in the vertical direction), the external work (in joules) performed on an inclined treadmill can be estimated from the product of the body weight [the product of body mass (m, in kg) and the acceleration of gravity (g = 9.8 m/s^2)] and the height to which the body weight was lifted during the exercise period. Height can be calculated by the product of the vertical velocity ($V\sin\theta$, in m/s) and exercise time (T, in s). Thus, work = mg $\cdot$ T $\cdot V\sin\theta$.

ENERGY COST OF WALKING (kcal/min)

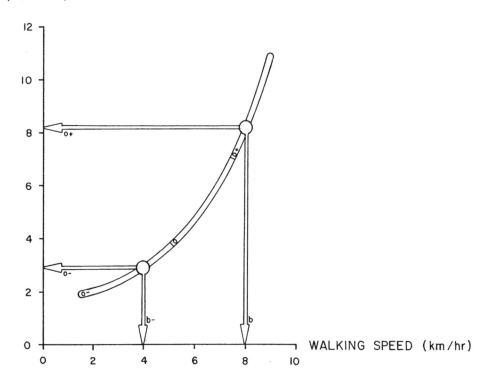

WALKING SPEED (km/hr)

Figure 3.30   Energy cost of walking. Color the line that plots the energy cost of walking (in kcal/min, determined by indirect calorimetry) against walking speed (in km/hr). Color the vertical and horizontal arrows, noting that a doubling of walking speed (from 4 to 8 km/hr) requires energy expenditure to more than double. Thus, the energy cost of walking (in kcal/min) increases disproportionately to walking speed. A relevant consequence of these findings is that the amount of energy (in kcal) needed to walk a given distance (in km) is higher during fast walking than during normal walking.

Economy of exercise

The *economy of exercise* is defined as the oxygen consumption associated with the performance of a given physical activity.

Economy of exercise can be regarded as an alternative measure of efficiency inasmuch as an observed increase in economy means that less oxygen is consumed in the performance of the same physical activity (Figure 3.31). The advantage of this measure of exercise performance is that it circumvents the technical difficulties associated with the quantification of external work.

OXYGEN CONSUMPTION (mL/kg·min)

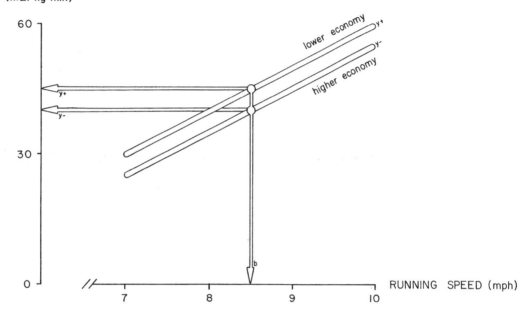

Figure 3.31   Economy of exercise. Color the lines that compare the oxygen consumption (in mL/kg · min) exhibited by two different individuals who were tested over the same range of running speeds (in mph). Observe that the line that corresponds to the higher economy runner falls below that of the lower economy runner. Color the vertical arrow that corresponds to a fixed running speed, and color the horizontal arrows that indicate the individual values of O₂ consumption associated with this speed. These findings demonstrate that a higher economy of running is associated with a lower O₂ consumption at any given running speed.

METs

Oxygen consumption is proportional to body mass in weight bearing exercises, such as walking and running; heavy persons consume more oxygen than light persons when walking or running at the same speed (Figure 3.32). Effects of differences in body mass on $\dot{V}O_2$ can be eliminated by expressing energy cost in terms of $\dot{V}O_2$ per kg of body mass, i.e., in units of $mLO_2/kg \cdot min$.

One *MET,* or metabolic equivalent, is defined as 3.5 $mLO_2/kg \cdot min$; it is assumed to be the normal resting value of oxygen consumption per kg body mass (Figure 3.33). Expressing $\dot{V}O_2$ in terms of METs enables the energy cost of any physical activity to be quantified as a multiple of the resting metabolic rate. For example, a physical activity for which the steady-state $\dot{V}O_2$ turns out to be 7 $mLO_2/kg \cdot min$ is said to be 2 METs of exercise, i.e., the energy cost of this particular activity is twice the energy cost of the resting state.

METs can be used to quantify work intensity. Light work can range from 1.6 to 4 METs, whereas heavy work can exceed 8 METs; most industrial jobs and household tasks require less than 3 METs of energy expenditure. METs can also be used to estimate the energy cost of occupational and recreational activities (Figure 3.33), as well as the energy cost of treadmill stress test protocols used in the evaluation of exercise performance (Figure 3.34).

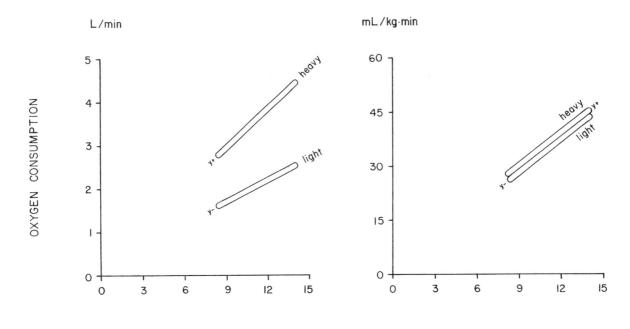

L/min

mL/kg·min

OXYGEN CONSUMPTION

RUNNING SPEED (km/hr)

Figure 3.32   Effect of body mass on oxygen consumption. Color the lines in the left panel that plot the absolute O_2 consumption (in L/min) of a heavy person (upper line) and a light person (lower line) against running speed (in km/hr). Observe that the O_2 consumption of the heavy person exceeds that of the light person at all running speeds. Repeat this process in the right panel in which the values of O_2 consumption (from the left panel) are divided by the body mass, and expressed in units of mL/kg · min. Note that this normalization of the data causes the line for the heavy person to coincide with the line for the light person. In other words, the effects of body mass on O_2 consumption are eliminated when O_2 data are expressed per kg of body mass.

Figure 3.33   METs. Color the vertical bar, noting the recreational and occupational activities that are associated with different levels of O_2 consumption, as quantified by METs.

METs

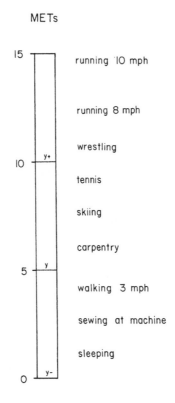

running 10 mph

running 8 mph

wrestling

tennis

skiing

carpentry

walking 3 mph

sewing at machine

sleeping

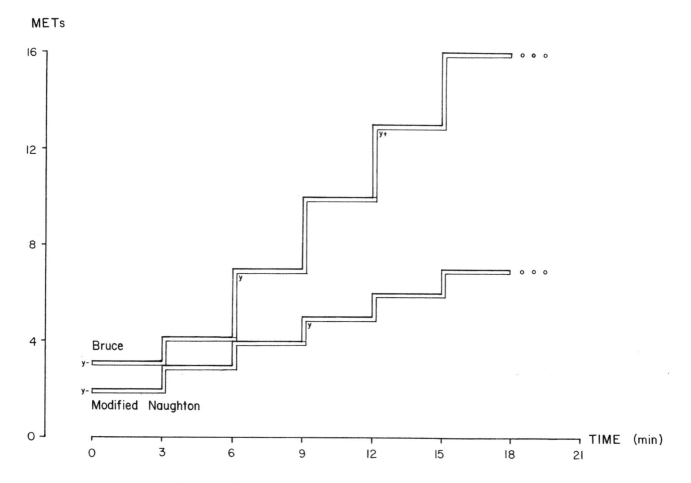

Figure 3.34 Energy cost of treadmill exercise protocols. This figure compares the energy cost of the Bruce and modified Naughton treadmill stress test protocols, also referred to as graded exercise tests. Both protocols increment the speed of the belt and the inclination of the treadmill (Figure 3.29) after every three-minute period, or stage; the energy cost of each stage is expressed in units of METs. Color the lines that correspond to each protocol, noting that the energy cost of the Bruce protocol exceeds that of the modified Naughton protocol. Compare the METs at each stage of these protocols with the activities itemized in Figure 3.33. The choice of a protocol used in a graded exercise test should take into account the health and fitness of the individual who is to be tested. Modified from P.S. Fardy et al. *Cardiac Rehabilitation, Adult Fitness, and Exercise Testing,* 2nd ed. Philadelphia: Lea & Febiger, 1988.

chapter **four**
skeletal muscle

Skeletal muscles permit the voluntary movement of exercise, maintain static and dynamic posture, and play a role in heat production.

Structure of skeletal muscle

Skeletal muscles consist of bundles of long, slender fibers whose ends fuse with tendons that insert into bone; this arrangement enables muscle contraction to move the skele-

ton. Muscle fibers are formed from bundles of myofibrils that, in turn, are made up of thick (myosin) and thin (actin) filaments that interdigitate (Figure 4.1).

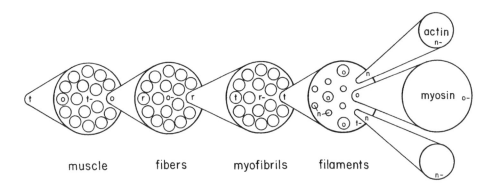

Figure 4.1   Structure of skeletal muscle. Color the picture from left to right, noting the relationships among the muscle, fibers, myofibrils, and filaments (also called myofilaments). Observe that the actin filaments form a hexagon that surrounds each myosin filament. Skeletal muscle also contains connective tissue (not shown). A thin layer of connective tissue called the endomysium surrounds each muscle fiber, a layer of perimysium surrounds each fasciculus (a bundle of ~150 muscle fibers), and a fibrous layer of epimysium surrounds the entire muscle to form a protective sheath that fuses at its distal ends with the connective tissue of the tendons.

Sarcomere

The *sarcomere* is the functional unit of skeletal muscle; it is the shortening of the sarcomere that causes the muscle to contract.

Each sarcomere consists of *actin* and *myosin* filaments that are connected to each other by cross-bridges that protrude from the myosin filaments (Figure 4.2). When viewed under

an electron microscope, the orderly arrangement of the filaments causes the myofibril to appear striated (striped), with alternating dark and light bands. The darker A, or anisotropic, bands contain myosin filaments, whereas the lighter I, or isotropic, bands do not contain myosin filaments (Figure 4.3). One end of each actin filament attaches to a structure called a Z disc; a sarcomere is that portion of the myofibril located between two successive Z discs.

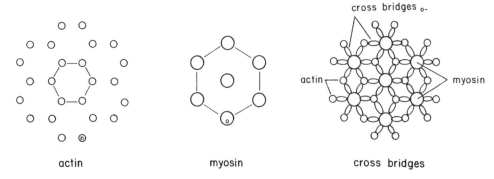

Figure 4.2   Arrangement of actin and myosin filaments. This figure shows the actin and myosin filaments as they would appear in a transverse section (cross section) of a sarcomere (Figure 4.3). Color the actin filaments in the left and right panels. Color the myosin filaments in the middle and right panels. Note that the right panel shows the actin filaments from the left panel superimposed on the myosin filaments from the middle panel. Note also that the actin and myosin filaments are oriented in such a way that they each form hexagons. Complete the picture by coloring the cross-bridges (formed by the myosin heads) that connect the actin and myosin filaments.

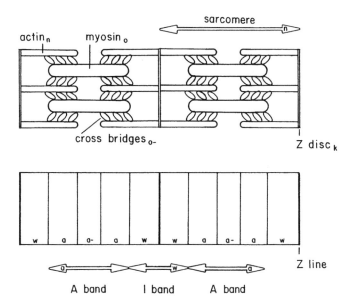

Figure 4.3   Sarcomere. This figure shows the actin and myosin filaments as they would appear in a longitudinal section of a sarcomere. Identify two sarcomeres and three Z discs in the figure. Color the actin and myosin filaments and the cross-bridges that connect them. Color the A bands and I band in the lower panel, noting that the darkness of the bands reflects the density of the myofilaments contained within them. Identify the location of the transverse sections that would produce each of the panels shown in Figure 4.2. Note that a myofibril consists of sarcomeres that are attached end-to-end at their Z discs (Figure 4.1). This arrangement enables the shortening of sarcomeres to shorten the muscle.

Structure of actin and myosin filaments

The myosin filament is composed of numerous myosin molecules that are bundled together with their globular protein heads protruding; it is these heads that attach to the active sites on the actin filaments (Figure 4.4). Each individual myosin molecule is made up of two heavy meromyosin chains and four light meromyosin chains that are wound together to form two heads at one end and a tail at the other. Each head contains two active sites—one binds with actin while the other binds with ATP; it is the high-energy bonds of ATP that supply the energy for muscle contraction (Figure 2.2).

The actin filament contains three different proteins—actin, tropomyosin, and troponin. Two helical strands of actin molecules are wound loosely together to form the backbone of the actin filament. A tropomyosin strand covers the active sites on each actin strand; this prevents the myosin heads from attaching to actin. Molecules of troponin are attached to the tropomyosin strands at regular intervals (Figure 4.4). Troponin is made up of three protein subunits—troponin A has an affinity for actin, troponin T has an affinity for tropomyosin, and troponin C has an affinity for calcium ions (Ca^{2+}).

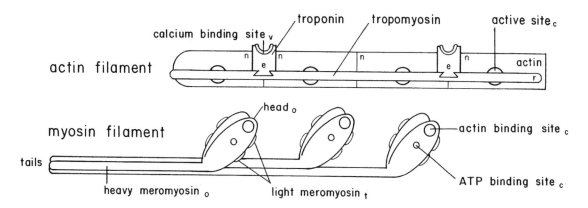

Figure 4.4   Structure of actin and myosin filaments. Identify and color each of the structures that comprise the actin and myosin filaments. Note that the myosin heads that make up the cross-bridges contain an ATP binding site. Observe that troponin molecules are attached to the tropomyosin strand at regularly spaced intervals, and that the tropomyosin strand covers the active sites on the actin strand; this prevents the attachment of the myosin heads to the actin filament.

Interaction between actin and myosin filaments

At rest, there is only a weak bond between the actin and myosin filaments, and the muscle can be stretched without much resistance. In the presence of calcium ions, however, actin and myosin bond strongly to one another. It is believed that the binding of calcium ions to troponin physically moves the troponin–tropomyosin complex so that the active sites on the actin filaments are exposed, thereby permitting the myosin heads to attach to them (Figure 4.5). This attachment causes the myosin head to tilt in a power stroke that pulls the actin filament across the myosin filament (Figure 4.6).

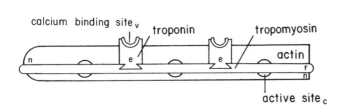
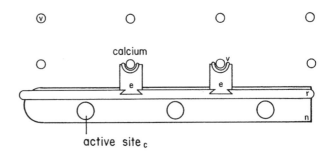

rest   contraction

Figure 4.5   Effect of calcium ions on actin filament. Color the structures in the left panel, which depicts conditions at rest. Observe that the calcium binding sites on the troponin molecules are empty and that the tropomyosin strand covers the active sites on the actin filament as in Figure 4.4. Color the structures in the right panel, which depicts conditions during muscle contraction. Observe that the calcium binding sites on the troponin molecules are occupied by some of the many calcium ions that have been released. Observe also that the tropomyosin strand is displaced and that the active sites on the actin strand are uncovered. Thus, the binding of calcium to troponin physically moves the troponin–tropomyosin complex so that the active sites on the actin filaments are exposed; thereby permitting the myosin heads to attach to them.

The energy for this process is provided by the breakdown of ATP into ADP and phosphate, a chemical reaction that is catalyzed by the enzymatic (ATPase) activity of the myosin heads (Figure 2.2). Numerous types, or isoforms, of myosin ATPase exist; they differ in terms of the rate at which they can break down ATP into ADP and phosphate. A muscle fiber that contains an isoform with a high ATPase activity can break down ATP more rapidly and therefore shorten faster than a fiber with a low ATPase activity. For this reason, differences in myosin ATPase isoforms give rise to differences in the contractile properties of muscle fibers (Table 4.1).

Following the power stroke, the head breaks away from the active site, returns to its normal configuration, and reattaches itself to the next active site farther down the actin filament (Figure 4.6). This repeated back-and-forth rotation of the myosin heads pulls the actin filaments across the myosin filaments. This process, which is called the *sliding filament hypothesis,* brings the Z discs closer together; the resultant shortening of sarcomeres causes the muscle to shorten.

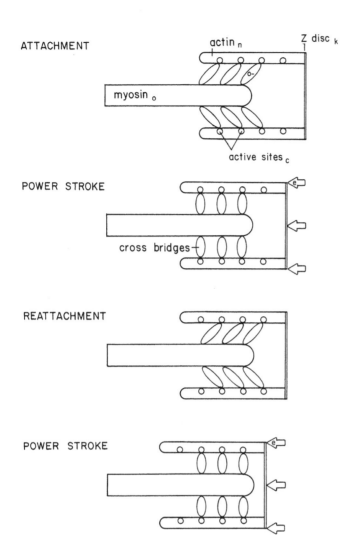

ATTACHMENT

actin $_n$ Z disc $_k$

myosin $_o$

active sites $_c$

POWER STROKE

cross bridges

REATTACHMENT

POWER STROKE

Figure 4.6   Interaction between actin and myosin filaments. This figure shows the interaction between the actin and myosin filaments that occurs when the active sites on the actin filaments are exposed and the myosin heads attach to them. Color the actin and myosin filaments, the cross-bridges, and the active sites in each panel. Note that the rotation of the cross-bridges to a vertical position during the power stroke pulls the actin filaments to the left and thereby shortens the sarcomere. Color the horizontal arrows that indicate the displacement of the Z disc that accompanies the shortening of a sarcomere. Note also that the actual lengths of the actin and myosin filaments remain unchanged when the sarcomere shortens. The energy released by the breakdown of ATP into ADP and phosphate is used to: (1) activate and reactivate the myosin cross-bridge prior to its binding with actin; (2) break the cross-bridge linkage between actin and myosin; and (3) remove calcium ions by an active transport mechanism called a reuptake pump (Figure 4.14). Compare this figure with Figure 4.3.

Effect of sarcomere length on muscle force

The initial length of the sarcomere determines the amount of overlap between the actin and myosin filaments and thus, the number of cross-bridges that participate in a given contraction. Since each cross-bridge contributes to the net force, sarcomeres generate their maximal force when they employ the maximal number of cross-bridges between the actin and myosin filaments. The length of the sarcomere that provides the maximal number of cross-bridges is called its *optimal length* (Figure 4.7).

Stretching a sarcomere to make it contract from a longer than optimal length decreases its contractile force by reducing the number of cross-bridges that participate in the contraction; passive insufficiency is a term that denotes muscle weakness due to overstretched sarcomeres. Shortening a sarcomere to make it contract from a less than optimal length also decreases its contractile force, but for different reasons. In a short sarcomere, force is reduced because the ends of the actin filaments abut each other. In a very short sarcomere, force is also reduced because the Z discs abut the ends of the myosin filaments. The variation in muscle force that results from changes in sarcomere length specifies the *length-tension relationship* of the muscle (Figure 4.8).

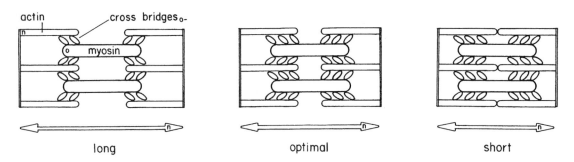

Figure 4.7 Effect of sarcomere length on filament interaction. Color the actin and myosin filaments in each panel. Color and count the cross-bridges in each panel. Note that the long sarcomere (left panel) generates less force than the optimal length sarcomere (middle panel) because it has fewer cross-bridges available to participate in the contraction. Note also that the short sarcomere (right panel) generates less force than the optimal length sarcomere because the actin filaments abut each other and interfere with the contraction.

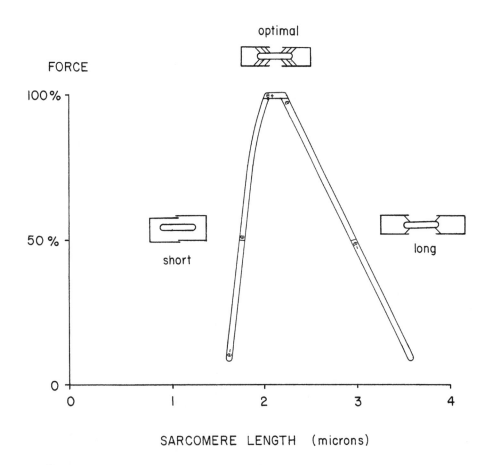

Figure 4.8 Length-tension relationship of skeletal muscle. The length–tension relationship of skeletal muscle describes how the fiber length of a muscle prior to its contraction influences the force (tension) that the muscle generates during its subsequent contraction. In this example, muscle force is measured during an isometric twitch in which the muscle is not permitted to shorten (Figure 4.15). Resting sarcomere lengths are varied by compressing or stretching the muscle prior to its contraction. Color the length–tension curve that shows how peak muscle force (expressed as a percentage of its maximal value) varies with sarcomere length [measured in microns (μm)]. Note that the muscle generates its maximal force when it contracts from an optimal sarcomere length (from 2.0 to 2.2 μm) and that force decreases considerably when the muscle contracts from a sarcomere length that is either too short or too long. Compare this figure with Figure 4.7.

Neural control of muscle contraction

Muscle contraction is regulated by the nervous system, which is organized as two main parts: the *central nervous system* (CNS), which consists of the brain and spinal cord, and the *peripheral nervous system* (PNS), which consists of nerve fibers (neurons) that transmit impulses to and from the CNS.

Afferent (sensory) nerve fibers are part of the PNS and carry impulses from peripheral sensory receptors to the CNS, while *efferent* (motor) nerve fibers carry impulses from the CNS to peripheral effector organs such as muscles or glands. The efferent nerve fibers that control skeletal muscle are part of the *somatic nervous system;* the efferent nerve fibers that control cardiac muscle, smooth muscle, and glands are part of the *autonomic nervous system* (Figure 4.9).

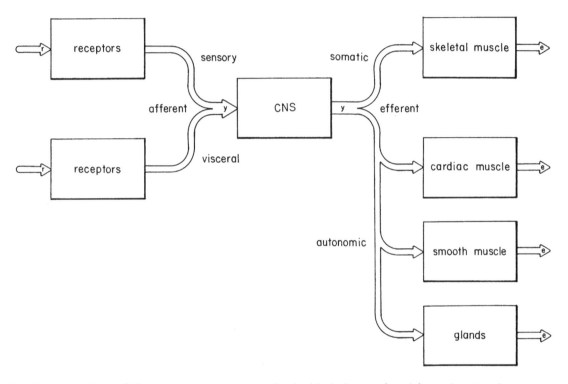

Figure 4.9 Organization of the nervous system. Color the block diagram from left to right. Note that responses (unlabeled arrows at right) to stimuli (unlabeled arrows at left) are mediated by the sequential action of sensory receptors, afferent nerve pathways, CNS centers, efferent nerve pathways, and effector organs (muscles or glands). Note that sensory receptors encode the intensity of their stimulation by the rate at which they generate action potentials. Thus, a small stimulus produces fewer action potentials than does a large stimulus. Observe that efferent nerves of the somatic nervous system innervate skeletal muscle, whereas efferent nerves of the autonomic nervous system innervate cardiac muscle, smooth muscle, and glands. The autonomic nervous system is subdivided into a parasympathetic and a sympathetic division that usually have opposite effects on their effector organs.

Innervation of skeletal muscle

Nerve fibers are classified according to their conduction velocity, which depends on the diameter of the fiber and the presence or absence of myelination (see below).

The efferent (motor) nerve fibers that innervate skeletal muscle are the *alpha* (α) *motor neurons* and the *gamma* (γ) *motor neurons* (Figure 4.10). The alpha motor neurons innervate the extrafusal muscle fibers, which are the force-generating fibers that make up most of the muscle, and the gamma motor neurons innervate the intrasfusal muscle fibers that are

part of the muscle spindle, a sensory receptor. Alpha motor neurons are controlled by nerve fibers that originate in different parts of the central nervous system, including the spinal cord, the lower regions of the brain, and the motor area of the cerebral cortex.

The afferent (sensory) nerve fibers that innervate skeletal muscle include the group Ia and group II afferent neurons that originate in muscle spindles and the group Ib afferent neurons that originate in Golgi tendon organs. *Muscle spindles* are sensory receptors that detect muscle length and play a role in the maintenance of posture (Figure 4.28), whereas

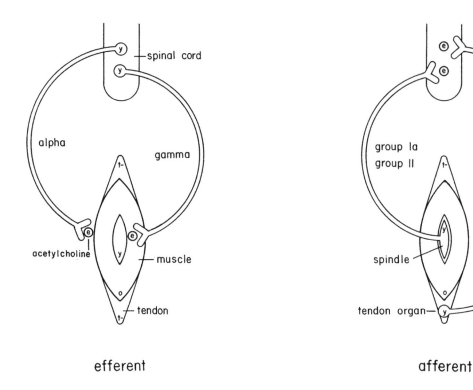

efferent

afferent

Figure 4.10   Innervation of skeletal muscle. Color the muscle, muscle spindle, efferent nerves, and afferent nerves. The efferent nerves (left panel) are also called motor nerves because they transmit neural signals from the central nervous system to the muscle. Alpha motor neurons are large-diameter myelinated fibers with high conduction velocities that regulate the contraction of the extrafusal (force-generating) fibers that make up most of the muscle. Gamma motor neurons are medium-diameter myelinated fibers with medium conduction velocities that regulate the contraction of intrafusal fibers that make up part of the muscle spindle, a sensory receptor in muscle. The afferent nerves (right panel) are also called sensory nerves because they transmit neural signals from sensory receptors in muscle to the central nervous system. Afferent pathways from muscle spindles (classified as group Ia and group II afferent nerve fibers) transmit information related to muscle length to the spinal cord, and afferent pathways from Golgi tendon organs (classified as group Ib afferent nerve fibers) transmit information related to muscle tension to the spinal cord. Group Ia and group Ib afferent nerve fibers are large-diameter myelinated fibers with high conduction velocities; group II afferent nerve fibers are medium-diameter myelinated fibers with medium conduction velocities. Muscle spindles and tendon organs initiate the stretch reflex (Figure 4.28) and the Golgi tendon reflex (Figure 4.29), respectively.

Golgi tendon organs are sensory receptors that detect muscle tension and play a role in the prevention of muscle injury (Figure 4.29).

Structure and function of nerve fibers

Neurons consist of a cell body, dendrites that respond to chemical, mechanical, or other stimuli, and an axon that transmits electrical impulses called action potentials (Figure 4.11). The axons have terminals that release chemical messengers called neurotransmitters. The neurotransmitter used by the somatic nervous system to regulate skeletal muscle contraction is *acetylcholine*. The autonomic nervous system regulates cardiac muscle, smooth muscle, and glands through the action of parasympathetic and sympathetic nerves. The neurotransmitter used by parasympathetic nerve fibers is acetylcholine and the neurotransmitter usually used by sym-

pathetic nerve fibers is *norepinephrine;* these neurotransmitters have opposite effects on effector organs. For example, acetylcholine decreases heart rate, whereas norepinephrine increases heart rate (Figure 5.12).

Action potentials in nerve fibers

Nerve cell membranes contain an active transport mechanism called a *sodium–potassium pump* that pumps three sodium ions (Na^+) outside the cell for every two potassium ions (K^+) that enter the cell. Since sodium and potassium have the same positive charge, the sodium–potassium pump removes an excess of positive charges from the interior of the cell. As a result, the interior of the cell becomes negatively charged with respect to the exterior and the membrane is said to be polarized (Figure 4.12).

This polarization of charges across the nerve cell membrane causes the resting membrane potentials of large motor neu-

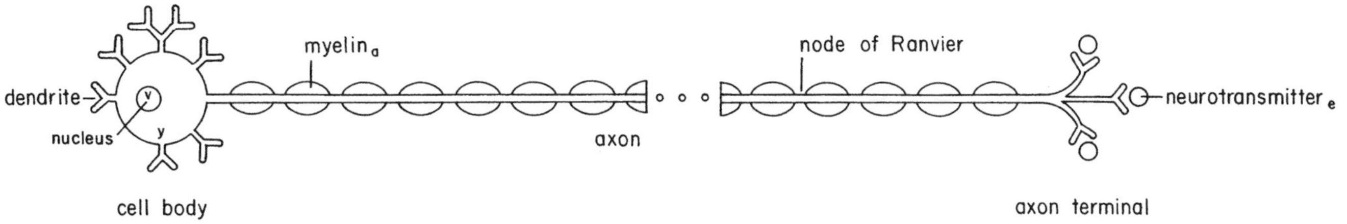

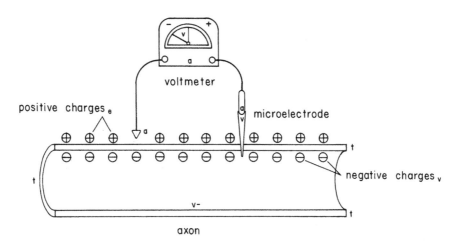

Figure 4.11   Structure of an alpha motor neuron. Color the diagram from left to right, identifying the structures as you go. Observe that an alpha motor neuron consists of a cell body, dendrites that respond to neurotransmitters, an axon that transmits action potentials, and axon terminals that release acetylcholine (neurotransmitter) at the neuromuscular junction. Observe that the axon is surrounded by myelin sheaths that are separated by unmyelinated segments called nodes of Ranvier; myelin increases the speed with which action potentials are transmitted. Nerve conduction velocities can range from ~100 m/s in alpha motor neurons (wide myelinated fibers) to 0.5 m/s in narrow unmyelinated fibers.

Figure 4.12   Membrane potentials in nerve cells. Color the membrane of the axon, the microelectrode, the voltmeter, and the charges on each side of the membrane. Observe that the voltmeter reading (in units of millivolts, mV) reflects the degree to which the inside of the axon is charged negatively with respect to the outside.

rons to be around −70 mV. Nerve signals are transmitted by *action potentials*, which are rapid changes in membrane potential that occur when the voltage across the nerve cell membrane rises from its resting level to a critical threshold level. Action potentials in nerve fibers are characterized by an initial rapid rise in membrane potential (*depolarization*) followed by a rapid return to the baseline level (*repolarization*) (Figure 4.13).

Transmission of action potentials in nerve fibers

Depolarization at one point on a nerve fiber creates local electrical currents that depolarize adjacent points. As a result, an action potential at any point on an axon initiates a wave of depolarization that travels the entire length of the fiber (Figure 4.11). Since large axons have less resistance to local current flow than small axons, the speed with which an action

potential travels along a nerve fiber is determined by the diameter of the nerve fiber—wide fibers exhibit higher conduction velocities than do narrow fibers.

The conduction velocity also depends on whether the axon is myelinated. Myelinated nerve fibers are those axons that are insulated by myelin sheaths that are separated by short unmyelinated segments called *nodes of Ranvier* (Figure 4.11). In myelinated axons, the action potential jumps from one unmyelinated node to the next in a process called *saltatory conduction*. Thus, two benefits of myelin are that it increases the speed at which action potentials are transmitted and it reduces the energy expended in their transmission.

Neuromuscular junction

Alpha motor neurons are large myelinated fibers that control the contraction of skeletal muscle by releasing molecules of acetylcholine at the *neuromuscular junction*, which is the in-

MEMBRANE POTENTIAL (mV)

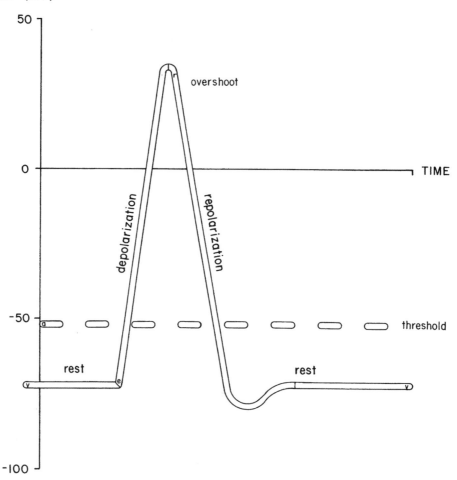

Figure 4.13   Action potentials in nerve fibers. Color the phases of the action potential that correspond to rest, depolarization, and repolarization. Depolarization is caused by a brief opening of sodium channels that allows sodium ions to flow rapidly down their concentration and voltage gradients to enter the nerve cell. These sodium channels can be activated by electrical (voltage-gated), chemical (ligand-gated) or mechanical stimuli. The resultant influx of positive charge causes the membrane potential to rise rapidly from the resting level of −70 mV to around +30 mV (overshoot). This phase of the action potential is called depolarization. Repolarization is caused by the closing of sodium channels and the opening of potassium channels that enable potassium ions to diffuse more rapidly out of the nerve cell, down their concentration gradient. This efflux of potassium ions removes positive charges from the interior of the cell and causes the membrane potential to return to its resting level of −70 mV. The overshoot corresponds to that portion of the action potential that appears above the abscissa (x-axis). The duration of an action potential in a nerve fiber is approximately 1 ms. Compare this figure with Figure 4.12.

terface between the motor neuron and the muscle fiber. The spread of an action potential over the axon terminal opens calcium channels in its membrane. The resultant influx of calcium ions causes a number of vesicles to undergo exocytosis and discharge the acetylcholine they contain into the synaptic cleft, which is the space between the nerve membrane and the muscle membrane (Figure 4.14).

Acetylcholine diffuses across the synaptic cleft to combine with receptors that open sodium channels in the muscle membrane. When open, these channels allow sodium ions to flow down their concentration and voltage gradients and

enter the muscle cell. The sudden influx of positive charge produces an action potential that spreads rapidly over the entire surface of the muscle membrane. Action potentials in muscle are characterized by an initial rapid rise in membrane potential (depolarization) followed by a return to the baseline level of around −90 mV (repolarization).

Excitation-contraction coupling

Excitation–contraction coupling refers to the process whereby an action potential (an electrical event) causes the

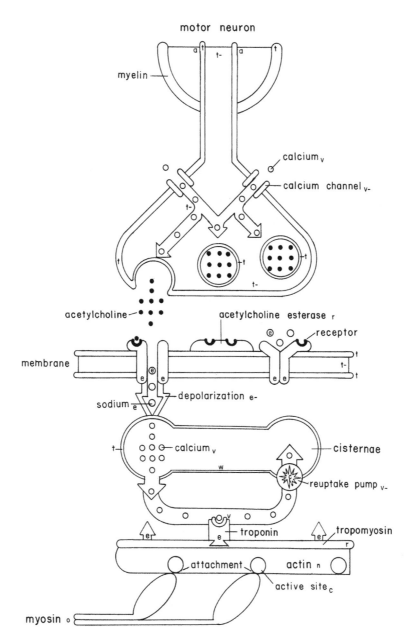

Figure 4.14 Neuromuscular transmission and excitation–contraction coupling. Begin at the top by coloring the myelin sheath, the membrane, and the calcium channels of the axon terminal of the alpha motor neuron. Color the calcium ions and note how they make contact with the vesicle that undergoes exocytosis, a process in which it ruptures and discharges its molecules of acetylcholine into the synaptic cleft, which is the space between the axon terminal and the muscle membrane. Color the membranes of the vesicles and identify the acetylcholine molecules that are the neurotransmitters at the neuromuscular junction; note the ones that are released into the synapse between the axon terminal and the muscle membrane. Color the membrane of the muscle, the sodium channels that span it, and the enzyme, acetylcholine esterase, that breaks down acetylcholine and prevents it from lingering too long in the synapse. Color the sodium ions that remain in the synapse; then color the ones that pass through the open channel to enter the muscle cell and depolarize it. Observe that the receptor in the open sodium channel is occupied by a molecule of acetylcholine. Color the depolarization arrow and note that it stimulates the release of calcium ions from the cisternae. Color the membrane of the cisternae and the calcium ions that are released. Note that the calcium ions are returned to the cisternae by a reuptake pump after they bind with troponin. Color the reuptake pump and the flash that indicates that it is an active transport mechanism that uses energy derived from the breakdown of ATP into ADP and phosphate. Note that the rate at which the reuptake pump removes calcium ions is an important determinant of muscle relaxation time. Color the troponin molecule and the tropomyosin strand and the vertical arrows indicating that the strand has been displaced from its resting position (Figure 4.5). Finish the picture by coloring the actin filament, the active sites that are uncovered, and the myosin filaments that attach to them as shown in Figure 4.6.

actin and mysoin filaments to generate tension (a mechanical event).

Action potentials in muscle spread rapidly to the central portions of the muscle through fast-conducting transverse tubules (T tubules) that penetrate the entire muscle fiber. The conduction of an action potential through the T tubules triggers the release of calcium ions that are stored in closed sacs, called cisternae, which are located within the sarcoplasmic reticulum, a specialized version of the endoplasmic reticulum. The released calcium ions bind to troponin and displace the tropomyosin strand, thereby uncovering the active sites on the actin filament, which, in turn, initiates a muscle contraction (Figure 4.14). The contraction ends when the calcium ions are returned to the cisternae by an active transport mechanism called a Ca^{2+} reuptake pump. The removal of calcium ions allows the troponin–tropomyosin complexes to return to their resting positions, where they again cover the active sites on the actin filaments.

Twitch

The *twitch* is the fundamental unit of muscle contraction; it is the contraction that is produced by a single action potential in a muscle fiber. A twitch can be characterized by: (1) a short delay called a *latent period;* (2) a period of contraction during which muscle tension (force) rises to its peak; and (3) a period of relaxation during which muscle tension returns to the baseline level (Figure 4.15).

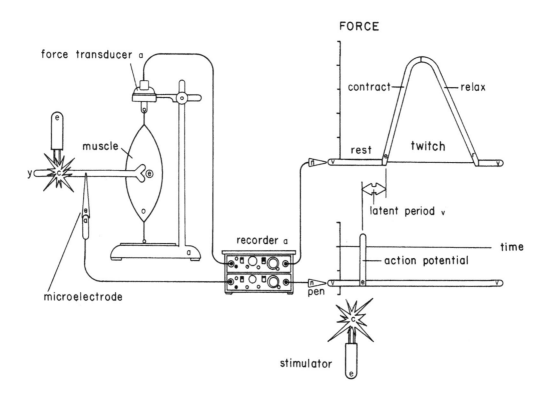

Figure 4.15   Muscle twitch. This figure describes a method for recording the force (tension) generated by a muscle during an isometric twitch (in which the muscle is not allowed to shorten). In this experiment, a nerve stimulator delivers a single shock to the motor nerve that produces an action potential in all of the muscle fibers simultaneously. Action potentials are recorded by a polygraph that amplifies and displays the voltage at the tip of a microelectrode positioned inside the nerve. The muscle is connected to an apparatus containing a force transducer (strain gauge), a device that converts muscle tension into an electrical signal that can be amplified and displayed by the polygraph recorder. Begin at the left by coloring the nerve stimulator and its electric shock, the motor nerve, the neurotransmitter, and the body of the muscle. Color the microelectrode, the force transducer, and the recorders. Color the stimulator, its shock, and the polygraph tracings of the action potential in the nerve and the twitch tension generated by the muscle. Note that the twitch is characterized by a short delay called a latent period, a period of contraction during which muscle tension rises to its peak, and a subsequent period of relaxation during which muscle tension returns to the baseline level. Color the arrow labeled latent period and note that it corresponds to the time delay between the delivery of the action potential to the nerve and the onset of the twitch in the muscle. Observe that the duration of the action potential is short in comparison to the duration of the twitch that it produces.

Types of muscle contractions

The term *contraction* is used here to mean the active generation of muscle tension (due to the interaction between the actin and myosin filaments); muscle contraction is not synonymous with muscle shortening. Types of muscle contractions (also referred to as muscle actions) include:

(1) *concentric contraction,* in which muscle length decreases during tension development; (2) *isometric contraction,* in which muscle length does not change during tension development; and (3) *eccentric contraction,* in which muscle length increases during tension development (Figure 4.16).

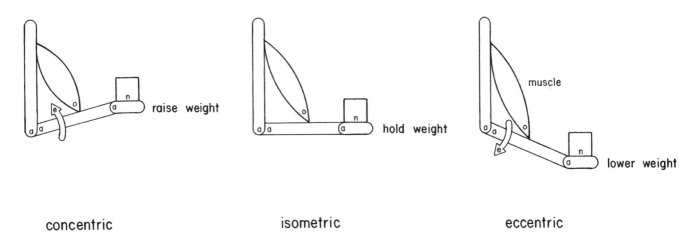

Figure 4.16   Types of muscle contractions. Color the panels from left to right. Observe that lifting a weight against gravity is a concentric contraction (muscle length decreases during tension development), holding a weight stationary is an isometric contraction (muscle length remains constant during tension development), and lowering a weight slowly is an eccentric contraction (muscle length increases during tension development).

The type of contraction depends on the magnitude of the force generated by the muscle in relation to the magnitude of the external force against which the muscle contracts. Thus, concentric contractions occur when muscle force is greater than external force, isometric contractions occur when muscle force equals external force, and eccentric contractions occur when muscle force is less than external force.

Effect of external load on muscle contraction

The tension developed by a muscle during a concentric contraction varies in accordance with the external load against which the muscle contracts. Heavier added weights prolong

the latent period, decrease the initial velocity of muscle shortening, and increase the peak tension (Figure 4.17).

Depending on the load, therefore, a given neural stimulation of muscle generates a high-force, low-velocity contraction against a heavy weight and a low-force, high-velocity contraction against a light weight. At the opposite ends of this range, a muscle generates its greatest force when it contracts against a load that is too heavy for it to move (its velocity is zero), and it generates its highest velocity (V_{max}) when it contracts against no load (its force is zero). The spectrum of all possible combinations of force and velocity, which can be obtained by using a range of weights, specifies the *force–velocity characteristic* of a muscle (Figure 4.18).

chapter **four**

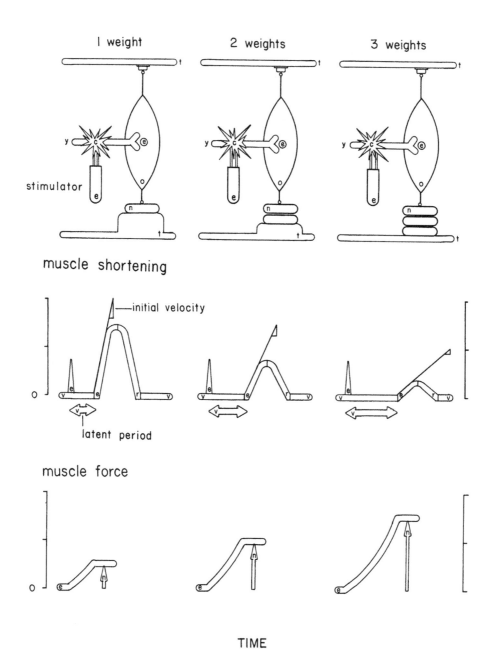

Figure 4.17   Effect of external load on concentric muscle contraction. This figure describes the concentric contraction of a muscle as it lifts three different weights. Color the top row, identifying the nerve stimulator, its shock, the motor nerve, and the muscle. Observe that the stimulation of the muscle and the initial fiber length of the muscle are identical in all three conditions. Color and count the weights beneath the muscle. Color the middle row, identifying the action potential (spike), latent period, and polygraph tracings that depict the time course of muscle shortening, shown as the absolute change in muscle length (in mm) plotted against time (in s). Because the slope of a line in a graph of distance (mm) vs. time (s) has the units of velocity (mm/sec), the initial slope of each tracing indicates the initial velocity of muscle shortening. Color the bottom row, noting that heavier weights, which require the muscle to generate more force to lift them, also prolong the latent period. The prolongation of the latent period is due in part to the extra time needed to stretch the muscle's internal elastic elements (connective tissue) by a greater amount. These findings demonstrate that heavier added weights increase muscle force and decrease the velocity of muscle shortening; this relationship between force and velocity is referred to as the force–velocity characteristic of skeletal muscle.

Figure 4.18 Force–velocity characteristic of skeletal muscle. The initial velocity of muscle shortening is plotted against the force generated by a muscle during concentric contractions against a range of fixed weights. The neural drive to the muscle and the initial muscle length are the same in all cases. Note that the three points indicate data obtained from Figure 4.17, where it was shown that a heavier weight causes the muscle to generate a higher force coupled with a lower velocity of shortening. Note that muscle force is greatest when its velocity is zero (isometric contraction, x-intercept of curve) and that muscle velocity is highest when its force is zero (unloaded contraction, y-intercept of curve). The spectrum of all possible combinations of force and velocity defines the force–velocity characteristic of a muscle.

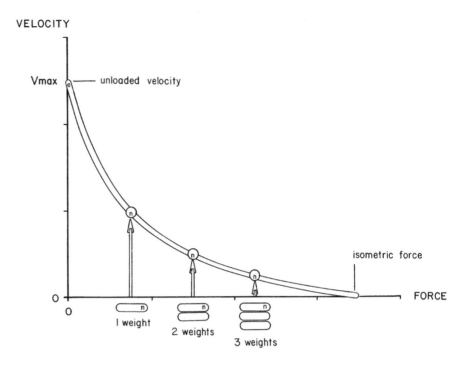

Motor unit

A *motor unit* is a single motor neuron plus all of the muscle fibers that the motor neuron innervates (Figure 4.19). Motor units of muscles involved in fine control (e.g., eye muscles) have few (3 to 6) muscle fibers per nerve fiber, whereas motor units of muscles involved in gross control (e.g., postural muscles of the leg) have hundreds of muscle fibers per nerve fiber.

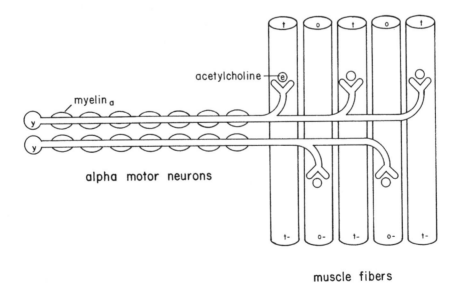

Figure 4.19 Motor unit. Identify two motor units; color each motor unit by coloring the alpha motor neurons and the individual muscle fibers they innervate, noting that the muscle fibers from different motor units are intermingled. Note that an α_2 motor neuron innervates slow-twitch muscle fibers and that an α_1 motor neuron innervates fast-twitch muscle fibers. The actual number of muscle fibers innervated by a single nerve fiber is called the innervation ratio; the innervation ratio is low in muscles involved in fine control (e.g., hand muscles) and large in muscles involved in gross control (e.g., leg muscles). Experiments in which the α_1 and α_2 motor neurons are switched surgically (a technique called cross-innervation) have found that this procedure causes muscle fibers to acquire the properties of their new motor neuron. In other words, cross-innervation can lead to a transformation of muscle fiber type. These findings indicate that the contractile properties of muscle fibers depend on the type of motor neuron that innervates them.

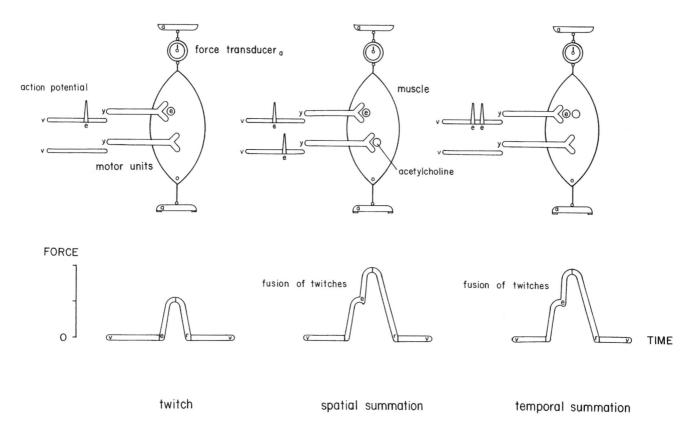

Figure 4.20 Spatial and temporal summation. Color the top row from left to right, identifying the action potentials, the two motor units, and the acetylcholine released in each condition; note that the initial muscle length is the same in all cases and that the force transducer detects the tension developed during isometric contractions. Color the bottom row from left to right, noting that the polygraph tracing depicts a recording of muscle force (in g, recorded by the force transducer) plotted against time in each condition. Note that a single action potential applied to one motor unit produces a twitch similar to that shown in Figure 4.15 (lower left panel). Observe that two action potentials (one to each motor unit), applied in rapid succession, produce twitches that fuse to yield a stronger contraction (middle panel). This summation of twitches due to the recruitment of motor units is called spatial summation. Also observe that two action potentials applied in rapid succession to the same motor unit produce twitches that fuse to yield a stronger contraction (right panel). The summation of twitches that is due to more frequent stimulation of a given motor unit is called temporal summation. Increases in muscle force during exercise are due both to spatial summation (a greater number of motor units are recruited) and temporal summation (a higher frequency of action potentials are delivered to individual motor units).

Motor units obey the all-or-none law, meaning that no muscle fiber in the motor unit contracts when a subthreshold stimulus is applied to the nerve fiber, and that every muscle fiber in the motor unit contracts when a suprathreshold stimulus is applied to the nerve fiber.

Spatial and temporal summation

Spatial and temporal summation are two different mechanisms that enable a whole muscle (which is made up of many motor units) to adjust the strength of its contraction. In *spatial summation,* an increase in muscle force is due to an increase in the number of motor units that are recruited to produce a contraction (Figure 4.20). Thus, weak contractions employ few motor units whereas strong contractions employ many motor units.

Temporal summation occurs when an increase in muscle force is due to an increase in the number of action potentials that are delivered to the same number of motor units. Since one action potential produces a twitch (Figure 4.15), frequent action potentials generate sequential twitches that fuse to produce a stronger contraction (Figure 4.20). Thus, weak contractions are produced by trains of low-frequency action potentials, whereas strong contractions are produced by trains of high-frequency action potentials. *Tetanus* is a condition in which the frequency of muscle stimulation is so high that there is no time for relaxation between successive stimuli and the individual twitches fuse to produce a steady contraction of maximal force (Figure 4.21).

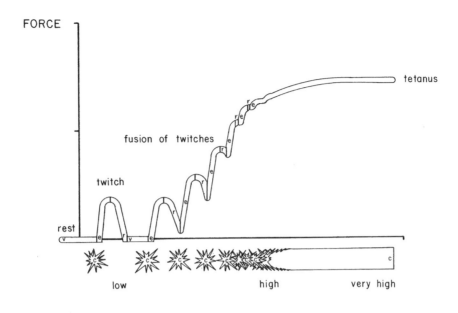

Figure 4.21   Tetanus. Color the shocks (flashes) and the graph that shows the isometric force developed by a skeletal muscle in response to repetitive stimulation at gradually increasing frequencies. As the frequency of stimulation increases, note that the twitches begin to fuse, the relaxation period between successive contractions shortens, and, at very high frequencies, the contraction becomes a complete or fused tetanus with no period of relaxation. Observe that the muscle generates its maximal force during a tetanic contraction.

Contractile and metabolic properties of muscle fibers

Muscle fiber types are classified in terms of their contractile properties and their metabolic characteristics. Based on their contractile properties, muscle fibers are characterized as *slow-twitch* fibers or *fast-twitch* fibers (Figure 4.22). Based on their metabolic characteristics, muscle fibers are classified as being oxidative (predominantly aerobic), glycolytic (predominantly anaerobic), or a combination of both oxidative and glycolytic. Since every muscle fiber derives energy from both aerobic and anaerobic sources, it is more accurate to envision the metabolic characteristics of different fibers within a muscle as a continuum, rather than to categorize them as discrete groups.

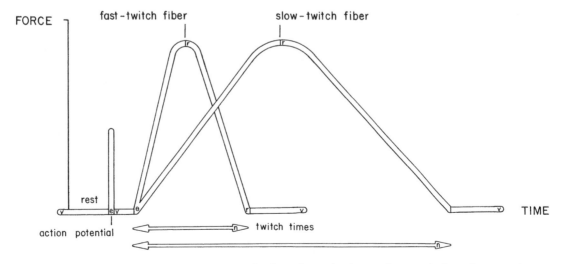

Figure 4.22   Effect of muscle fiber type on twitch duration. This figure plots muscle force (expressed as a percent of its maximal value) against time during an isometric twitch in a slow-twitch and a fast-twitch muscle fiber. Color the action potential, the contraction phase, the relaxation phase, and the twitch time (horizontal arrow) for each fiber; observe that the fast-twitch fiber has a shorter twitch time than does the slow-twitch fiber. Note that absolute differences in peak tension are not visible when force data are normalized as a percentage of their maximal values. Compare this figure with Figure 4.15.

95

Muscle fiber types

Type I fibers refer to the slow-twitch, fatigue-resistant fibers that derive most of their energy from aerobic sources of ATP (the oxidative system, Figure 3.1). They are also called oxidative fibers, or slow oxidative (SO) fibers.

Table 4.1 shows that type I fibers contain abundant mitochondria, high levels of oxidative enzymes, and a high density of capillaries that enable them to obtain an adequate supply of fuels and oxygen from the blood. They also contain high concentrations of myoglobin—myoglobin is similar to hemoglobin in that it binds oxygen and acts as a shuttle for oxygen between the cell membrane and the mitochondria, where it is ultimately utilized. High myoglobin concentrations therefore improve the delivery of oxygen from the capillaries to the mitochondria. The structural, functional, and metabolic characteristics of type I muscle fibers make them well-adapted for activities that require endurance, such as cross-country skiing or marathon running.

Type II fibers refer to the fast-twitch, fatigable fibers that derive much of their energy from anaerobic sources of ATP (the ATP-PCr and glycolytic systems, Fig. 3.1). Type II fibers are subdivided into type IIa and type IIb fibers. The type IIa fibers are also called fast oxidative glycolytic (FOG) fibers because they derive their energy from both aerobic (oxidative system) and anaerobic (ATP-PCr and glycolytic systems) sources of ATP. The type IIb fibers are also called glycolytic fibers, or fast glycolytic (FG) fibers, because they derive their energy predominantly from anaerobic sources of ATP.

Table 4.1 shows that, in comparison to type I fibers, type IIb fibers have fewer mitochondria, higher levels of glycolytic enzymes, and a lower density of capillaries. They also release calcium ions at a higher rate and have a higher myosin ATPase activity. These features enable fast-twitch fibers to break down ATP more quickly and therefore contract faster than slow-twitch fibers. The structural, functional, and metabolic characteristics of type II muscle fibers make them well-adapted for activities that require short bursts of high-power output, such as sprinting or weight lifting.

Contractile properties of slow-twitch and fast-twitch motor units

Fast-twitch muscle fibers have larger diameters than slow-twitch muscle fibers because they contain a greater amount of contractile protein. A nerve fiber in a fast-twitch motor unit also innervates a greater number of muscle fibers than does a nerve fiber in a slow-twitch motor unit. For these reasons, fast-twitch motor units generate more force and shorten faster against any given load than do slow-twitch motor units (Figure 4.23, top row). These differences between the con-

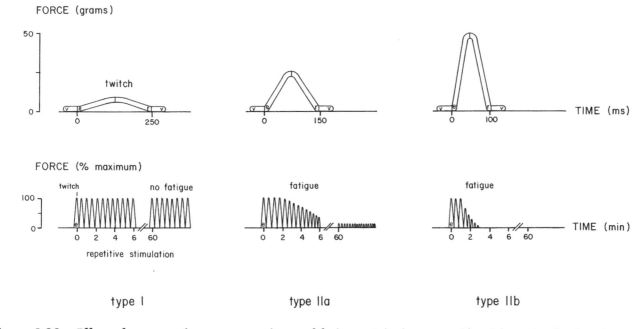

Figure 4.23   Effect of motor unit type on tension and fatigue. Color the top panel from left to right, identifying the contraction and relaxation phases associated with each twitch. Compare their absolute magnitudes and durations, noting that the peak force (in g) increases and the twitch time (in ms) decreases from type I (slow-twitch, fatigue-resistant) to type IIa (fast-twitch, fatigue-resistant) to type IIb (fast-twitch, fatigable) motor units. Color the bottom panel from left to right, noting that each spike represents the twitch (normalized as a percentage of the maximal value shown in the top panel) observed during a period (in min) of repetitive stimulation. Observe that the onset of fatigue can be identified as the point at which the muscle becomes unable to maintain the same level of force during repeated contractions. Examine the patterns of twitches to compare the fatigablity of type I, type IIa, and type IIb motor units. Compare this figure with Figure 4.22.

tractile properties of slow-twitch and fast-twitch muscle fibers manifest themselves as corresponding differences in their force–velocity characteristics (Figure 4.24).

Fatigability of slow-twitch and fast-twitch muscle fibers

The type I muscle fibers that rely on aerobic sources of ATP for their energy are referred to as *fatigue-resistant fibers,* whereas the type IIb fibers that rely on anaerobic sources of ATP for their energy are referred to as *fatigable fibers.* The type IIa fibers, which rely on both aerobic and anaerobic

sources, exhibit an intermediate degree of fatigability; they are more fatigable than the type I fibers but less fatigable than the type IIb fibers (Fig. 4.23, bottom row).

Types of fatigue

Fatigue, which can be regarded as an inability to maintain the same level of force output during repeated contractions, could be due to: (1) *central fatigue,* defined as a failure of the nervous system to maintain the same level of neural output to contracting muscles; or (2) *peripheral fatigue,* defined as a failure of contracting muscles to maintain the same conversion of neural drive into force.

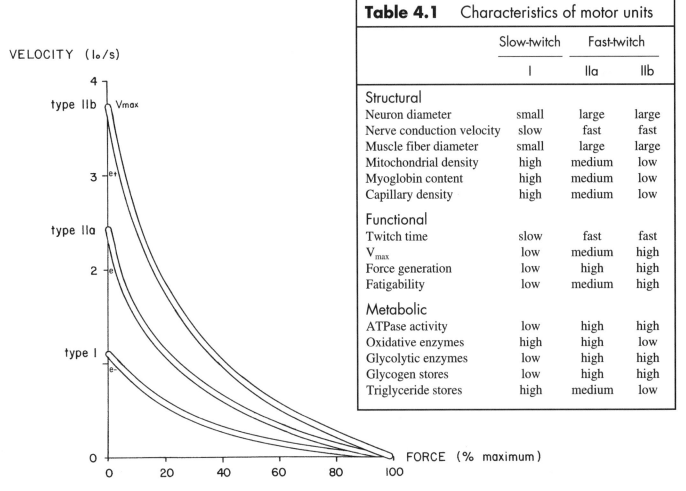

Table 4.1	Characteristics of motor units		
	Slow-twitch	Fast-twitch	
	I	IIa	IIb
Structural			
Neuron diameter	small	large	large
Nerve conduction velocity	slow	fast	fast
Muscle fiber diameter	small	large	large
Mitochondrial density	high	medium	low
Myoglobin content	high	medium	low
Capillary density	high	medium	low
Functional			
Twitch time	slow	fast	fast
V_{max}	low	medium	high
Force generation	low	high	high
Fatigability	low	medium	high
Metabolic			
ATPase activity	low	high	high
Oxidative enzymes	high	high	low
Glycolytic enzymes	low	high	high
Glycogen stores	low	high	high
Triglyceride stores	high	medium	low

VELOCITY (l_o/s)

Figure 4.24   Effect of muscle fiber type on force-velocity characteristic. Color and compare the individual force–velocity characteristics of type I, type IIa , and type IIb muscle fibers that were obtained under conditions similar to those described in Figure 4.18. Initial velocity of shortening is expressed in units of resting muscle length (l_o) per sec, and force is expressed in units of percentage maximum (isometric) force. Observe that the maximal velocity of muscle shortening (V_{max}, y-intercept) is highest in the type IIb muscle fiber, intermediate in the type IIa fiber, and lowest in the type I fiber (Table 4.1). Observe also that at any given level of force (as indicated by any given vertical line), the velocity of muscle shortening is also highest in the type IIb muscle fiber, intermediate in the type IIa muscle fiber, and lowest in the type I muscle fiber. Because power is given by the product of force and velocity, these observations demonstrate that power output is greatest in the type IIb fibers, intermediate in the type IIa fibers, and lowest in the type I fibers. These observations explain why a higher percentage of fast-twitch fibers in a given muscle is associated with the capacity to generate more power and therefore shorten faster against any given load.

Central fatigue can be caused by a dysfunction in the nerve cells of the central nervous system. It could also be due to psychological factors, such as motivation, or to physiological factors, such as pain, both of which could cause a decline in voluntary effort. Peripheral fatigue could be due to a dysfunction either in the peripheral nervous system or in the ex-

ercising muscles (Figure 4.25). Possible causes of peripheral fatigue include any factor that impairs: (1) the transmission of signals across the neuromuscular junction; (2) the release or binding of calcium ions in the excitation–contraction process; or (3) the ability of the actin and myosin filaments to generate force.

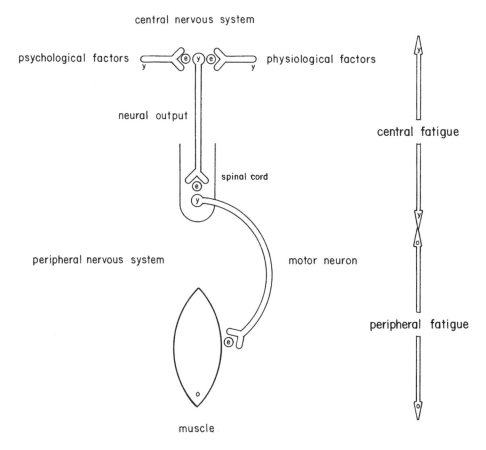

Figure 4.25   Central and peripheral fatigue. Color the nerves labeled psychological factors, physiological factors, and neural output, noting that these nerves are part of the central nervous system (brain and spinal cord, Figure 4.9). Observe that central fatigue is characterized by a failure of the central nervous system to maintain the same level of neural output during repetitive muscle contractions. Also observe that this type of fatigue could be due to dysfunction in the nerve cells of the central nervous system, psychological factors (motivation), or physiological factors (pain), any one of which could lead to a decline in voluntary effort. Color the nerve labeled motor neuron, the acetylcholine that it releases, and the muscle that it innervates. Observe that peripheral fatigue is characterized by a failure to maintain the same conversion of neural drive into force during repeated contractions. Also observe that this type of fatigue could be due to any factor that impairs the transmission of signals across the neuromuscular junction, the excitation–contraction process, or the ability of actin and myosin filaments to generate force. It follows from these considerations that muscle fatigue during exercise could be due to a variety of factors.

With regard to this last possibility, metabolic alterations that impair the ability of the actin and myosin filaments to generate force include: (1) depletion of energy sources, such as ATP, PCr (phosphocreatine, Figure 3.2), and glycogen; or (2) accumulation of metabolites, such as the hydrogen and lactate ions produced by anaerobic glycolysis (Figure 2.17), ammonia produced by protein breakdown, and phosphate

produced by the breakdown of ATP into ADP and phosphate. A decrease in intracellular pH interferes with the excitation-contraction coupling mechanism because excessive levels of hydrogen ions (H^+) displace calcium ions (Ca^{2+}) and impair actin-myosin cross-bridge formation; this is the major factor limiting performance during short-term maximal exercise.

During long-term maximal exercise, however, fatigue is primarily related to the depletion of energy sources, particularly muscle glycogen. A mechanism that has been proposed to explain why muscle glycogen depletion causes fatigue is based on the premise that low levels of glycogen cause low levels of pyruvate. Consequently, those intermediate compounds in the Krebs cycle that are derived from pyruvate are also low, which, in turn, inhibits Krebs cycle activity and thereby limits the ability of the oxidative system to produce ATP for muscle contraction. These considerations can explain why high-carbohydrate diets, which promote glycogen synthesis (Figure 10.7), delay the onset of fatigue during prolonged physical activities.

Relative distributions of muscle fiber types

Although all of the muscles of the body contain both slow-twitch and fast-twitch fibers, the distribution of fiber types can vary among different muscles in the same individual and in the same muscle among different individuals. In a given individual, for example, the percentages of slow-twitch and fast-twitch fibers in different muscles vary with the function of the muscle. Thus, a leg muscle that is used to maintain posture, such as the soleus, contains a higher percentage of slow-twitch fibers than a leg muscle that is used in jumping, such as the gastrocnemius.

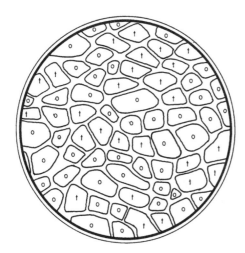

Figure 4.26 Distribution of muscle fiber types. Color the individual fibers in this cross section of a muscle and note the relative numbers of slow-twitch and fast-twitch fibers. The relative percentages of slow-twitch and fast-twitch fibers can vary among the same muscle in different individuals and among different muscles in the same individual. The metabolic properties of individual muscle fibers are determined by staining for key enzymes in the muscle specimen. For example, high levels of phosphofructokinase (an enzyme of glycolysis, Figure 3.4) are found in fast-twitch fibers and high levels of succinate dehydrogenase (an enzyme of the Krebs cycle) are found in slow-twitch fibers.

Studies on identical twins suggest that the relative numbers of each fiber type in a given muscle is determined primarily by genetic factors. However, the findings that strength training enhances the glycolytic capacity of muscle (Figure 9.15), and that endurance training enhances the oxidative capacity of muscle (Figure 9.26), demonstrate that training protocols can alter the metabolic characteristics of muscle fibers. These findings suggest that some transformation of fiber type might be possible under extreme conditions, such as chronic and specific types of physical activities.

Distribution of muscle fiber types in elite athletes

Muscle biopsies performed on the leg muscles of elite long distance runners and elite sprint swimmers reveal considerable differences between the relative distributions of slow-twitch and fast-twitch fibers (Figure 4.26). Slow-twitch fibers predominate in the leg muscles of highly trained long distance runners and fast-twitch fibers predominate in the leg muscles of highly trained sprinters.

The relationship between exercise performance and muscle fiber composition can also be studied in elite athletes by comparing the maximum oxygen consumption ($\dot{V}O_2$max) attained during a specific sport with the percentage of slow-twitch fibers in the muscles that are activated during the sport. Highly trained endurance athletes who exhibit the highest $\dot{V}O_2$max, such as cross-country skiers, have the highest percentage of slow-twitch fibers in their trained muscles. Conversely, highly trained athletes who exhibit the highest levels of power output, such as sprinters, have the highest percentage of fast-twitch fibers in their trained muscles. These findings indicate that muscle fiber distribution is a determinant of maximal performance in physical activities that require strength, power, or endurance.

Recruitment patterns of motor units

All of the muscle fibers within a given motor unit have the same contractile properties; any particular motor unit contains only slow-twitch fibers or only fast-twitch fibers, and not a mixture of the two fiber types (Figure 4.19). Because motor units are activated in size order, a given muscle produces identical forces on different occasions by the orderly recruitment of the same motor units.

There are two categories of alpha motor neurons that innervate skeletal muscle—α_1 and α_2. The α_1 motor neurons are the larger nerve fibers that control the fast-twitch motor units, whereas the α_2 motor neurons are the smaller nerve fibers that control the slow-twitch motor units. Because smaller motor neurons have lower excitation thresholds than do larger motor neurons, differences in nerve size can explain why slow-twitch motor units are preferentially activated at low exercise intensities and why slow-twitch and fast-twitch motor units are both activated at high exercise intensities (Figure 4.27).

Given that slow-twitch fibers rely on aerobic metabolism and that fast-twitch fibers rely on anaerobic metabolism, any given pattern of motor unit recruitment is accompanied by a corresponding pattern of metabolic activity. It follows that the relative contributions of aerobic and anaerobic metabolism to the net energy expenditure reflect the relative contributions of slow-twitch and fast-twitch muscle fibers to the total work. Thus, the energy for low work rates can be derived primarily from the aerobic pathways of slow-twitch fibers, but the energy for high work rates must be derived from both the aerobic pathways of slow-twitch fibers and the anaerobic pathways of fast-twitch fibers. Because anaerobic glycolysis is a major pathway which leads to the formation of lactic acid (Figure 2.17), these considerations help explain why low levels of exercise intensity are associated with low levels of blood lactate and high levels of exercise intensity are associated with high levels of blood lactate (Figure 3.12).

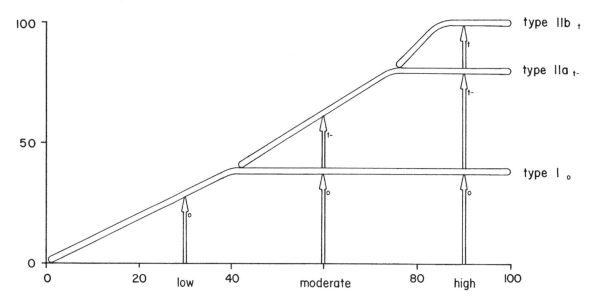

ACTIVE MUSCLE FIBERS (%)

EXERCISE INTENSITY (% $\dot{V}O_2$max)

Figure 4.27   Recruitment patterns of motor units. Color the individual lines that depict the activation of type I, type IIa, and type IIb muscle fibers at different exercise intensities (in % $\dot{V}O_2$max). Observe that the pattern of motor unit recruitment varies with exercise intensity. Color the vertical arrows that correspond to low, moderate, and high levels of exercise intensity. Observe that low levels of exercise intensity recruit only type I muscle fibers, moderate levels of exercise intensity recruit type I and type IIa muscle fibers, and high levels of exercise intensity recruit type I, type IIa and type IIb muscle fibers. This pattern of motor unit recruitment explains why the energy for low exercise intensities can be derived primarily from the aerobic pathways of the slow-twitch muscle fibers, but the energy for high exercise intensities must be derived from both the aerobic pathways of the slow-twitch muscle fibers and the anaerobic pathways of the fast-twitch fibers. Modified from K.B. Pandolf. *Exercise and Sports Sciences Reviews*, vol 15, New York: McGraw Hill, 1987.

Components of a reflex arc

A *reflex* can be regarded as a rapid, involuntary response to a stimulus that is mediated by the sequential operation of a sensory receptor, an afferent pathway, a coordinating center, an efferent pathway, and an effector organ (Figure 4.9). The sensory receptor translates the stimulus into a coded neural signal that is transmitted along an afferent pathway to a coordinating center in the central nervous system. The neural output from the coordinating center is then transmitted along an efferent nerve pathway to the effector organ, which could be a muscle or gland. The resultant action of the effector organ constitutes the response.

Reflex control of skeletal muscle contraction

The alpha motor neuron output to skeletal muscle is modulated by reflexes that originate in sensory receptors, including: (1) muscle spindles, which detect muscle length;

(2) Golgi tendon organs, which detect muscle tension; and (3) Pacinian corpuscles, which detect sudden changes in muscle pressure (vibration).

Muscle spindles

The muscle spindle is a sensory receptor that assists in the maintenance of static and dynamic posture and in the maintenance of muscle tonus, which is a state of low-level contraction at rest. The density of muscle spindles is high in muscles involved in fine control, such as hand muscles, and low in muscles involved in gross control, such as leg muscles. The fibers of the muscle spindle (called intrafusal fibers) are arranged in parallel with the force-generating (extrafusal) muscle fibers. Muscle spindles contain two types of intrafusal fibers—the nuclear bag fibers and the nuclear chain fibers.

The sensory innervation of the muscle spindle consists of group Ia afferent nerves, which originate in both the nuclear bag fibers and the nuclear chain fibers, and group II afferent nerves, which originate in only the nuclear chain fibers. Group Ia afferent nerves transmit information related to the rate at which muscle length increases (an expression of velocity of muscle lengthening), while group II afferent nerves transmit information related to the absolute muscle length (an expression of muscle position). These features of muscle spindles enable them to transmit feedback related to muscle length to the central nervous system. This information is used in the regulation of static and dynamic posture.

Stretch reflex

The *stretch reflex,* also called the myotatic reflex, plays an important role in the maintenance of posture. The stretch reflex is called a *monosynaptic reflex* because there is only one synapse between the afferent nerve fibers (group Ia and group II nerve fibers) and the efferent nerve fibers (alpha motor neurons) (Figure 4.28).

The knee-jerk reflex is an example of the stretch reflex in which a sudden stretch of the quadriceps tendon reflexively causes the muscle to contract and thereby oppose its stretch. The reflex is initiated by muscle spindles that generate action potentials when they are stretched. These action potentials are transmitted to the spinal cord via afferent nerve fibers. More specifically, group Ia and group II afferent nerve fibers synapse with alpha motor neurons of the same muscle in which the spindles reside. Thus, when muscle spindles are stimulated by a sudden stretch of the muscle, the alpha motor neuron output increases and the muscle reflexly contracts to oppose its stretch (Figure 4.28).

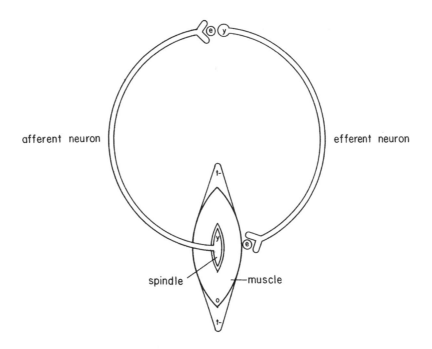

afferent neuron   efferent neuron

spindle   muscle

Figure 4.28   Stretch reflex. Begin at the muscle spindle and proceed in a clockwise direction, coloring the structures as you go. Observe that the stretch reflex is mediated by the sequential operation of a sensory receptor (muscle spindle), afferent pathway (group Ia and group II afferent nerve fibers), coordinating center (monosynaptic connection in the spinal cord), efferent pathway (alpha motor neuron), and effector organ (skeletal muscle). The stretch reflex plays an important role in the maintenance of posture. Compare this figure with Figures 4.9 and 4.10.

Golgi tendon organs

The Golgi tendon organs (GTOs), which are encapsulated sensory receptors located in the tendons of the muscle, are arranged in series with the fibers of the muscle. This arrangement enables these receptors to detect the tension generated by the muscle, rather than the length of the muscle. Golgi tendon organs are stimulated by an increase in muscle tension that occurs during an active contraction of the muscle or during a passive stretch of the muscle.

Golgi tendon reflex

The Golgi tendon reflex plays an important role in the protection of muscle from injury caused by excessive levels of muscle tension. It is called a *disynaptic reflex* because there are two synapses between the afferent (group Ib fibers) and efferent (alpha motor neurons) nerve pathways. More specifically, the group Ib afferent fibers synapse with inhibitory interneurons, which then synapse with the alpha motor neurons of the same muscle in which the tendon organ resides. Thus, when an increase in muscle tension stimulates the Golgi tendon organs, the alpha motor neuron output to the same muscle is reflexly inhibited and muscle tension is thereby decreased (Figure 4.29).

Summary of factors that influence muscle force

Factors that influence muscle force include:

1. The size of the muscle
2. The initial fiber length of the muscle (Figure 4.8)
3. The type of muscle contraction (Figure 4.16)
4. The load against which the muscle contracts (Figure 4.17)
5. The number of motor units that participate in the contraction (Figure 4.20)
6. The frequency with which each of the motor units is stimulated (Figures 4.20 and 4.21)
7. The types of motor units that participate in the contraction (Figure 4.23)
8. The effects of central or peripheral fatigue (Figure 4.25)
9. The modulation of alpha motor neuron output by excitatory (Figure 4.28) and inhibitory (Figure 4.29) reflexes

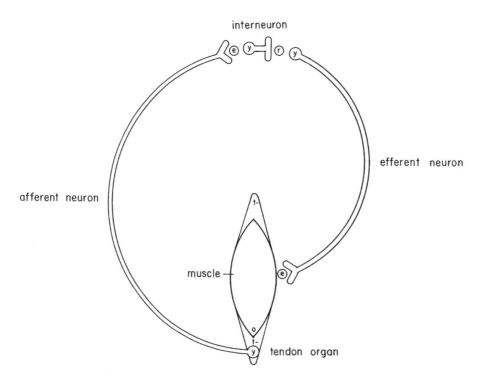

Figure 4.29   Golgi tendon reflex. Begin at the Golgi tendon organ and continue in a clockwise direction, coloring the structures as you go. Observe that the Golgi tendon reflex is mediated by the sequential operation of a sensory receptor (tendon organ), afferent pathway (group Ib afferent nerve fiber), coordinating center (disynaptic connection in the spinal cord), efferent pathway (alpha motor neuron), and effector organ (skeletal muscle). The Golgi tendon reflex plays an important role in the protection of muscle from injury. Compare this figure with Figures 4.9, 4.10, and 4.28.

chapter **five**
cardiovascular system

The cardiovascular system transports essential substances to cells, removes metabolic waste products from cells, and helps maintain body temperature.

Cardiovascular responses to exercise represent the combined action of mechanical, neural, and humoral mechanisms that regulate the contraction of cardiac muscle in the heart and the contraction of vascular smooth muscle in the blood vessels. These adjustments in cardiac function and vascular tone increase the blood flow to exercising muscles in order to satisfy their greater needs for fuels and oxygen.

Components of the cardiovascular system

The *cardiovascular system* contains two pumps (the right and left hearts) and two circulations (the pulmonary and systemic circuits), which are connected in series (Figure 5.1). Each side of the heart consists of a thin-walled *atrium* that serves as a reservoir for blood and a thick-walled *ventricle* that performs the work needed to pump blood through its respective circuit.

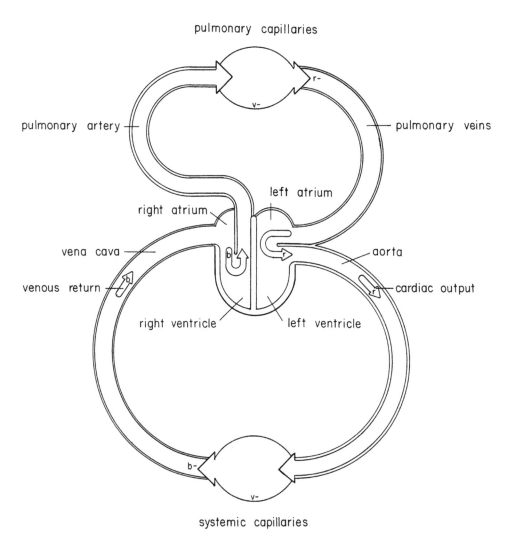

Figure 5.1   Components of the cardiovascular system. Color the blood in the pulmonary veins, noting that it is fully oxygenated. Proceed in a clockwise direction, identify the left heart chambers, the aorta, and the systemic capillaries, noting that this is the site where oxygen is removed from the blood and carbon dioxide is added to the blood. Color the systemic capillaries and the mixed venous blood that leaves them; identify the vena cava, right heart chambers and the pulmonary artery. Finish the picture by coloring the pulmonary capillaries; the site where oxygen is added to the blood and carbon dioxide is removed from the blood.

The right heart pumps mixed venous blood from the tissues into the pulmonary circulation, where oxygen is added to the blood and excess carbon dioxide is removed from the blood. The left heart then pumps the oxygenated blood into the systemic circulation where O_2, fuels, and hormones are delivered to the tissues while CO_2 and other metabolic byproducts are picked up from the tissues (Figure 6.1).

Cardiac output is defined as the rate at which the left ventricle pumps blood into the aorta, expressed in units of L/min. *Venous return* is defined as the rate at which the systemic circuit delivers blood to the right atrium, also expressed in L/min. Given that fluid is incompressible, blood normally flows into and out of the systemic circulation at the same average rate; consequently, cardiac output and venous return are equal (Figure 5.1).

Action potentials in cardiac muscle fibers

Action potentials in cardiac muscle fibers are characterized by an initial period of depolarization, during which positively charged ions enter the cell, and a subsequent period of repolarization, during which positively charged ions exit the cell.

The shapes of the action potentials in cardiac muscle differ from those in skeletal muscle. Fibers of the *sinoatrial* (SA) *node,* in the right atrium, exhibit spontaneous depolarization, and fibers of the ventricles exhibit a long plateau phase during which they remain completely depolarized (Figure 5.2). The *plateau phase* is due to open calcium channels in the muscle membrane and it represents an absolute refractory period during which the ventricular fibers cannot be restimulated. This long refractory period prevents cardiac muscle from being tetanized (Figure 4.21), a potentially lethal condition in which the heart would be incapable of pumping blood.

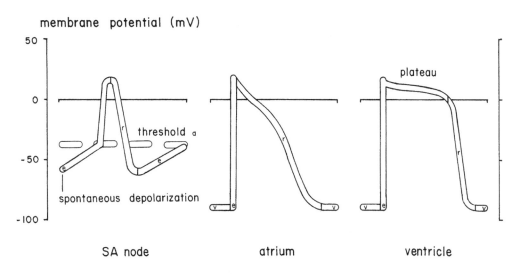

Figure 5.2 Action potentials in cardiac muscle fibers. Color the action potentials in each cardiac muscle fiber, noting that they are characterized by a period of depolarization (segments labeled e) followed by a period of repolarization (segments labeled r). Identify the prolonged plateau phase of the ventricular fiber and the resting membrane potentials of the atrial and ventricular fibers (segments labeled v). Color the threshold and note that pacemaker cells of the SA node differ from atrial and ventricular cells in that they exhibit spontaneous depolarization. Compare this figure with Figure 4.13.

Cardiac muscle contraction

Action potentials in cardiac muscle fibers trigger the release of intracellular calcium ions that initiate a series of events that culminate in a muscle contraction (Figure 4.14).

The duration of the action potential is short in comparison to the twitch that it produces in skeletal muscle (Figure 4.15); this is not the case in cardiac muscle. Ventricular muscle fibers, which only begin to develop tension at the onset of the depolarization phase, actually develop their maximum tension around the end of their repolarization phase (Figure 5.3). The magnitude of the developed tension depends on a number of factors, including: (1) the initial length of the muscle fibers (*preload*); (2) the load against which the muscle fibers contract (*afterload*); and (3) the *contractility,* or strength, of the muscle fibers.

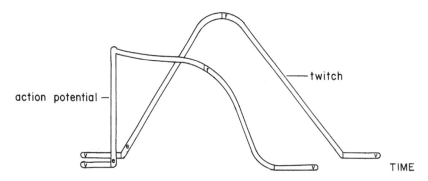

Figure 5.3   Relationship between action potential and twitch tension in cardiac muscle. Color the action potential, which is a recording of the changes in voltage that occur across the membrane of a ventricular muscle fiber, and identify the depolarization and repolarization phases. Color the twitch tension, which is a recording of the changes in ventricular force that occur during the corresponding twitch, and identify the contraction and relaxation phases. Note that the onset of depolarization coincides with the beginning of tension development and that maximal tension occurs during repolarization. Compare this figure with Figure 4.15, noting that the action potential in a ventricular muscle fiber is very long in comparison to that in a skeletal muscle fiber.

Effect of initial fiber length on cardiac muscle contraction

A fundamental property of cardiac muscle fibers is that they contract more forcefully if they are stretched prior to their contraction (Figure 5.4).

This property permits the ventricles to generate more tension and therefore develop higher ventricular pressures when they contract from a larger ventricular volume (an expression of ventricular fiber length) (Figure 5.5). The volume of blood in the ventricle at the onset of its contraction is sometimes called the preload because it is this volume that determines the initial length of the ventricular muscle fibers from which they contract. This intrinsic property of cardiac muscle, which causes the heart to contract more forcefully when it is filled more completely, enables the heart to pump all the blood it receives from the veins.

Figure 5.4 Effect of fiber length on force–velocity characteristic. Color the force–velocity characteristics of a cardiac muscle studied at two different initial fiber lengths (obtained by stretching the muscle prior to its contraction). Observe that the force–velocity curve of the longer fiber appears above that of the shorter fiber, indicating that stretching cardiac muscle fibers causes them to shorten faster against any given external load. Observe also that the x-intercept of the curve for the longer fiber exceeds that of the shorter fiber, indicating that stretching cardiac muscle fibers causes them to generate a higher isometric force. These findings demonstrate that ventricular fibers contract more forcefully when they are stretched prior to their contraction. Finally, observe that the y-intercept (V_{max}) of the two curves is the same, indicating that longer and shorter fibers exhibit the same initial velocity of shortening against no load. Because V_{max} can be regarded as an index of muscle contractility, these findings indicate that stretching a ventricular muscle fiber does not influence its contractility. Compare this figure with Figure 4.24.

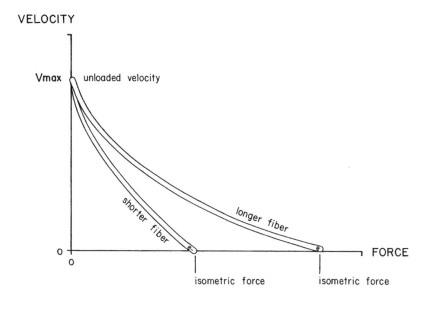

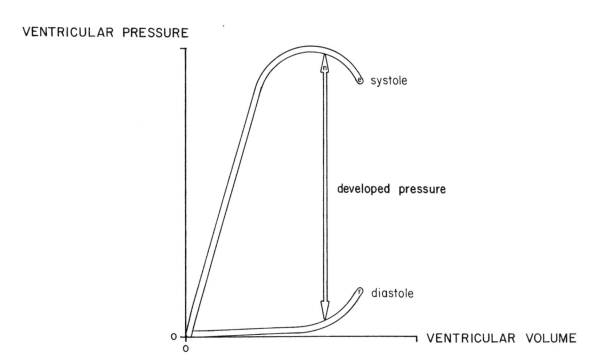

Figure 5.5 Effect of fiber length on ventricular pressures. Color the lines that depict the pressure measured inside the ventricle during contraction (systole) and relaxation (diastole) at different ventricular volumes (fiber lengths). Observe that the peak systolic pressure increases with increasing ventricular volume until it attains a maximum value; this behavior can be accounted for by intrinsic properties of cardiac muscle fibers that enable them to contract more forcefully when they are stretched prior to their contraction. Observe also that peak systolic pressure falls with further increases in ventricular volume. This behavior could be due to a decline in ventricular muscle tension that could occur when its sarcomeres are stretched beyond their optimal fiber length (Figure 4.8) and/or to changes in the geometry of the ventricle; a given muscle tension produces a smaller ventricular pressure when the heart is dilated (enlarged). Observe also that the diastolic pressure remains low in the face of considerable increases in volume, indicating that the relaxed ventricle is easily distended. Note that the pressure developed by the contracting ventricle at any given volume can be visualized by the vertical distance between the systolic and diastolic pressures.

Effect of external load on cardiac muscle contraction

The force developed by cardiac muscle fibers also depends on the external load against which they contract. Heavier added loads prolong the latent period, decrease the initial velocity of shortening, and increase the maximal developed tension in cardiac muscle fibers; this behavior is similar to that observed in skeletal muscle fibers (Figure 4.17).

A twitch in cardiac muscle can therefore range from a high-force, low-velocity contraction against a heavy load to a low-force, high-velocity contraction against a light load. The force generated by the muscle is maximum when it contracts against a load that is too heavy for it to move (an isometric contraction) and the velocity of shortening is maximum when it contracts against no load. The spectrum of all possible combinations of force and velocity specifies the force–velocity characteristic of cardiac muscle (Figure 5.6).

Since the ventricles pump blood into their respective arteries (Figure 5.1), arterial blood pressure is sometimes called the afterload because it reflects the force against which the ventricles contract. For this reason, arterial pressure is a factor that influences the amount of work that the ventricles perform during the course of their contraction (Figure 5.22).

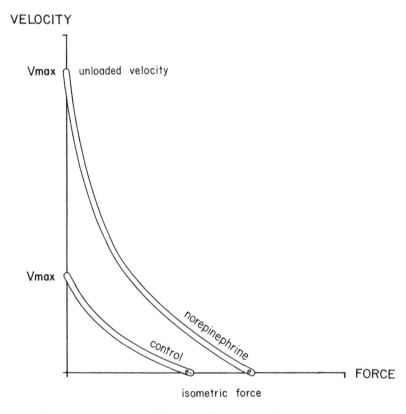

Figure 5.6   Force–velocity characteristic of cardiac muscle. Color the force–velocity characteristics of a cardiac muscle studied in the presence and absence (control) of norepinephrine, a catecholamine released by the sympathetic nervous system. Note that the force–velocity curve for norepinephrine appears above that of the control curve, indicating that norepinephrine causes cardiac muscle to shorten faster against any given load. Observe that the x-intercept of the norepinephrine curve exceeds that of the control curve, indicating that norepinephrine causes cardiac muscle to generate a higher isometric pressure. Observe also that the y-intercept of the norepinephrine curve exceeds that of the control curve, indicating that norepinephrine causes cardiac muscle to exhibit a higher V_{max}; this result demonstrates that norepinephrine increases myocardial contractility. Compare this figure with Figure 5.4.

Electrical activity of the heart

Cardiac muscle fibers are connected to each other by intercalated discs, which are highly permeable cell membranes that function as gap junctions between adjacent fibers. This feature of cardiac muscle permits an action potential that is initiated in one cell to spread throughout the muscle, thereby enabling the heart to contract as a single unit. The heart also contains a specialized conducting system that helps synchronize the contraction of its muscle fibers. The conduction system consists of internodal fibers, the atrioventricular (AV) node, the bundle of His, the right and left bundle branches, and the Purkinje fibers (Figure 5.7).

Action potentials that originate in the *pacemaker cells* of the SA node initiate a wave of depolarization that spreads over the atria and through the internodal pathways to the AV node, which is normally the only pathway between the atria and the ventricles. Because action potentials initiate muscle contractions (Figure 5.3), this wave of atrial muscle depolarization (an electrical event) is followed by a wave of atrial muscle contraction (a mechanical event) that pumps blood from the atria into the ventricles.

The impulse is delayed as it travels through the slow-conducting fibers of the AV node; this allows sufficient time for the atria to complete their contraction before the impulse is delivered to the ventricles via the fast-conducting fibers of the bundle of His, the right and left bundle branches, and the Purkinje fibers (Figure 5.8). These fast-conducting fibers rapidly spread the impulse to all the ventricular fibers so that they can depolarize, and therefore contract, simultaneously; this synchrony among the ventricular fibers makes the heart an effective pump.

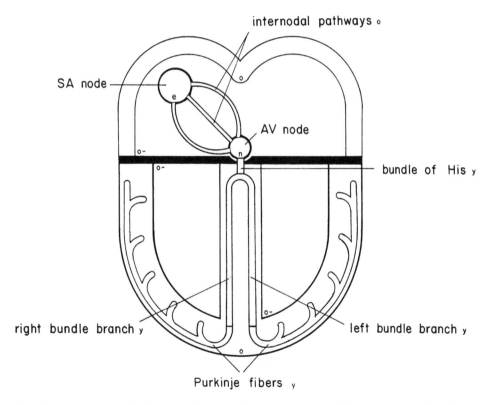

Figure 5.7 Conduction system of the heart. Color the SA node, the internodal pathways, and the AV node. Note that the impulse originates in the SA node (Figure 5.2) and that the fibers of the AV node are normally the only connection between the atria and ventricles. Color the bundle of His, the right and left bundle branches, and the Purkinje fibers. Finish the picture by coloring the walls and chambers of the heart.

Figure 5.8 Electrical activity of the heart. Begin coloring at the top, noting that the cardiac cycle begins when the pacemaker cells of the SA node depolarize while the atria and ventricles are in the resting (polarized) state. Continue coloring clockwise, noting that the spread of the action potential through the atria causes them to depolarize before the ventricles depolarize. Continue clockwise, observing that the atria repolarize when the ventricles depolarize, and that the atria are in their resting state when the ventricles repolarize. Thus, the electrical activity of the heart can be viewed as a wave of depolarization followed by a wave of repolarization. Compare this figure with Figure 5.2.

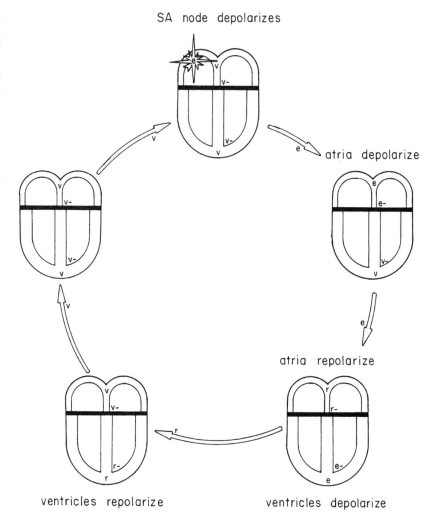

SA node depolarizes

atria depolarize

atria repolarize

ventricles depolarize

ventricles repolarize

The electrocardiogram (ECG)

The *electrocardiogram* is a recording of the electrical activity of the heart that can be obtained by measuring the voltage between surface electrodes that are placed on the limbs (bipolar leads) (Figure 5.9). Electrocardiograms can also be obtained with electrodes that are placed on the anterior chest wall (chest leads) to observe the electrical activity of the cardiac muscle directly beneath the electrode (Figure 5.10).

The normal ECG is characterized by a P wave, a QRS complex, and a T wave. The P wave corresponds to atrial depolarization, the QRS complex corresponds to ventricular depolarization, and the T wave corresponds to ventricular repolarization (Figure 5.9). The low-amplitude wave of atrial repolarization is obscured by the high-amplitude QRS complex.

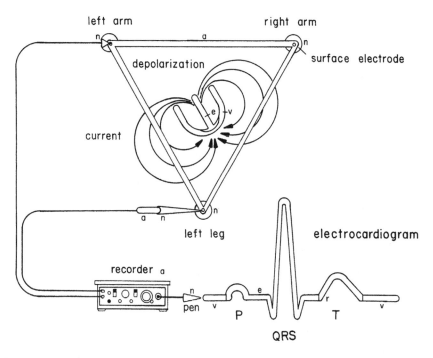

Figure 5.9 Normal electrocardiogram. Begin by coloring the heart, noting that it is in a phase in which only a portion of it is depolarized. Identify the current that flows from the depolarized fibers to the resting fibers, noting that the voltage created by the flow of ions in the body can be recorded by electrodes placed on the body surface. Identify and color the surface electrodes, the recorder and its probe, and the electrocardiogram. Note that the ventricle remains completely depolarized during the S-T segment, the period between the end of the QRS complex and the beginning of the T wave. This segment of the ECG corresponds to the plateau phase of the ventricular fibers shown in Figure 5.2. Heart rate (HR, in beats/min) is determined by the period (T, in s) between successive QRS complexes, i.e., HR = 60/T. Thus, a period of 1 s corresponds to a heart rate of 60 beats/min and a period of ½ s corresponds to a heart rate of 120 beats/min.

Figure 5.10 Chest leads. Color the diagram, noting that six chest leads, also called precordial leads, are obtained from surface electrodes placed at specific landmarks on the anterior chest wall to record the electrical activity of different parts of the heart. The recordings obtained from these leads are designated as V_1, V_2, V_3, V_4, V_5, and V_6. The electrocardiogram records the difference between the voltage at a chest electrode and an indifferent electrode, which is connected by resistors (5 kΩ) to each of the electrodes positioned at the right arm, left arm, and left leg (Figure 5.9). Because the surface of the heart is close to the chest, each chest lead records mainly the electrical activity of the cardiac muscle just beneath the electrode. As a result, relatively minute abnormalities in the anterior ventricular wall can frequently be detected by alterations in the electrocardiogram recorded by chest leads.

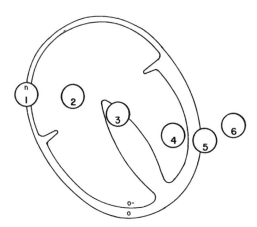

Autonomic control of cardiac function

The autonomic nervous system modulates cardiac function by releasing neurotransmitters that modify heart rate (chronotropic effects) and myocardial contractility (inotropic effects) (Figure 5.11).

Chronotropic effects are due to changes in the pattern of spontaneous depolarization of the pacemaker cells in the SA node (Figure 5.2). Parasympathetic nerve fibers that travel in the vagus nerve (cranial nerve X), also called *vagal fibers,* release acetylcholine at the SA node. Acetylcholine decreases heart rate by prolonging the period between successive pacemaker action potentials (Figure 5.12, left panel). In contrast, sympathetic nerve fibers release norepinephrine at the SA node. Norepinephrine increases heart rate by shortening the period between successive pacemaker action potentials (Figure 5.12, right panel). *Bradycardia* and *tachycardia* are terms that are used to denote abnormally low (<60 beats/min, or bpm, at rest) and abnormally high (>100 bpm at rest) heart rates, respectively.

Figure 5.11 Autonomic innervation of the heart. Color the heart and the autonomic nerves that innervate it. Note that the parasympathetic nerves inhibit the heart, while the sympathetic nerves stimulate the heart. Parasympathetic stimulation releases acetylcholine, which decreases heart rate and mildly depresses myocardial contractility (the parasympathetic innervation of the ventricular myocardium shown is intended to illustrate a functional relationship—essentially all of the cardiac parasympathetic fibers innervate the SA node or AV node). In contrast, sympathetic stimulation increases heart rate and strongly enhances myocardial contractility (Figure 5.6).

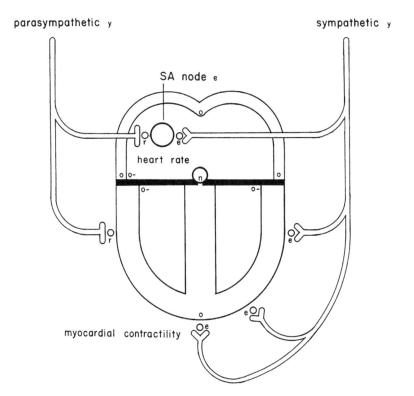

Figure 5.12 Autonomic control of heart rate. Color the threshold and the membrane potentials from the pacemaker cells of the SA node, noting that they are similar to those shown in Figure 5.2. Observe that acetylcholine (ACh) released by parasympathetic stimulation decreases the rate of spontaneous depolarization and thereby prolongs the period between successive action potentials (left panel). Observe also that norepinephrine released by sympathetic stimulation increases the rate of spontaneous depolarization and thereby shortens the period between successive action potentials (right panel). For these reasons, parasympathetic stimulation decreases heart rate and sympathetic stimulation increases heart rate.

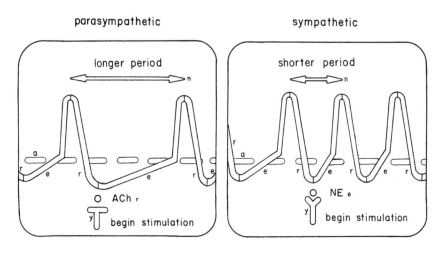

Inotropic effects are due to changes in the contractility of the myocardial fibers. Stimulation of parasympathetic nerve fibers mildly decreases myocardial contractility, whereas stimulation of sympathetic nerve fibers strongly increases myocardial contractility. Changes in contractility modify the force–velocity characteristic of cardiac muscle. An increase in contractility causes cardiac muscle to exhibit a higher isometric force as well as a higher velocity of muscle shortening under unloaded (V_{max}) and loaded conditions (Figure 5.6). Because power is given by the product of force and velocity, an increase in contractility manifests itself as an increase in power output. Conversely, a decrease in contractility causes cardiac muscle to exhibit a lower velocity of muscle shortening against any given load. For these reasons, an increase in contractility amplifies the force–velocity characteristic, whereas a decrease in contractility attenuates it.

Cardiac cycle

The cardiac cycle consists of a period of *systole,* during which the ventricles contract, and a period of *diastole,* during which the ventricles relax. One-way valves between the atria and ventricles (AV valves) prevent the retrograde (backward) flow of blood when ventricular pressure rises during systole. Similarly, one-way valves between the ventricles and arteries (semilunar valves) prevent the retrograde flow of blood when ventricular pressure falls during diastole (Figure 5.13).

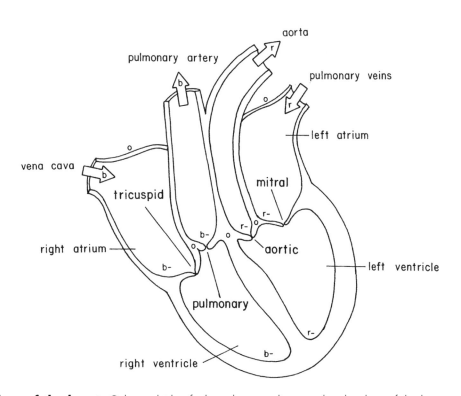

Figure 5.13   Valves of the heart. Color and identify the valves, cardiac muscle, chambers of the heart, and the blood vessels they supply. The tricuspid and mitral valves are known as atrioventricular (AV) valves, and the pulmonary and aortic valves are known as semilunar valves. Note that the pulmonary artery and aorta have been displaced from their normal anatomical positions in this schematic diagram.

Cardiac valves contain flaps, or cusps, that open and close in accordance with the pressures that develop across them. The pressures on both sides of an open valve are essentially equal because an open valve normally does not constitute a measurable impediment to blood flow. The opening and closing of the heart valves further divides the *cardiac cycle* into four distinct phases: (1) filling; (2) isovolumic (isovolumetric) contraction; (3) ejection; and (4) isovolumic relaxation (Figure 5.14). Diastole coincides with the phases of isovolumic relaxation and filling, while systole coincides with the phases of isovolumic contraction and ejection.

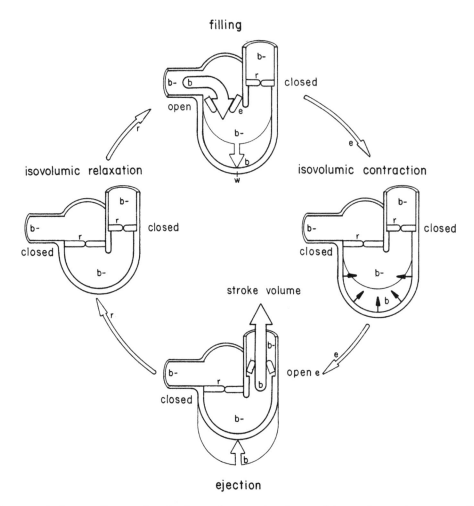

Figure 5.14 **Phases of the cardiac cycle.** This figure illustrates the phases of the cardiac cycle on one side of the heart. Begin coloring at the top and work clockwise, noting the flow of blood (arrows) and the opening and closing of the valves. The first heart sound corresponds to the closure of the AV valves; its vibration is low in pitch and relatively prolonged. The second heart sound occurs when the aortic and pulmonary valves close; its vibration is high in pitch and relatively short because these valves close rapidly. Note that the stroke volume is equal to the change in ventricular volume that occurs during ejection, i.e., the difference between the volume in the ventricle at the end of the filling phase (end-diastolic volume) and at the end of the ejection phase (end-systolic volume).

Pressure and volume changes during the cardiac cycle

The patterns of the pressure and volume changes during the phases of the cardiac cycle are similar in the right and left sides of the heart; left ventricular pressures are approximately seven times higher than right ventricular pressures. Only the events in the left heart are described below.

During the filling phase, the mitral valve is open and blood flows from the left atrium into the left ventricle, thereby increasing ventricular volume (Figure 5.14). Atrial pressure and ventricular pressure are equal because the mitral valve is open. The volume from which the ventricle contracts, which

is termed the preload, is therefore determined by atrial pressure. The aortic valve is closed during this phase because aortic pressure exceeds ventricular pressure (Figure 5.15).

The phase of isovolumic contraction begins when the mitral valve closes because the pressure in the contracting ventricle exceeds the pressure in the atrium (Figure 5.14). Throughout this phase, ventricular pressure is higher than atrial pressure but lower than aortic pressure. Consequently, both the mitral and aortic valves are closed and blood can neither enter nor leave the ventricle. The rise in ventricular pressure therefore occurs at a constant ventricular volume (an isometric contraction, Figure 4.16). For this reason, isovolumic contraction is sometimes referred to as isometric contraction (Figure 5.15).

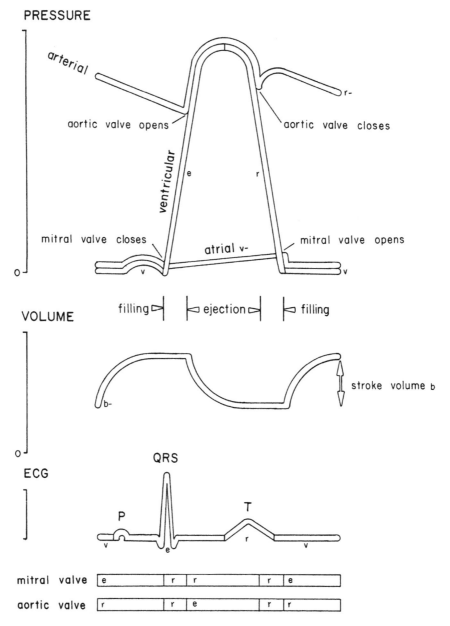

PRESSURE

arterial

aortic valve opens   aortic valve closes

ventricular   e   r

mitral valve closes   atrial v-   mitral valve opens

0

filling ▷| |◁ ejection ▷| |◁ filling

VOLUME

stroke volume b

b-

0

ECG

QRS

P   T

          r

v   e   r   v

mitral valve	e		r	r		r	e
aortic valve	r		r	e		r	r

Figure 5.15   Pressure and volume changes during the cardiac cycle. Begin by coloring the left ventricular pressure tracing in which pressure is plotted against time. Identify the contraction (segment labeled e) and relaxation (segment labeled r) phases. Color the arterial pressure tracing and note that it coincides with the ventricular pressure tracing when the aortic valve is open (throughout the ejection phase). Color the atrial pressure tracing and note that it coincides with the ventricular pressure tracing when the mitral valve is open (throughout the filling phase). Color the ventricular volume tracing, noting that ventricular volume increases during filling and decreases during ejection. Note also that the stroke volume is determined by the difference between the volume in the ventricle at the end of the filling phase (end-diastolic volume) and the end of the ejection phase (end-systolic volume). Color the ECG, noting its relationship to the ventricular pressure tracing. Finish the picture by coloring the horizontal bands that indicate the opening and closing of the mitral and aortic valves. Note that the mitral and aortic valves are never open at the same time. Compare this figure with Figure 5.14.

The ejection phase begins with the opening of the aortic valve (Figure 5.14). During this phase, the ventricle propels blood into the aorta, thereby decreasing ventricular volume. Ventricular pressure and aortic pressure are equal because the aortic valve is open. Aortic pressure can therefore be regarded as the load against which the ventricle contracts, i.e., the afterload. The volume of blood ejected by the ventricle during this phase is called the *stroke volume* (SV); it is the difference between the volume of blood in the ventricle at the end of the filling phase (end-diastolic volume, or EDV) and at the end of the ejection phase (end-systolic volume, or ESV), i.e., SV = EDV – ESV (Figure 5.15). The magnitude of the stroke volume depends on the preload (an expression of the initial fiber length), afterload (an expression of the force opposing ventricular contraction), and myocardial contractility (an expression of muscle strength) (Figure 5.16).

The phase of isovolumic relaxation begins when the aortic valve closes (Figure 5.14). Throughout this phase, both the aortic and mitral valves are closed because the pressure in the relaxing ventricle is lower than aortic pressure but higher than atrial pressure. The fall in ventricular pressure therefore occurs at a constant ventricular volume (an isometric relaxation). For this reason, isovolumic relaxation is sometimes referred to as isometric relaxation. When ventricular pressure falls to the point where it matches the rising atrial pressure, the mitral valve opens and the next filling phase begins (Figure 5.15).

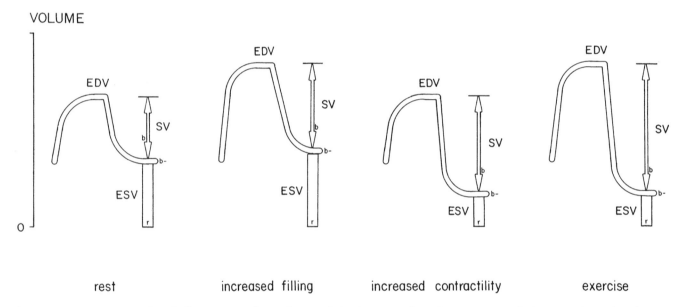

VOLUME

rest   increased filling   increased contractility   exercise

Figure 5.16   Factors that influence stroke volume. Color the ventricular volume tracings, which are similar to that shown in Figure 5.15. Identify and compare the end-diastolic volume (EDV), end-systolic volume (ESV), and stroke volume (SV) in each condition. Observe that increases in stroke volume occur during increased filling (higher EDV), increased contractility (lower ESV), and exercise (higher EDV and lower ESV). Note that the increase in stroke volume during exercise is due to increases in venous return, which increase EDV, and to increases in myocardial contractility, which decrease ESV.

Ejection fraction

The *ejection fraction* (EF) is a measure of the degree to which the ventricle empties during systole (Figure 5.17, left panel). It is calculated by dividing the stroke volume by the end-diastolic volume, and expressing the ratio as a percent, i.e., EF (%) = SV · 100/ EDV.

The ejection fraction, which is normally around 60% at rest, increases when myocardial contractility is enhanced by sympathetic stimulation, circulating catecholamines, or inotropic drugs such as digitalis (Figure 5.17, middle panel). Conversely, the ejection fraction decreases when myocardial contractility is depressed by a reduction in sympathetic stimulation or by very low levels of oxygen in blood (hypoxemia) (Figure 5.17, right panel).

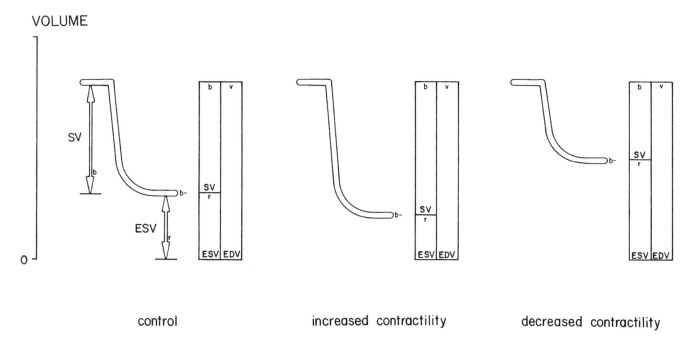

VOLUME

control   increased contractility   decreased contractility

Figure 5.17   Effect of myocardial contractility on ejection fraction. Color the ventricular volume tracings, which are similar to those shown in Figure 5.16, and the bar graphs that depict the end-diastolic volume (EDV), end-systolic volume (ESV), and stroke volume (SV) in each condition. Note that the stroke volume is given by the difference between the end-diastolic and end-systolic volumes, i.e., SV = EDV − ESV. Observe that increased myocardial contractility causes an increase in stroke volume coupled with a corresponding decrease in end-diastolic volume, indicating that the ventricle empties itself to a greater extent (middle panel). Also observe that decreased myocardial contractility causes a decrease in stroke volume coupled with a corresponding increase in end-systolic volume, indicating that the ventricle empties itself to a lesser extent (right panel). These findings demonstrate that myocardial contractility influences stroke volume and ejection fraction [EF (%) = SV·100/EDV]. These considerations explain why ejection fraction increases when myocardial contractility is enhanced and decreases when myocardial contractility is depressed. They also explain why a low ejection fraction is a sign of ventricular muscle weakness.

Effect of heart rate and stroke volume on cardiac output

Cardiac output (CO, in L/min) is determined by the product of *heart rate* (HR, in beats/min) and stroke volume (SV, the volume of blood ejected per beat, in mL), i.e., CO = HR · SV. For example, a typical resting cardiac output of 5 L/min is given by the product of the resting values of heart rate (72 beats/min) and stroke volume (70 mL), i.e., 5 L/min = 5000 mL/min ≈ 72 · 70 mL /min.

The four factors that determine cardiac output are heart rate plus three factors that determine stroke volume, namely preload (an expression of ventricular fiber length), myocardial contractility (an expression of cardiac muscle strength), and afterload (an expression of the load against which the ventricles contract) (Figure 5.18).

Increases in cardiac output during continuous exercise (Figure 5.19, left panel) are due to increases in both heart rate and stroke volume. The magnitudes of the heart rate and stroke volume responses to exercise vary with exercise intensity and thus, the rate at which oxygen is consumed by the body. Heart rate varies linearly with oxygen consumption ($\dot{V}O_2$) over the range from rest to maximal exercise (middle panel) whereas stroke volume increases over the range from rest to moderate exercise but does not change appreciably over the range from moderate to maximal exercise (right panel).

Figure 5.18 Determinants of cardiac output. Color the diagram, noting that the four factors that determine cardiac output are: (1) heart rate (determined by the pacemaker, Figure 5.12); (2) preload (initial ventricular fiber length, determined in part by venous return); (3) myocardial contractility (the strength of cardiac muscle, determined by ventricular muscle mass and inotropic influences); and (4) afterload (the load against which the ventricle contracts, determined by arterial blood pressure, Figure 5.15). These considerations demonstrate that cardiac output is determined both by the ability of the venous circuit to return blood to the heart and by the ability of the heart to pump blood.

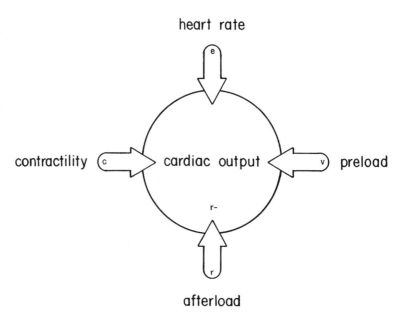

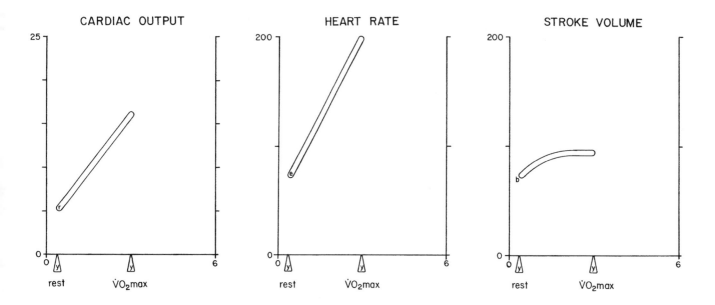

OXYGEN CONSUMPTION (liters/min)

Figure 5.19 Heart rate and stroke volume responses to exercise. Color the lines that depict the responses of cardiac output (in L/min, left panel), heart rate (in beats/min, middle panel), and stroke volume (in mL, right panel) to continuous exercise at different levels of exercise intensity, as indicated by measurements of oxygen consumption ($\dot{V}O_2$, in L/min). Observe that cardiac output and heart rate in this example are shown to increase linearly with oxygen consumption over the range from rest (left endpoints of lines) to maximal exercise ($\dot{V}O_2$max, right endpoints of lines). This behavior explains why heart rate can be used as an indicator of exercise intensity. Observe also that stroke volume increases over the range from rest to moderate exercise (~ 50% $\dot{V}O_2$max) but does not change appreciably over the range from moderate to maximal exercise. Thus, increases in cardiac output during exercise are mediated by the combined effects of increases in both heart rate and stroke volume. Endurance training can increase an individual's maximal values of cardiac output, oxygen consumption, and stroke volume (Figure 9.23).

Stroke work

The work performed by the ventricle during systole is called the *stroke work,* and it can be determined by plotting the ventricular pressure against the corresponding ventricular volume throughout each of the four phases of the cardiac cycle (Figure 5.14). This procedure yields a closed loop (Figure 5.20). Because work is determined by the product of pressure and volume (Figure 1.6), the area enclosed by this loop is a quantitative measure of stroke work (Figure 5.21). The cumulative amount of work done over a one-minute period (work/min, an expression of power) is given by the product of the stroke work (work/beat) and heart rate (beats/min).

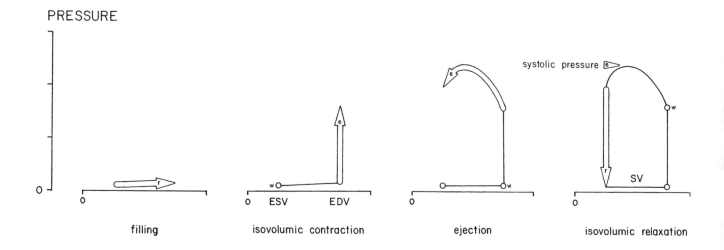

Figure 5.20 **Ventricular pressure–volume relationships during the cardiac cycle.** Color the figure from left to right, noting that the arrow in each panel depicts left ventricular pressure (in mmHg) plotted against left ventricular volume (in mL) during each of the four phases of the cardiac cycle. Observe that ventricular pressure remains low while volume increases (nearly horizontal arrow) during filling, pressure rises while volume remains constant (upward arrow) during isovolumic contraction, pressure rises and falls while volume decreases (curved arrow) during ejection, and that pressure falls while volume remains constant (downward arrow) during isovolumic relaxation. Identify the end-diastolic volume (EDV), end-systolic volume (ESV), stroke volume (SV), and systolic blood pressure. Identify which arrows correspond to systole and which arrows correspond to diastole. Note that the ventricular pressure–volume relationship for a single cardiac cycle forms a closed loop. Compare this figure with Figure 5.15.

This analysis shows that a higher arterial blood pressure (hypertension) or a larger stroke volume increases stroke work; this requires the heart to perform more work per beat (Figure 5.22, middle panels). This analysis also shows that stroke work increases during exercise because arterial blood pressure is higher and stroke volume is larger (right panel).

VENTRICULAR PRESSURE (mmHg)

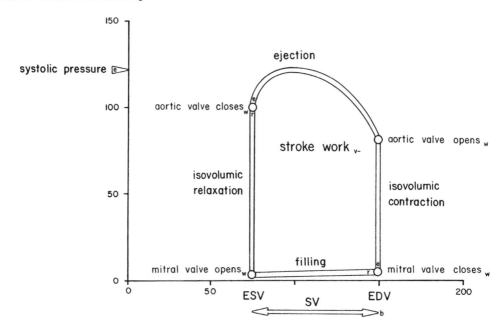

VENTRICULAR VOLUME (mL)

Figure 5.21   Determination of stroke work. Color the left ventricular pressure–volume loop associated with a single cardiac cycle; identify the four phases of the cardiac cycle and the points at which the mitral and aortic valves open and close. Identify the end-diastolic volume (EDV), end-systolic volume (ESV), stroke volume (SV), and systolic pressure. Observe that the stroke volume determines the width of the loop and that systolic pressure determines the maximal height of the loop. Color the interior of the loop, noting that this area is a quantitative measure of stroke work. Compare this figure with Figures 1.6 and 5.20.

PRESSURE (mmHg)

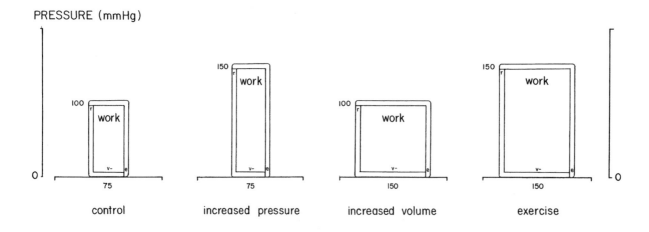

VOLUME (mL)

Figure 5.22   Effects of arterial blood pressure and stroke volume on stroke work. Color the simplified ventricular pressure–volume loops for each of the conditions, noting that the area of each rectangle is given by the product of stroke volume (base of rectangle, in mL) and systolic pressure (height of rectangle, in mmHg). Color the interior areas of the rectangles, noting that the ventricle performs more stroke work when it pumps the same stroke volume against a higher pressure (panel labeled increased pressure) or when it pumps a larger stroke volume against the same arterial pressure (panel labeled increased volume). Thus, hypertension (high blood pressure) increases the work of the heart. Observe that the increase in stroke work during exercise is due both to larger stroke volumes and to higher arterial pressures (panel labeled exercise). Compare this figure with Figure 5.21.

Double product

The *double product,* also known as the rate–pressure product (RPP), is calculated by multiplying the systolic blood pressure (in mmHg) by heart rate (in beats/min); this parameter has been found to correlate well with myocardial oxygen consumption (in mLO_2/min). Typical values of double product range from 6,000 at rest (50 bpm · 120 mmHg) to 40,000 during intense exercise (200 bpm · 200 mmHg).

The levels of heart rate and blood pressure during upper-extremity exercise are higher than those observed when the same work rate is achieved during lower-extremity exercise. The higher double product associated with upper-extremity exercise indicates that the performance of a given amount of external work is associated with higher levels of myocardial oxygen consumption and therefore myocardial work. In light of these considerations, upper-extremity exercise may pose a greater risk for people with compromised myocardial O_2 supply, as can occur in coronary heart disease.

Measurement of blood pressure by sphygmomanometry

The pulsatile nature of blood flow causes arterial blood pressure to rise during systole and fall during diastole. Arterial blood pressure is therefore expressed in terms of its maximum *systolic* and minimum *diastolic* values. For example, normal arterial blood pressure is said to be 120/80, where 120 and 80 are the systolic and diastolic pressures in mmHg, respectively (Figure 5.15).

Blood pressure in the brachial artery can be measured by *sphygmomanometry,* a method that employs an inflatable pressure cuff that is wrapped around the arm and connected to a mercury manometer (Figure 5.23). When the cuff is inflated to a pressure that exceeds systolic pressure, the cuff occludes (collapses) the artery, blood flow stops, and a brachial pulse cannot be felt (palpated) or heard (auscultated) downstream from the occlusion (upper left panel). The

Figure 5.23   Measurement of arterial blood pressure by sphygmomanometry. Color the cuff pressure and arterial blood pressure tracings, noting that the artery collapses when the cuff pressure outside the artery exceeds the arterial pressure inside the artery (upper left panel). Color the remaining panels, noting the changes in blood flow that occur when the cuff pressure is slowly reduced; the number in each panel indicates cuff pressure in mmHg. Note also that sound can be heard when cuff pressure interrupts blood flow for only some portion of the cycle; no sounds are heard when blood flows continuously.

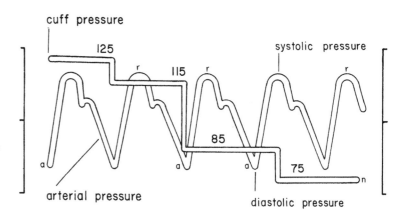

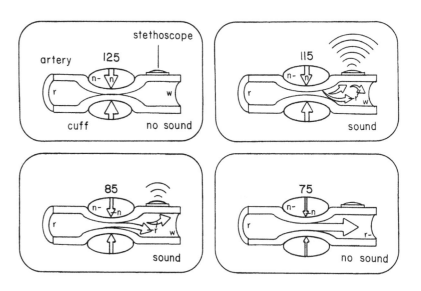

pressure in the cuff is then reduced slowly until the first faint sounds of turbulent blood flow can be heard (upper right panel). Cuff pressure at this point is taken as systolic pressure. Cuff pressure is reduced further (lower left panel) until the muffled sounds of interrupted blood flow just disappear (lower right panel). Cuff pressure at this point is taken as diastolic pressure.

Mean arterial pressure and pulse pressure

Arterial blood pressure can be characterized by two components; one component is called the mean arterial pressure and the other is called the pulse pressure.

The *pulse pressure* (PP, Figure 5.24) is a measure of the amount by which arterial pressure fluctuates during the cardiac cycle; it is calculated by subtracting the diastolic pressure (P_d) from the systolic pressure (P_s) and expressing the difference in units of mmHg, i.e., $PP = P_s - P_d$. For example, the pulse pressure is 40 mmHg when the systolic pressure is 120 mmHg and the diastolic pressure is 80 mmHg, i.e., $40 = 120 - 80$.

The *mean arterial pressure* (MAP, Figure 5.24) represents the average pressure over the entire cardiac cycle. If the blood pressure wave shape were symmetrical, MAP could be calculated from the average of its minimum and maximum values. However, given the asymmetrical shape of the arterial blood pressure wave form, MAP is usually estimated by adding one-third of the pulse pressure to the diastolic pressure, i.e., $MAP = P_d + (P_s - P_d)/3$. For example, the mean arterial pressure is approximately 93 mmHg when the systolic pressure is 120 mmHg and the diastolic pressure is 80 mmHg, i.e., $93 = 80 + (120 - 80)/3$.

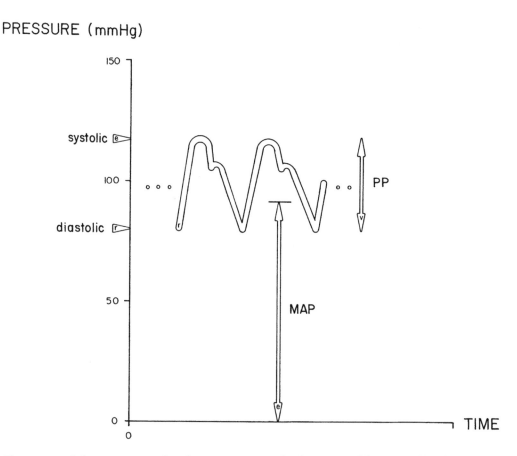

Figure 5.24   Mean arterial pressure and pulse pressure. Color the tracing of the arterial blood pressure wave form, noting its similarity to that shown in Figure 5.15. Color the arrows depicting the pulse pressure (PP) and mean arterial pressure (MAP). Note that pulse pressure is given by the difference between the systolic and diastolic pressures, and that mean arterial pressure is greater than diastolic pressure but less than systolic pressure. Pulse pressure depends on stroke volume and arterial compliance, a measure of the amount by which the vessels are distended (widened) by a given increment in pressure. Thus, pulse pressure increases in the face of larger stroke volumes and/or stiffer blood vessels. The functional significance of mean arterial blood pressure is that it can be regarded as the driving force that propels blood through the systemic circuit.

Systemic circulation

The mean arterial pressure is the driving force that pumps blood through the *vascular beds,* which are networks of branching blood vessels that perfuse the tissues of the body. The vascular beds from different organs in the systemic circulation are arranged in parallel (Figure 5.25). This arrangement enables each vascular bed to receive its own supply of arterial blood from a common high-pressure arterial line and drain its venous blood into a common low-pressure venous line. This arrangement also enables the same pressure gradient to appear across each vascular bed: the magnitude of this pressure gradient (ΔP) is determined by the amount by which the mean arterial pressure (MAP) exceeds the venous pressure (P_v), which is normally small by comparison, i.e., $\Delta P = MAP - P_v \approx MAP$.

Hemodynamic principles dictate that the rate at which blood flows through any given vascular bed (Q, in L/min) is equal to the pressure gradient across the bed (ΔP, in mmHg) divided by the vascular resistance of the bed (R, in mmHg·min/L), i.e.,

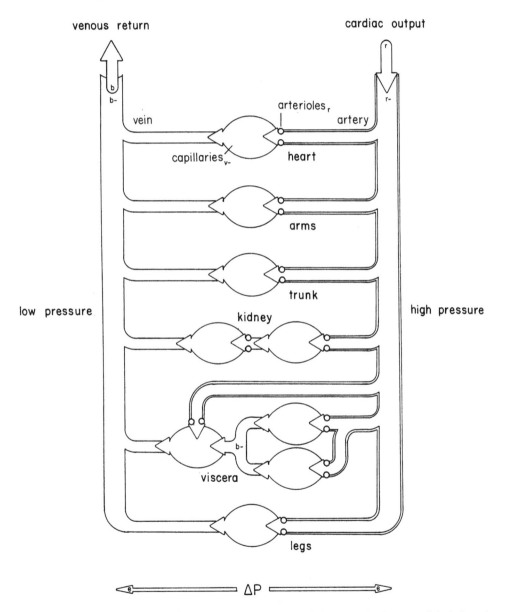

Figure 5.25   Arrangement of vascular beds in the systemic circulation. Color the arrow labeled cardiac output. Color the arterial blood supply and each vascular bed, depicted as a serial connection of arteries, arterioles, capillaries, and veins. Color the arrow labeled venous return, noting that it represents the mixing of venous blood from all of the vascular beds. Observe that the vascular beds are arranged in parallel and that this arrangement enables each vascular bed to receive its own supply of blood from a common high-pressure arterial line and drain its blood into a common low-pressure venous line. Thus, the pressure gradient across each vascular bed (ΔP) is given by the amount by which mean arterial pressure (MAP, Figure 5.24) exceeds venous pressure (P_v), which is small by comparison, i.e., $\Delta P = MAP - P_v \approx MAP$. Observe that this arrangement enables individual organs to determine their own flow by regulating the constriction of their arterioles.

123

$Q = \Delta P/R$. An increase in blood flow to an individual vascular bed could therefore be due to an increase in arterial pressure or a decrease in its vascular resistance. Since arterial pressure is held reasonably constant by the action of the blood pressure regulating mechanisms described below, the regulation of blood flow to individual vascular beds is achieved primarily by neural, hormonal, and chemical mechanisms that adjust the resistance of vascular beds in accordance with the needs of the tissues they supply. More blood flows to a vascular bed when its resistance decreases and less blood flows to a vascular bed when its resistance increases.

Types of blood vessels

Four different types of blood vessels are found in each vascular bed: (1) *arteries,* which transport blood at high pressure; (2) *arterioles,* which regulate the amount of blood that flows through them; (3) *capillaries,* which allow exchange of substances between the blood and the cells that surround them; and (4) *venules and veins,* which not only conduct blood back to the heart but also serve as a reservoir for blood (Figure 5.26).

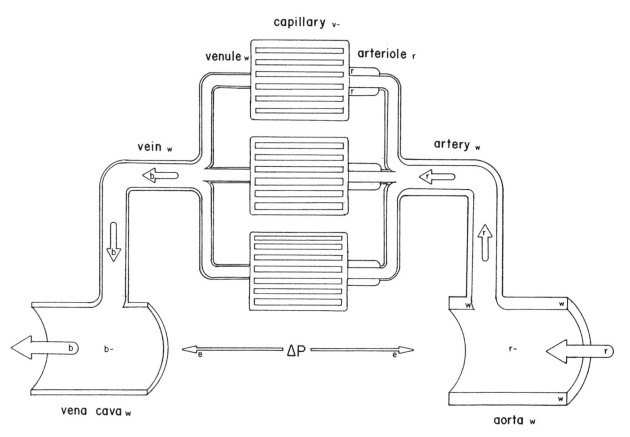

Figure 5.26   Arrangement of blood vessels in a vascular bed. Color the blood and the vessels from right to left. Note the relative numbers, sizes, and shapes of the different types of blood vessels. Note also that the pressure gradient across the vascular bed (ΔP) is determined by the amount by which mean arterial blood pressure (MAP) exceeds venous pressure (P_v). Compare this figure with Figure 5.25.

These different types of blood vessels differ in terms of their relative proportions of endothelium, smooth muscle, elastic tissue, and fibrous tissue. Arteries have a high percentage of elastic tissue, arterioles are made primarily of smooth muscle, and capillaries are made entirely of endothelial cells. The types of blood vessels also differ in terms of their number, their internal diameter, and the relative thickness of their walls (Figure 5.27).

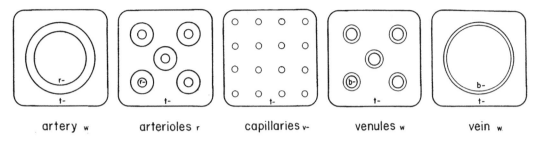

Figure 5.27 Types of blood vessels. Color the blood vessels and the blood they contain in this cross-sectional view. Note the relative numbers, sizes, and shapes of the different types of blood vessels and compare them with those shown in Figure 5.26.

Functional differences among types of blood vessels

These anatomical and structural differences among the types of blood vessels give rise to the following functional differences: (1) the blood pressure is highest in the arteries; (2) the resistance to blood flow is greatest in the arterioles; (3) the velocity of blood flow is lowest in the capillaries; and (4) the volume of blood is largest in the veins (Figure 5.28).

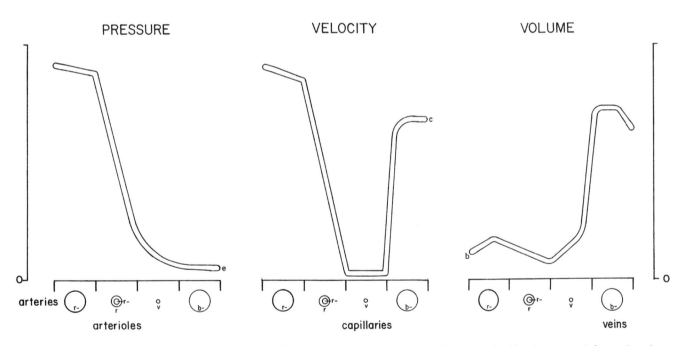

Figure 5.28 Functional differences among blood vessels. Color the lines that depict the blood pressure (left panel), velocity of blood flow (middle panel), and blood volume (right panel) associated with the different types of blood vessels. Note that blood pressure is highest in the arteries. Note also that the drop in blood pressure is greatest across the arterioles, indicating that the arterioles account for most of the resistance of the vascular bed. For this reason, the blood flow to individual vascular beds can be regulated by adjusting the diameter of the arterioles. Observe that the velocity of blood flow is lowest in the capillaries, indicating that the cross-sectional area of the capillaries is greatest. This allows sufficient time for exchange of substances between the blood and the tissues. Also observe that the volume of blood is greatest in the veins. These functional differences among the blood vessels play an important role in the regulation of blood flow. Compare this figure with Figure 5.27.

Determinants of vascular resistance

Poiseuille's law states that for a homogeneous fluid undergoing streamline flow (no turbulence) through a rigid pipe of length L and radius r, the hydraulic resistance (R) of the pipe is given by

$$R = 8\eta L/\pi r^4$$

where η represents the viscosity of the fluid, a measure of its lack of slipperiness.

Poiseuille's law shows that the resistance of a pipe depends on both the geometry of the pipe and the viscosity of the fluid that flows through it. The viscosity of blood, which is normally three times that of water, depends on its plasma proteins and its *hematocrit*, defined as the percent of blood volume occupied by red blood cells (Figure 5.29). The hematocrit of blood and therefore, the resistance of the vascular beds through which it flows, is decreased in *anemia* (low volume of red blood cells) and increased in *polycythemia* (high volume of red blood cells). A consequence of the effects of hematocrit on resistance is that the work required to pump a given cardiac output through the circulatory system is also decreased in anemia and increased in polycythemia.

Poiseuille's law also states that the resistance of a rigid pipe varies inversely with the fourth power of the radius ($1/r^4$). For a fixed pressure gradient, for example, halving the radius of a pipe would increase its resistance sixteen-fold and thereby

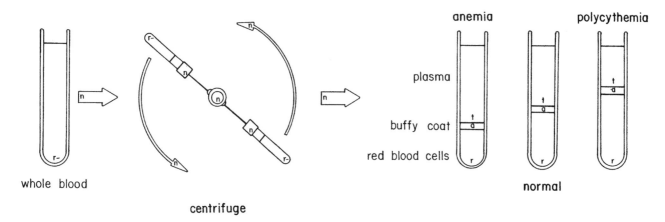

Figure 5.29 Constituents of blood. Color the diagram from left to right, noting that whole blood can be separated into three distinct layers by spinning it at high speed in a centrifuge. The layers correspond to red blood cells, white blood cells (buffy coat), and plasma. Color the tubes at the right, noting that the normal value for hematocrit, defined as the percent of the blood volume occupied by red blood cells, is 42 in men and 38 in women. Observe that the hematocrit is decreased in anemia (left tube) and increased in polycythemia (right tube). Since hematocrit is an important determinant of blood viscosity, the resistance of blood vessels is also decreased in anemia and increased in polycythemia.

decrease flow to one-sixteenth of its initial value. Conversely, doubling the radius would decrease its resistance to one-sixteenth of its initial value and thereby increase flow sixteen-fold (Figure 5.30). These theoretical findings explain why small adjustments in vessel diameter can lead to large changes in vessel resistance.

Even though the simplifying assumptions underlying Poiseuille's law are not strictly applicable to blood flowing through distensible blood vessels, the law does provide a theoretical framework to explain why the resistance to blood flow of a vascular bed is exquisitely sensitive to changes in the caliber of its blood vessels. Since the arterioles are the major site of the resistance within a vascular bed (Figure 5.28), the blood flow to any given vascular bed can be regulated by adjusting the internal diameter of its arterioles.

Figure 5.30 Effect of radius on resistance to fluid flow. Color the fluid in the reservoir. Note that the port at the left has a radius (2R) that is twice that (R) of the port at the right and that the pressure at each of the ports (height of fluid in reservoir) is the same. Observe that the rate at which fluid flows through the wide port is sixteen times that of the narrow port. Color and compare the volume of fluid in each of the graduated cylinders. These findings demonstrate that the radius of a blood vessel is an important determinant of its resistance to blood flow.

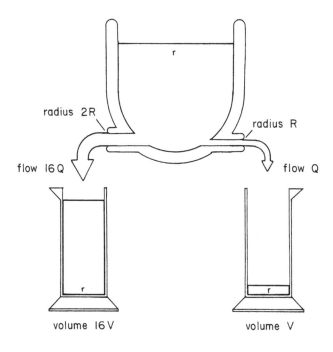

Mechanisms that regulate the caliber of arterioles

The internal diameter of an arteriole is regulated by neural, hormonal, and chemical mechanisms that control the contraction of the vascular smooth muscle fibers that are arranged circumferentially within its wall (Figure 5.31). *Vasoconstriction* is a term that denotes a narrowing of an arteriole caused by the contraction of its smooth muscle; *vasodilation* denotes a widening of an arteriole caused by the relaxation of its smooth muscle.

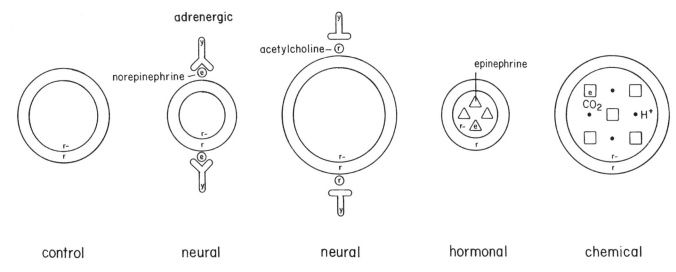

Figure 5.31 Mechanisms that regulate the caliber of arterioles. Color the panels from left to right, noting that the diameter of an arteriole depends on the competition between neural, hormonal, and chemical factors. Neural factors include sympathetic adrenergic fibers that release norepinephrine and cause vasoconstriction (narrowing of arterioles). Neural factors also include sympathetic cholinergic fibers that release acetylcholine and cause vasodilation (widening of arterioles). Hormonal factors include the effects of: (1) epinephrine, a hormone released by the adrenal medulla; (2) angiotensin, a hormone whose activation in the blood is stimulated by renin, a protein released by the kidney; and (3) antidiuretic hormone (ADH), a hormone released by the posterior pituitary gland. Chemical factors that cause vasodilation include a low level of oxygen (hypoxemia), a high level of carbon dioxide (hypercarbia), and a low pH (acidosis). Since the arterioles are the major site of resistance in a vascular bed, the blood flow to individual vascular beds can be regulated by these factors.

Neural control of vascular smooth muscle is achieved by neurotransmitters that are released by the sympathetic nervous system (Figure 5.31). The two types of sympathetic fibers are the *sympathetic adrenergic fibers,* which release norepinephrine, and the *sympathetic cholinergic fibers,* which release acetylcholine. Norepinephrine binds to alpha adrenergic receptors of vascular smooth muscle and causes vasoconstriction. In contrast, acetylcholine binds to cholinergic receptors of vascular smooth muscle and causes vasodilation.

Hormonal control of vascular smooth muscle is achieved by vasoactive hormones that are released by the endocrine system (Figure 5.31). These hormones include epinephrine (Figure 7.19), a hormone that is secreted by the adrenal medulla; angiotensin, a hormone whose activation in the blood is stimulated by renin, a protein released by the kidney; and antidiuretic hormone (ADH), a hormone that is released by the posterior pituitary gland.

Chemical control of vascular smooth muscle is achieved by the prevailing levels of oxygen, carbon dioxide, and acidity (pH) of the local blood supply (Figure 5.31). Arterioles of the systemic circulation dilate when they are exposed to blood that has a low level of oxygen (hypoxemia), a high level of carbon dioxide (hypercarbia), or a low pH (acidosis)—conditions that occur when vascular beds do not supply enough blood to meet the metabolic needs of the tissues they perfuse. In contrast, arterioles of the pulmonary circulation constrict when exposed to these same stimuli; this serves to improve gas exchange in the lung by redirecting blood from underventilated alveoli (where O_2 levels are low) to better ventilated alveoli (where O_2 levels are higher).

Autoregulation

Autoregulation is the process whereby systemic vascular beds regulate their blood flow in accordance with the metabolism of the tissues they supply. When blood flow is insufficient to meet the metabolic needs of a tissue, the cells remove more oxygen from a given volume of blood and *hypoxemia* (low O_2 levels in blood) occurs. The cells also add more carbon dioxide to this volume of blood and *hypercarbia* (high CO_2 levels in blood) occurs. As noted above, these alterations in local blood chemistry dilate the arterioles, decrease their resistance, and thereby increase blood flow through the vascular bed. The increased blood flow, in turn, supplies more oxygen to and removes more carbon dioxide from the tissues, thereby helping to restore the normal levels of oxygen and carbon dioxide in the tissues (Figure 5.32).

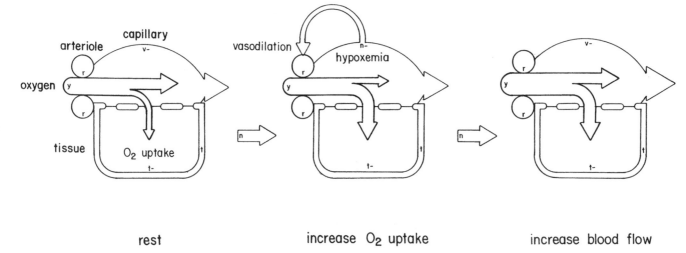

Figure 5.32 Autoregulation. For each panel, color the tissue, arteriole, capillary bed, and the arrow depicting the rate at which oxygen is delivered to the vascular bed. Observe that the O_2 supply is divided into two portions: one that is taken up by the tissues (downward arrowhead) and one that remains in the blood (horizontal arrowhead). Observe that an increase in O_2 uptake by the tissue causes hypoxemia (low O_2 levels in blood) and that hypoxemia is a chemical factor that dilates the arterioles that regulate the amount of blood that flows to the vascular bed (middle panel). Also observe that vasodilation increases the blood flow and therefore the O_2 supply; this helps restore normal O_2 levels (right panel). Thus, autoregulation is a mechanism whereby vascular beds can regulate their blood flow in accordance with the metabolic rate of the tissues they supply. Compare this figure with Figure 6.14.

Model of the systemic circuit

A simple but useful model of the systemic circulation is a thin cylindrical reservoir that is connected by a narrow-bore tube to a wide cylindrical reservoir (Figure 5.33). The thin cylinder represents the arteries, the narrow-bore tube represents the arterioles, and the wide cylinder represents the veins. This model embodies the salient features of the systemic circulation—pressure is highest in the arteries, resistance is greatest in the arterioles, and volume is largest in the veins (Figure 5.28).

The value of this model is that the relationships among pressure, flow, and volume in the model are the same as those in the actual systemic circulation. For example, the blood pressures in the arteries and veins can be visualized from the heights of the fluid in their respective reservoirs. The model therefore explains why blood pressure is raised by an increase in blood volume and lowered by a decrease in blood volume (Figure 5.33).

The model also shows that arterial pressure provides the driving force that pumps the entire cardiac output through the *total peripheral resistance*. The model therefore explains why arterial blood pressure is raised by an increase in cardiac output or total peripheral resistance and lowered by a decrease in cardiac output or total peripheral resistance (Figure 5.33).

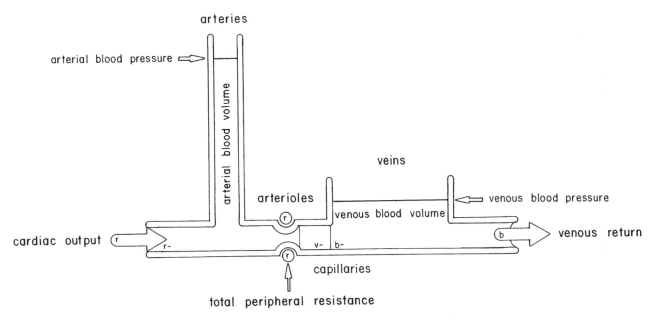

Figure 5.33   Model of the systemic circuit. Color the simplified model of the systemic circuit from left to right, identifying the structures as you go. Observe that the arteries are shown as a thin cylindrical reservoir (a small capacitance), the arterioles are shown as a narrow orifice (a large resistance), and the veins are shown as a wide cylindrical reservoir (a large capacitance). Note that the hydrostatic pressure at any point can be visualized from the vertical distance between that point and the fluid surface. Observe that this model embodies the salient features of the circulation—blood pressure is highest in the arteries, resistance is greatest in the arterioles, and blood volume is largest in the veins (Figure 5.28). Observe also that arterial blood pressure will be raised by factors that increase cardiac output, total peripheral resistance, or arterial blood volume. Arterial blood pressure can therefore be controlled by mechanisms that adjust cardiac output, total peripheral resistance, and blood volume. Note that resistance (R) specifies a relationship between pressure (P) and flow (Q), i.e., $R = P/Q$, whereas capacitance (C) specifies a relationship between volume (V) and pressure (P), i.e., $C = V/P$.

Regulation of arterial blood pressure

Arterial blood pressure is maintained at a reasonably constant level by the action of physiological mechanisms and control systems that adjust the factors that determine blood pressure, namely cardiac output, total peripheral resistance, and blood volume (Figure 5.33).

Short-term regulation of blood pressure is provided by baroreceptor reflexes that adjust cardiac output and total peripheral resistance. Intermediate-term mechanisms include the capillary fluid shift mechanism, which adjusts blood volume, and the renin-angiotensin system, which adjusts total peripheral resistance and blood volume. Long-term regulation of blood pressure is provided by the kidney–body fluid system, which adjusts blood volume.

chapter **five**

Baroreceptor reflexes

A *baroreceptor reflex* is an example of a reflex arc in which a response is mediated by the sequential operation of sensory receptors, afferent pathways, coordinating centers, efferent pathways, and effector organs (Figure 4.9).

Arterial *baroreceptors* are sensory receptors that respond to the stretch of the arterial walls in which they reside. They are located at the carotid sinus (the input to the brain) and the aortic arch (the output of the heart). They generate neural signals related to the prevailing level of arterial blood pressure

and transmit these signals along afferent pathways to the cardiovascular control centers in the medulla (Figure 5.34). When arterial blood pressure suddenly rises, for example, nerve impulses from the baroreceptors inhibit the cardiovascular control centers that, in turn, increase the parasympathetic output to the heart and decrease the sympathetic output to the heart and to the blood vessels. These alterations in neural output decrease cardiac output and total peripheral resistance, thereby eliciting a compensatory drop in blood pressure (Figure 5.35). Conversely, a sudden fall in arterial blood pressure gives rise to opposite changes in neural output which then elicit a compensatory rise in blood pressure.

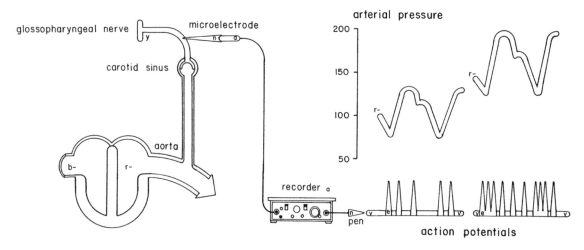

Figure 5.34 Transduction characteristics of arterial baroreceptors. Color the blood in the heart; note that the carotid sinus baroreceptors are exposed to arterial blood pressure. Color the glossopharyngeal nerve (cranial nerve IX), the microelectrode, and the recorder. Color the arterial blood pressure tracings and the corresponding action potentials generated by baroreceptors. Observe that the frequency of action potentials increases when arterial blood pressure rises. This feature of baroreceptor function enables them to transmit information related to blood pressure to the cardiovascular control centers in the brain.

Figure 5.35 Block diagram of a baroreceptor reflex. Color the block diagram. Observe that the setpoint (generated by a neural network in the cardiovascular control center) provides neural information related to the desired level of arterial blood pressure to a comparator, which also consists of a neural network in the cardiovascular control center. Note that the comparator also receives neural information related to the actual level of arterial blood pressure from baroreceptors (feedback loop). The difference between the two neural signals produces an error signal which causes the cardiovascular system (heart plus circuit) to adjust cardiac function (heart rate and myocardial contractility) and vascular tone (vasoconstriction) in such a way as to restore the normal level of arterial blood pressure. Thus, the operation of this system can be regarded as a negative feedback control system that maintains a normal level of arterial blood pressure in the face of naturally occurring disturbances in homeostasis.

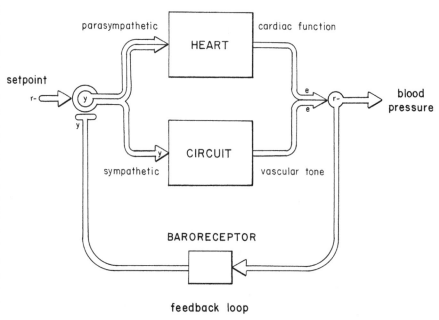

Capillary fluid shift mechanism

Starling's law states that the net flow of fluid across a capillary wall (Q, in mL/min) depends on the permeability of the membrane (K) and the balance between the hydrostatic (P) and osmotic (Π) pressures in the capillary and in the interstitial space just outside the capillary, i.e.,

$$Q = K \cdot [(P_c - P_i) - (\Pi_c - \Pi_i)]$$

where P_c and P_i are the *hydrostatic pressures* inside and outside the capillary, respectively, and Π_c and Π_i are the *osmotic*

pressures inside and outside the capillary, respectively (Figure 5.36). These osmotic pressures are due to the presence of nondiffusible particles, such as protein molecules that are too large to pass through the capillary wall.

Figure 5.36 Capillary fluid shift mechanism. The magnitude and direction of fluid flow across a capillary membrane depends on the balance between the inward and outward forces. Color the arrows that depict the rate at which water flows across the membrane by filtration (hydrostatic pressures, indicated by unmarked arrows in the left panel) and osmosis (osmotic pressures, indicated by hatched arrows in the right panel); note that the length of an arrow represents the magnitude of its effect. Examine the magnitude and direction of each arrow and identify its corresponding hydrostatic (P) or osmotic (Π) pressure. Finish the picture by coloring the background areas on both sides of the membrane. Plasma osmotic pressure (Π_c), a major inward force, is due to nondiffusible plasma proteins, such as serum albumin (mw ~69,000). Interstitial hydrostatic pressure (P_i) is shown as an outward force because it is normally negative (subatmospheric). Note that a high capillary pressure (P_c, an outward force) or a low plasma osmotic pressure (an inward force) would promote the flow of water from the capillary bed into the interstitial space outside the capillary.

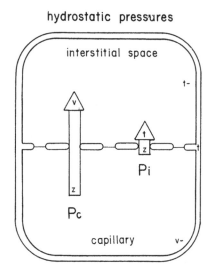 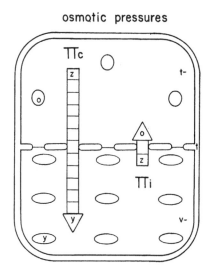

Capillary pressure is considered to be an outward force because it causes fluid to flow from the inside of the capillary to the interstitial space outside the capillary. During exercise, for example, capillary pressure in the vascular beds of exercising muscles increases because arterial blood pressure rises and because the arterioles dilate as a result of local changes in blood chemistry (autoregulation, Figure 5.32). These

higher capillary pressures cause fluid to filter out of the capillaries and thereby reduce plasma volume. Since red blood cells are too large to pass through the capillary wall, the same number of red blood cells will be suspended in a smaller plasma volume; this yields a higher concentration of red blood cells in the blood (hemoconcentration) (Figure 5.37).

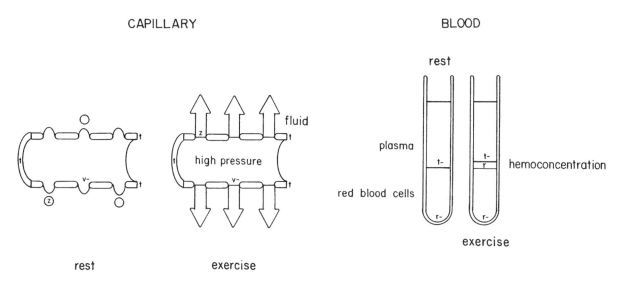

Figure 5.37   Hemoconcentration during exercise. Color the capillaries from left to right, comparing the rest condition (for which capillary pressure is low) with the exercise condition (for which capillary pressure is high). Note that high capillary pressures (an outward force, Figure 5.36) cause excessive filtration of fluid across the capillary wall, a condition that leads to a smaller plasma volume. High capillary pressures do not change the number of red blood cells in the blood because these cells are too large to cross the capillary wall. Color the centrifuged blood samples in the right panel, noting that hemoconcentration (higher hematocrit, Figure 5.29) occurs when the same number of red blood cells are suspended in a smaller plasma volume. These considerations explain why strenuous exercise can cause hemoconcentration.

Kidney-body fluid mechanism

Long-term regulation of arterial blood pressure is provided by the kidney–body fluid system, which increases blood volume when arterial pressure is low (*hypotension*) and decreases blood volume when arterial pressure is high (*hypertension*). These changes in blood volume help restore the normal level of arterial blood pressure (Figure 5.33).

The kidney–body fluid system relies on the operation of *nephrons*, which are the functional units of the kidney. Each nephron is made up of a system of blood vessels that consists of two capillary beds that are connected in series, and a system of kidney tubules. The pressure in the first capillary bed, which is called the *glomerulus*, provides the driving force that filters fluid through the glomerular membrane and into the kidney tubules (Figure 5.38). This fluid (called glomeru-

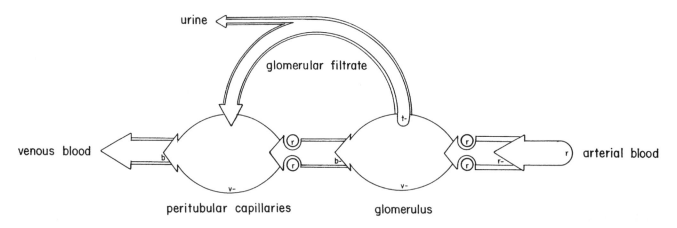

Figure 5.38   Renal circulation. Color the diagram from right to left, noting that the renal circulation consists of two arterioles and two capillary beds that are connected in series. Arterial blood enters the first capillary bed, which is called the glomerulus, through the afferent arteriole, and leaves the glomerulus through the efferent arteriole. From there, it flows through the second capillary bed, which is called the peritubular capillaries, before it returns to the venous circuit. Fluid that filters through the glomerular membrane, called glomerular filtrate, passes through kidney tubules (not shown) that are surrounded by the peritubular capillaries. Color the arrow labeled glomerular filtrate, noting that most of the glomerular filtrate (>99%) is returned to the blood in the peritubular capillaries while the remaining fraction (<1%) is excreted as urine. Thus, the kidney controls blood volume by regulating the amount of fluid excreted in urine. The actual amount of urine excreted by the kidney varies with arterial pressure, i.e., urine output increases when arterial pressure is high (hypertension) and decreases when arterial pressure is low (hypotension).

lar filtrate) then continues through the kidney tubules where most of it is returned to the blood via the second capillary bed (called the *peritubular capillaries*). The portion of the glomerular filtrate that is not returned to the blood is excreted from the body as urine.

Hypertension raises glomerular capillary pressure and increases the rate at which fluid filters through the glomerular membrane. The higher glomerular filtration rate increases urine output which, in turn, decreases blood volume and helps restore the normal level of arterial blood pressure (Figure 5.39). Conversely, hypotension lowers the glomerular capillary pressure and decreases the glomerular filtration rate. The lower glomerular filtration rate decreases urine output which, in turn, increases blood volume and helps restore the normal level of arterial blood pressure.

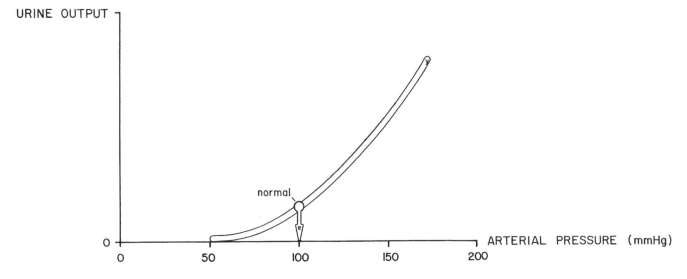

Figure 5.39   Effect of arterial blood pressure on urine output. Color the line that shows the effect of arterial blood pressure on urine output; identify the normal operating point (arterial pressure = 100 mmHg). Observe that a doubling of arterial pressure (to 200 mmHg) causes an eight-fold increase in urine output and that a halving of arterial pressure (to 50 mmHg) causes a complete cessation of urine output. These findings demonstrate that urine output is high during hypertension (high blood pressure) and low during hypotension (low blood pressure). These adjustments in urine output alter blood volume in such a way as to help maintain a normal level of arterial blood pressure. The strong dependency of urine output on arterial blood pressure explains how the kidney–body fluid system provides long-term regulation of blood pressure. Compare this figure with Figure 5.38.

Cardiovascular reflexes during exercise

During exercise, the cardiovascular control centers in the medulla are stimulated by a central command, which consists of nerve impulses originating in higher brain centers that control muscle activity (Figure 5.40).

At the beginning of exercise, the central command causes the cardiovascular control centers to decrease the parasympathetic output and increase the sympathetic output. The changes in neural output to the heart increase both heart rate and myocardial contractility, which improves the pumping capability of the heart. The changes in neural output to the systemic circulation cause both vasoconstriction in the vascular beds of visceral organs, which shunts more blood to exercising muscle, and generalized venoconstriction, which promotes venous return by mobilizing blood contained in the veins.

The blood flow to exercising muscles increases to meet their greater metabolic requirements for fuels and oxygen. This circulatory adaptation to exercise is due both to a higher cardiac output (Figure 5.19) and to an increase in the fraction of the cardiac output that is directed to exercising muscles (Figure 5.41).

As exercise continues, the neural output to the heart and blood vessels is modulated by nerve impulses that are transmitted to the cardiovascular control centers from a variety of peripheral sensory receptors (Figure 5.40), including: (1) arterial baroreceptors, which monitor blood pressure (Figure 5.34); (2) chemoreceptors, which sense the chemical composition of arterial blood (Figure 6.34); and (3) skeletal muscle mechanoreceptors, which detect muscle length and muscle tension (Figure 4.10).

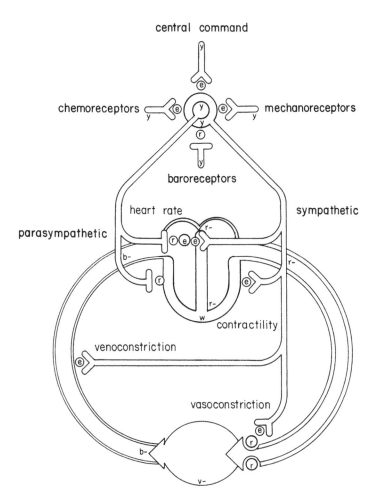

Figure 5.40 Cardiovascular reflexes during exercise. Color the cardiovascular control center and its inputs from higher centers (labeled central command), chemoreceptors (which detect blood levels of CO_2, O_2, and H^+, Figure 6.34), baroreceptors (which detect blood pressure, Figure 5.34), and mechanoreceptors (which detect mechanical stimuli, such as muscle length and tension, Figure 6.45). Color the parasympathetic efferent pathways, noting that stimulation of these fibers decreases heart rate and mildly decreases myocardial contractility. Color the sympathetic efferent pathways, noting that stimulation of these fibers increases heart rate and myocardial contractility and causes contraction of smooth muscle in the arterioles (vasoconstriction) and veins (venoconstriction) of the systemic circuit. Vasoconstriction increases total peripheral resistance and venoconstriction decreases venous capacitance. Thus, autonomic control of cardiovascular function is mediated by parasympathetic nerves that innervate the heart and by sympathetic nerves that innervate the heart and the systemic circulation. Compare this figure with Figures 5.11 and 5.35.

Cardiac function curves

Cardiac muscle fibers contract more forcefully when they are stretched prior to their contraction (Figure 5.4). This intrinsic property of cardiac muscle accounts for Starling's original observation that a denervated heart can pump more blood and do more work simply by operating from a longer initial fiber length (Figure 5.42). This property of cardiac muscle can be expressed graphically by a *cardiac function curve* in which cardiac output is plotted against some index of fiber length (preload), such as filling pressure, atrial pressure, or ventricular end-diastolic volume. Cardiac function curves are characterized by a steep portion and a flat, nearly horizontal, portion (Figure 5.43).

The steep portion of the cardiac function curve corresponds to a range of fiber lengths over which higher filling pressures yield higher cardiac outputs. Over this range, the heart pumps all of the blood it receives from the veins. The flat portion of the cardiac function curve corresponds to a range of filling pressures over which the cardiac output remains constant at its maximum value. An important ramification of these considerations is that at rest and during mild exercise, cardiac output is determined by peripheral factors that limit venous return, whereas during strenuous exercise, cardiac output is determined by cardiac factors that limit the ability of the heart to pump blood.

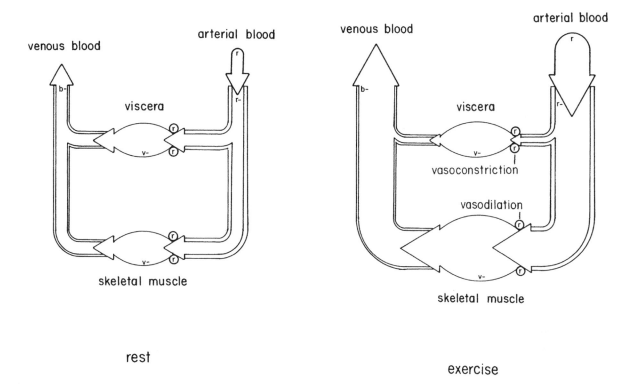

Figure 5.41 Redistribution of cardiac output during exercise. Color the arterial blood, vascular beds, and venous blood in both panels; note from the size of the arrow labeled arterial blood that cardiac output is higher during exercise (right panel) than at rest (left panel). Compare the constriction of the arterioles in the rest and exercise conditions, noting that the arterioles of the visceral vascular bed are constricted (due to sympathetic adrenergic fibers) while the arterioles of the skeletal muscle vascular bed are dilated (due to autoregulation and sympathetic cholinergic fibers) (Figure 5.31). Observe that these adaptations increase blood flow to exercising muscle while decreasing blood flow to visceral organs. This redistribution of cardiac output enables exercising muscles to enjoy a larger share of the cardiac output; this promotes the delivery of fuels and oxygen to exercising muscles. Compare this figure with Figure 5.25.

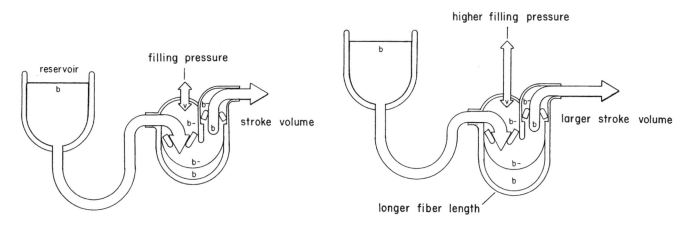

Figure 5.42 Law of the heart. Color the panels from left to right, noting the vertical arrows that denote filling pressure. Observe that a higher filling pressure (elevated reservoir in right panel) results in a larger stroke volume. Observe also that the stroke volume is equal to the volume displaced by ventricular contraction. This behavior, which is also called the Frank–Starling mechanism, can be explained by intrinsic properties of cardiac muscles that enable them to contract more forcefully when they are stretched prior to their contraction. This mechanism enables the heart to pump all of the blood that it receives from the veins. Compare this figure with Figures 5.14 and 5.16.

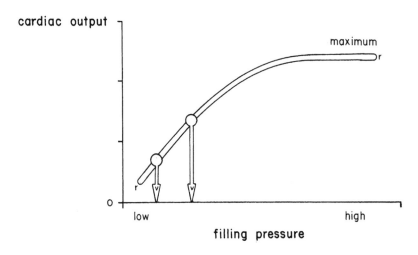

Figure 5.43   Cardiac function curve. Color the line that shows how cardiac output varies with filling pressure, an expression of ventricular fiber length (Figure 5.5). Observe that the cardiac function curve is characterized by a steep portion in which cardiac output increases with increasing filling pressure, and a flat portion in which cardiac output is at its maximum value, independent of filling pressure. Color the vertical arrows that correspond to the conditions shown in Figure 5.42, noting that a higher filling pressure results in a larger cardiac output.

Factors that modify the cardiac function curve

The cardiac function curve is amplified by any factor that increases the pumping capability of the heart (Figure 5.44). Factors that render the heart hypereffective include enhanced

myocardial contractility (due to sympathetic stimulation and/or circulating catecholamines) and cardiac hypertrophy (increased cardiac muscle mass). These factors increase exercise capacity because they raise the maximal level of cardiac output.

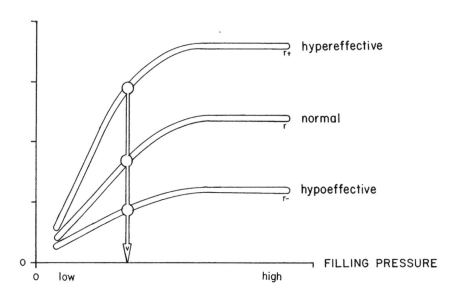

Figure 5.44   Factors that modify the cardiac function curve. Color each of the curves, noting that the normal curve is identical to that shown in Figure 5.43. Observe that the cardiac function curves for the hypereffective and hypoeffective hearts fall above and below the cardiac function curve for the normal heart, respectively. Color the vertical line that indicates a fixed filling pressure and thus, the same ventricular fiber length. Observe that the cardiac output associated with this fiber length is high in the hypereffective heart, intermediate in the normal heart, and low in the hypoeffective heart.

On the other hand, the cardiac function curve is attenuated by any factor that decreases the pumping capability of the heart (Figure 5.44). Some factors that render the heart hypoeffective are decreased heart rate, diminished myocardial contractility, cardiac anoxia (due to very low oxygen levels in arterial blood), congenital heart disease, and valvular heart disease. These factors decrease exercise capacity because they lower the maximal level of cardiac output.

Vascular function curves

Vascular function curves, which are graphs of venous return plotted against right atrial pressure, quantify the ability of the systemic circulation to return blood to the heart. Vascular function curves are also characterized by a steep portion and a flat, nearly horizontal, portion (Figure 5.45).

The steep portion of the vascular function curve corresponds to positive right atrial pressures. Over this range, a given increment in right atrial pressure has been found to cause a proportional decrement in venous return. The steep portion of the vascular function curve therefore forms a straight line that can be specified by numerical values for its slope and x-intercept (Figure 5.45).

The slope defines a parameter called the *resistance to venous return* (R_{vr}) and the x-intercept defines a parameter called the *mean systemic pressure* (P_{ms}). Any factor that alters R_{vr} modifies the slope of the vascular function curve, and any factor that alters P_{ms} modifies its x-intercept. Thus, this analysis permits the effect of any factor on vascular function to be analyzed by determining the extent to which the factor modifies the slope (R_{vr}) and x-intercept (P_{ms}) of the vascular function curve.

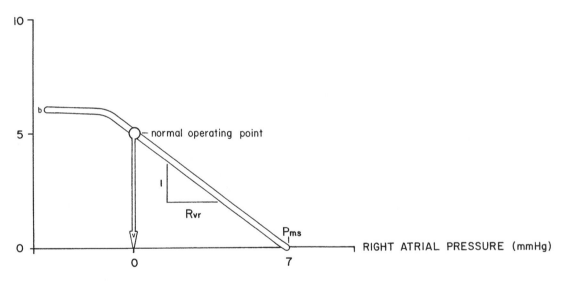

Figure 5.45 **Vascular function curve.** Color the vascular function curve, which depicts the effects of right atrial pressure (P_{ra}, in mmHg) on venous return (in L/min) and identify the normal operating point ($P_{ra} = 0$). Observe that the vascular function curve is characterized by a steep, linear portion in which venous return decreases with increasing right atrial pressure; note also that venous return ceases when right atrial pressure equals P_{ms} (the x-intercept, normally 7 mmHg). The linear portion of the vascular function curve can be specified by numerical values of its slope ($1/R_{vr}$, where R_{vr} is defined as the resistance to venous return and expressed in units of mmHg · min/L) and its x-intercept (P_{ms}, in mmHg). Redrawn from A. C. Guyon et al., 1973 (recommended reading).

Mean systemic pressure

Mean systemic pressure has been measured experimentally by fibrillating the heart (to prevent it from beating), and clamping both the aorta and vena cava so that blood can nei-

ther enter nor leave the systemic circuit. Under these conditions, blood initially flows from the arteries, where pressure is highest, into the veins, where pressure is lowest (Figure 5.46). This redistribution of blood volume causes arterial pressure to fall and venous pressure to rise until the pressures

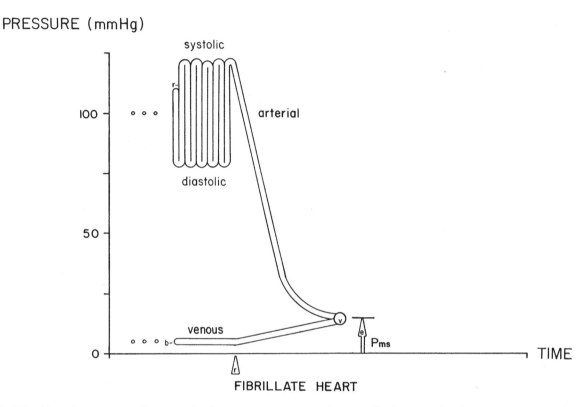

Figure 5.46 Blood pressure changes during measurement of P$_{ms}$. Color the arterial and venous blood pressure tracings. Observe that ventricular fibrillation, which prevents the heart from pumping blood, causes arterial pressure to fall and venous pressure to rise until the two pressures equilibrate at the same pressure; this equilibrium pressure defines the mean systemic pressure (P$_{ms}$). Note that the fall in arterial pressure is greater than the rise in venous pressure. This difference in pressure change reflects corresponding differences in arterial and venous capacitance; the capacitance of the veins (C$_v$) is approximately 20 times that of the arteries (C$_a$).

in the arteries and veins equilibrate at the same level; this equilibrium pressure was originally defined by Guyton as the mean systemic pressure (P$_{ms}$) (Figure 5.47).

The magnitude of P$_{ms}$ depends on the volume of blood in the systemic circuit relative to its capacitance (Figure 5.33). In other words, P$_{ms}$ can be regarded as a measure of the degree of filling of the systemic circuit. Thus, P$_{ms}$ increases when more blood occupies the same blood vessels (same capaci-

tance) or when the same volume of blood occupies smaller vessels (smaller capacitance).

The functional significance of this parameter is that P$_{ms}$ determines the x-intercept of the vascular function curve. Therefore, factors that increase P$_{ms}$ shift the vascular function curve to the right whereas factors that decrease P$_{ms}$ shift the vascular function curve to the left.

Figure 5.47 Blood volume changes during measurement of P_{ms}. Color the top diagram, noting the plugs that prevent blood from flowing into and out of the systemic circuit. Observe that arterial pressure (height of fluid in arterial reservoir) initially exceeds venous pressure (height of fluid in venous reservoir); this pressure gradient causes fluid to flow from the arterial reservoir (where pressure is higher) to the venous reservoir (where pressure is lower). Color the bottom diagram, noting that the translocation of blood from the arterial circuit to the venous circuit ceases when arterial pressure equilibrates with venous pressure. This equilibrium pressure is defined as P_{ms} and it can be regarded as a measure of the degree of filling of the systemic circuit. Another measure of the degree of filling of the circulation is the mean circulatory pressure (P_{mc}), defined as the pressure that would be measured at all points in the entire circulatory system if the heart were stopped suddenly and blood was redistributed in such a way that pressures in all parts of the pulmonary and systemic circulations were equal. Compare this figure with Figure 5.46.

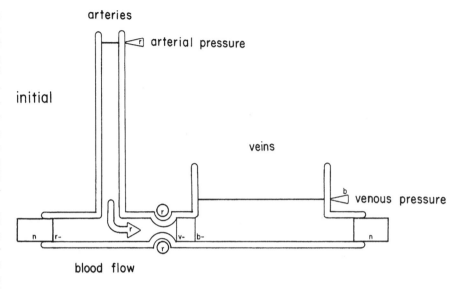

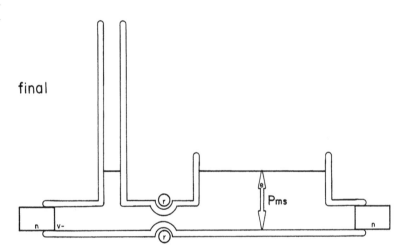

Determinants of mean systemic pressure

Because mean systemic pressure reflects the degree of filling of the systemic circuit, P_{ms} varies directly with blood volume and inversely with venous capacitance (C_v).

If venous capacitance remained constant, an increase in blood volume, as can occur with a transfusion, would raise P_{ms} and thereby shift the vascular function curve to the right. Conversely, a decrease in blood volume, as can occur from a hemorrhage, dehydration, or excessive filtration of fluid across the capillary membranes, would lower P_{ms} and shift the vascular function curve to the left.

If blood volume remained constant, a decrease in C_v, as occurs during *venoconstriction* would raise P_{ms} and shift the vascular function curve to the right. Conversely, an increase in C_v, as occurs during *venodilation,* would lower P_{ms} and shift the vascular function curve to the left (Figure 5.48). Venous capacitance decreases when the vascular smooth muscle in the walls of the venules and veins contracts (venoconstriction), as can occur in response to neurotransmitters released by the sympathetic nervous system or to circulating catecholamines released by the adrenal medulla. Venous capacitance also decreases when skeletal muscles contract and mechanically compress the venules and veins that perfuse them. In summary, venous capacitance, and therefore P_{ms}, can be altered by mechanical, neural, and humoral mechanisms (Figure 5.49).

VENOUS RETURN (liters/min)

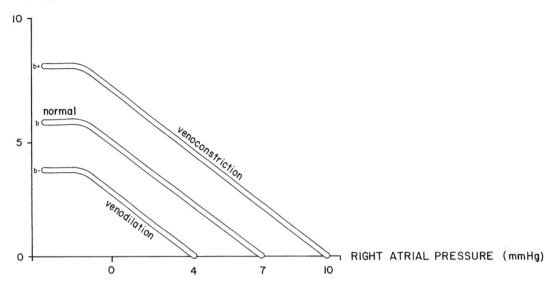

Figure 5.48   Effects of venomotor tone on vascular function curve. Color the individual vascular function curves for each condition, noting that the normal vascular function curve is identical to that shown in Figure 5.45. Observe that venoconstriction (upper curve) is associated with an increase in P_{ms} (to 10 mmHg) and that venodilation (lower curve) is associated with a decrease in P_{ms} (to 4 mmHg). Observe also that the slopes of the three curves are the same, indicating that alterations in the capacitance of the venous circuit do not have any appreciable effect on its resistance. Because P_{ms} defines the x-intercept of the vascular function curve, it follows that changes in venous capacitance modify the x-intercept of the vascular function curve. Thus, the effects of venomoter tone on vascular function can be accounted for by changes in the x-intercept of the vascular function curve. For this reason, skeletal muscle contraction and increased sympathetic stimulation during exercise manifest themselves as a vascular function curve that is shifted to the right. Redrawn from A.C. Guyton et al., 1973 (recommended reading).

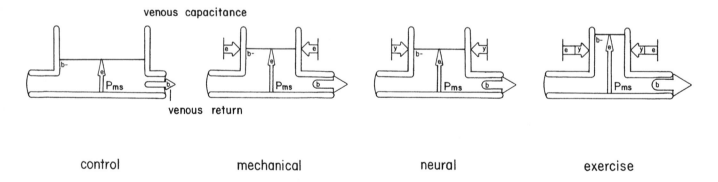

Figure 5.49   Mechanical and neural factors that influence P_{ms}. Color the diagram from left to right, identifying the venous capacitance, mean systemic pressure (P_{ms}), and arrow depicting venous return. Color the horizontal arrows that show the compression of veins: this decreases venous capacitance. Observe that venous capacitance can be decreased by mechanical factors (skeletal muscle contraction), neural factors (venoconstriction), and exercise (skeletal muscle contraction coupled with venoconstriction). Observe also that compression of the veins leads to an increase in P_{ms} (indicated by the height of the fluid in the venous reservoir) which, in turn, increases venous return (arrow at right of each panel). Because the heart normally pumps all the blood it receives from the veins, increases in venous return lead to corresponding increases in cardiac output. Thus, compression of the veins and the consequent mobilization of blood from the veins promotes ventricular filling (preload) and thereby increases cardiac output.

Resistance to venous return

The resistance to venous return (R_{vr}) reflects the resistance of the venules and veins, which is normally small in comparison to the resistance of the arterioles (Figure 5.28). As a result, changes in venous resistance do not normally have any appreciable effect on the total peripheral resistance, which depends primarily on the caliber of the arterioles.

The resistance to venous return increases when the vascular smooth muscle in the walls of venules and veins contracts or when the hematocrit is increased by polycythemia. An increase in R_{vr} decreases the slope of the steep portion of the vascular function curve. Conversely, the resistance to venous return decreases when the vascular smooth muscle relaxes or when the hematocrit is decreased by anemia. A decrease in R_{vr} increases the slope of the steep portion of the vascular function curve (Figure 5.50).

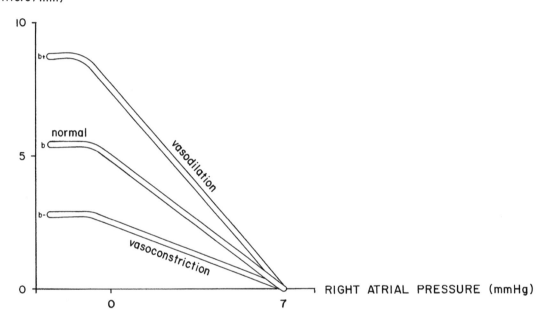

Figure 5.50   Effects of vasomotor tone on vascular function curve. Color the individual vascular function curves for each condition, noting that the normal vascular function curve is identical to that shown in Figure 5.45. Observe that vasodilation (upper curve) is associated with an increase in the slope of the vascular function curve and that vasoconstriction (lower curve) is associated with a decrease in the slope. Observe also that the x-intercept of the three curves are the same, indicating that alterations in the resistance of the venous circuit do not have any appreciable effect on its capacitance (Figure 5.48). Thus, the effects of alterations in the resistance of blood vessels on vascular function can be accounted for by changes in the slope of the vascular function curve. For this reason, metabolic vasodilation during exercise manifests itself as an increase in the slope of the vascular function curve. Redrawn from A.C. Guyton et al., 1973 (recommended reading).

Equating cardiac function and vascular function curves

The positive slope of the cardiac function curve indicates that the behavior of the heart causes cardiac output to increase with increasing right atrial pressure. The negative slope of the vascular function curve indicates that the behavior of systemic circulation causes venous return to decrease with increasing right atrial pressure. Since cardiac output and venous return are equal, the point at which the two curves intersect specifies equilibrium values for cardiac output and right atrial pressure that satisfy the constraints imposed by the heart and by the systemic circulation (Figure 5.51).

CARDIAC OUTPUT (liters/min)

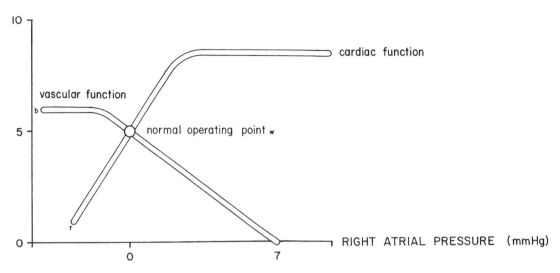

Figure 5.51 **Equating cardiac function and vascular function curves.** Color the cardiac function curve from Figure 5.43 and the vascular function curve from Figure 5.45 and identify the normal operating point as the point at which the two curves intersect. Observe also that the operating point specifies unique values for cardiac output and right atrial pressure that satisfy the constraints imposed by the heart (cardiac function curve) and the constraints imposed by the systemic circuit (vascular function curve). Note that changes in either curve will modify the point at which they intersect and that the new operating point defines the values of cardiac output and right atrial pressure that would occur as a result of these changes. Thus, the beauty of this analysis is that the effects of alterations in cardiac function (Figure 5.44) can be separated from the effects of alterations in vascular function (Figs. 5.48 and 5.50). Redrawn from A. C. Guyton et al., 1973 (recommended reading).

Regulation of cardiac output during exercise

The increase in cardiac output during exercise is mediated by the combined action of mechanical, neural, and humoral mechanisms that modify both cardiac function and vascular function. These adjustments in cardiac and vascular function modify their corresponding curves and thereby displace the equilibrium point at which the two curves intersect. The value of this analysis is that the displaced equilibrium point specifies new values of cardiac output and right atrial pressure that are consistent with the given alterations in cardiac and vascular function.

At rest, the intersection of the resting cardiac function and vascular function curves depicts the cardiac output and right atrial pressure in a healthy subject prior to the onset of exercise (point A, Figure 5.52). During exercise, the cardiac function curve is amplified by increases in both heart rate and myocardial contractility. This enhancement of cardiac function is due to the combined effects of an increased sympathetic output, a decreased parasympathetic output (neural effects), and increased blood levels of catecholamines re-

leased by the adrenal medulla (humoral effects). At the same time, the vascular function curve is displaced to the right by an increase in mean systemic pressure. This increase in P_{ms} is due to the effects of skeletal muscle contraction on P_{ms} (mechanical effects) and to the effects of venoconstriction on P_{ms} (neural and humoral effects). The improvement of cardiac function (which increases the ability of the heart to pump blood) in conjunction with the improvement in vascular function (which increases the ability of the systemic circuit to return blood to the heart) both make significant contributions to the net increase in cardiac output (Point B). As exercise continues, further increases in cardiac output can be attributed to the decrease in R_{vr} that accompanies metabolic vasodilation (point C).

During moderate exercise (left panel), point C is located on the steep portion of the cardiac function curve, whereas during maximal exercise (right panel), point C is located on the flat portion of the cardiac function curve. These considerations demonstrate that, during moderate exercise, cardiac output is determined by peripheral factors that limit venous return, whereas during strenuous exercise, cardiac output is determined by cardiac factors that limit the pumping capability of the heart.

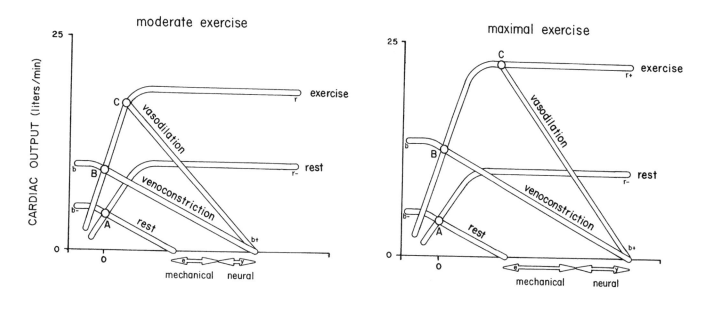

Figure 5.52 Cardiovascular responses to exercise. Color the cardiac function and vascular function curves at rest in both panels, noting that these curves are identical to those shown in Figure 5.51. Color the cardiac function curves labeled exercise, noting that the heart is hypereffective (Figure 5.44). Color the vascular function curves labeled venoconstriction, noting that they have been displaced to the right by the combined action of mechanical and neural mechanisms that increase P_{ms} (Figure 5.49). Color the vascular function curves labeled vasodilation, noting that the steeper slopes of these lines enable them to intersect the cardiac function curve at a point that corresponds to a higher cardiac output. Compare the magnitudes of the responses in the two panels, observing that the cardiac function curve is higher during maximal exercise and that the x-intercept of the vascular function curve is greater during maximal exercise. Also observe that the final operating point lies on the steep portion of the cardiac function curve during moderate exercise but on the flat portion of the cardiac function curve during maximal exercise. These findings demonstrate that cardiac output during moderate exercise is determined by peripheral factors that limit venous return, whereas cardiac output during maximal exercise is determined by cardiac factors that limit the pumping capability of the heart. Redrawn from A. C. Guyton et al., 1973 (recommended reading).

chapter **six**
respiratory
system

The respiratory system supplies oxygen to, and removes excess carbon dioxide from, the blood (Figure 6.1).

Respiratory responses to exercise represent the combined action of mechanical, neural, and humoral mechanisms that regulate the ventilation of the lung in order to keep pace with the higher rates of oxygen consumption and carbon dioxide production that occur during exercise.

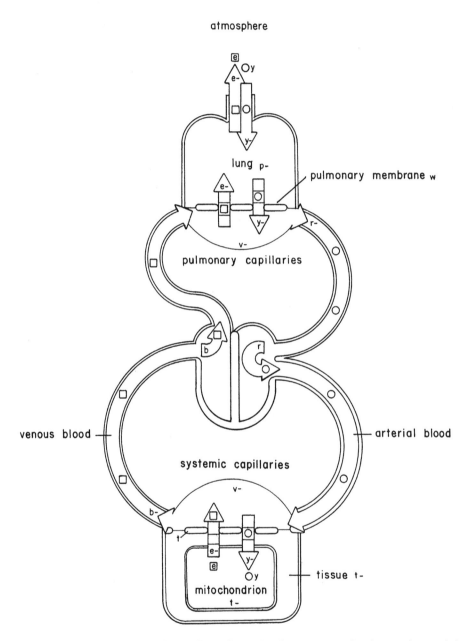

Figure 6.1   Transport of oxygen and carbon dioxide. Color the oxygen molecules (circles) and their arrows as they are transported from the atmosphere through the blood and into the mitochondrion, the site where O_2 is consumed and CO_2 is produced by the oxidative system (Figure 3.6). Color the carbon dioxide molecules (squares) and their arrows as they are transported in the opposite direction, from the mitochondrion to the atmosphere. Note that gas exchange between the lung and blood and between the blood and tissues occurs across capillary membranes by diffusion (hatched arrows; ignore hatches when coloring). Finish the picture by coloring the background areas of the lung, cardiovascular system, tissue, and mitochondrion. Compare this figure with Figure 5.1.

Gas exchange in the lung

Gas exchange between air and blood in the lung occurs across the *pulmonary membrane*, which is the boundary between alveolar gas and capillary blood, by the passive process of diffusion (Figure 6.2). Oxygen diffuses from the alveolus into the blood while carbon dioxide diffuses simultaneously from the blood into the alveolus (Figure 6.3).

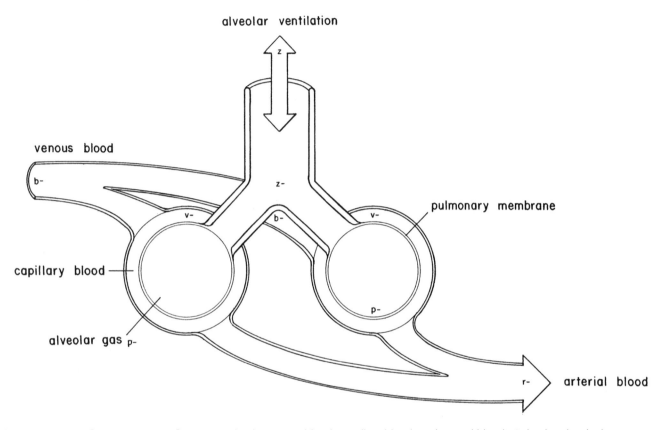

Figure 6.2 Pulmonary membrane. Color the venous blood, capillary blood, and arterial blood. Color the alveoli, their airways, and the arrow labeled alveolar ventilation, which depicts the rate at which the alveoli are ventilated by inspired air. Note that the pulmonary membrane is the boundary between alveolar gas and pulmonary capillary blood, and that gas exchange occurs across this membrane by the passive process of diffusion.

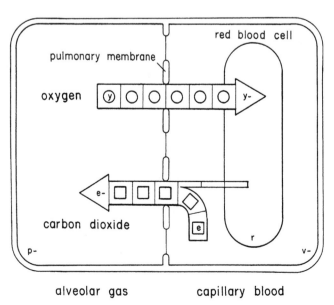

Figure 6.3 Diffusion of gases across the pulmonary membrane. Color the oxygen molecules (circles) and their diffusion arrow, noting that oxygen diffuses from alveolar gas into the red blood cell. Color the carbon dioxide molecules (squares) and their diffusion arrow, noting that carbon dioxide diffuses in the opposite direction, from pulmonary capillary blood into alveolar gas. Color the background area on both sides of the pulmonary membrane. Note that all of the oxygen is carried in the red blood cell while most of the carbon dioxide is carried in blood plasma, the fluid that surrounds the red blood cells. Compare this figure with Figure 6.2.

Fick's law of diffusion states that the rate at which a gas diffuses across an ideal membrane ($\dot{V}_{gas}$, in molecules/s) is determined by the product of three different factors: (1) the diffusion constant of the gas (D); (2) the ratio of the area of the membrane to the thickness of the membrane (A/T); and (3) the partial pressure gradient of the gas across the membrane (ΔP), i.e.,

$$\dot{V}_{gas} = D \cdot (A/T) \cdot \Delta P$$

Diffusion constants for oxygen and carbon dioxide

The first factor in the above diffusion equation is the *diffusion constant* (D), which is a measure of how easily the gas passes through the membrane. The diffusion constant for any particular gas in the lung depends on its solubility and its molecular weight. Light molecules diffuse faster than do heavy ones in the alveolus (gas phase), and more soluble molecules diffuse faster than less soluble molecules in the pulmonary membrane (liquid phase). Combining both factors, carbon dioxide diffuses twenty times faster than oxygen, even though it is a heavier molecule, because of its much greater solubility in the pulmonary membrane.

Geometry of the pulmonary membrane

The second factor in the diffusion equation is a geometric term representing the membrane's area-to-thickness ratio (A/T) (Figure 6.4). The pulmonary membrane is ideally suited for diffusion because it has a very large surface area ($A \approx 80$ m^2) and it is extremely thin ($0.1 < T < 1.0$ µm). Two examples of conditions that decrease the rate at which gases diffuse through the pulmonary membrane are *emphysema,* which decreases the area of the membrane, and *pulmonary edema,* which increases the thickness of the membrane.

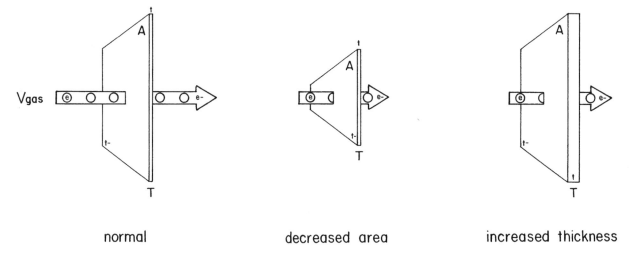

normal   decreased area   increased thickness

Figure 6.4   Effect of membrane geometry on diffusion. Color the molecules of gas, their diffusion arrow, and the membrane in each condition. Observe that the rate at which molecules diffuse across the membrane (length of arrow labeled $\dot{V}_{gas}$) decreases when the area of the membrane is decreased (middle panel) or the thickness of the membrane is increased (right panel). These results show that the geometry of a membrane is an important determinant of the rate at which gases can diffuse through it.

Tracheobronchial tree

The branches of the *tracheobronchial tree* bifurcate, meaning that they each divide into two smaller branches, a total of twenty-three times. The tracheobronchial tree terminates in the 300 million alveoli whose membranes make up most of the pulmonary membrane (Figure 6.5).

In the first sixteen bifurcations, or divisions, the walls of the tracheobronchial tree are too thick for gases to diffuse through them. The volume of this region of the lung where no gas exchange takes place is called the *anatomical dead space* (V_D). In the remaining divisions, the airway walls are thin enough for gas exchange to occur between the airways and the blood vessels that surround them; the volume of this region of the lung is called the *alveolar volume* (Figure 6.5).

Figure 6.5 Tracheobronchial tree. Color the schematic tracheobronchial tree, and its simplified model at the right. Note that the volume of the first sixteen generations of the tracheobronchial tree corresponds to the anatomical dead space, the part of the lung where no gas exchange takes place. Note also that the volume of the remaining generations corresponds to the alveolar volume, the part of the lung where gas exchange does take place.

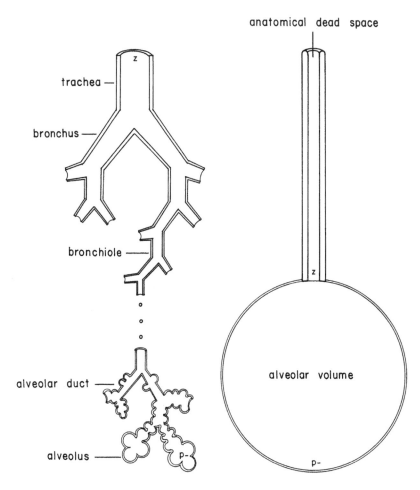

Partial pressure gradients

The third factor in the diffusion equation is the *partial pressure gradient* of the gas across the membrane (ΔP). Partial pressure gradients, rather than concentration gradients, provide the driving force for diffusion in systems that have air–liquid interfaces. Gases in the lung therefore diffuse from a region of higher partial pressure to one of lower partial pressure. At *equilibrium,* net diffusion ceases when the partial pressures of a gas on the two sides of the pulmonary membrane are equal. In other words, equilibrium occurs when the partial pressure of the gas in the alveolus (one side of the pulmonary membrane) is the same as that in the blood (the other side of the pulmonary membrane).

Partial pressures of oxygen and carbon dioxide

Ambient air is a mixture of nitrogen (N_2, 79.04%), oxygen (O_2, 20.93%), carbon dioxide (CO_2, 0.03%), water vapor (H_2O, which varies with humidity), and minute amounts of inert gases. Dalton's law states that the total pressure of a mixture of gases is given by the sum of the partial pressures of each of its constituents (Figure 6.6). *Barometric pressure* (P_B), which is 760 mmHg (760 Torr) at sea level, is therefore equal to the sum of the partial pressures of nitrogen (PN_2), oxygen (PO_2), carbon dioxide (PCO_2), and water vapor (PH_2O), i.e.,

$$P_B = PN_2 + PO_2 + PCO_2 + PH_2O$$

Inspired air is completely saturated with water vapor in the mouth and pharynx. Since the partial pressure of water vapor (PH_2O) at body temperature is 47 mmHg, the partial pressure of oxygen in inspired air (P_IO_2) can be calculated from the product of its fractional concentration in dry air, which is 20.9%, and ($P_B - 47$), i.e., $P_IO_2 = 20.9\% \cdot (760 - 47) \approx 150$ mmHg. Similarly, the partial pressure of carbon dioxide in inspired air (P_ICO_2) can be calculated from the product of its fractional concentration, which is 0.03%, and ($P_B - 47$), i.e., $P_ICO_2 = 0.03\% \cdot (760 - 47) \approx 0$ mmHg (Figure 6.7).

149

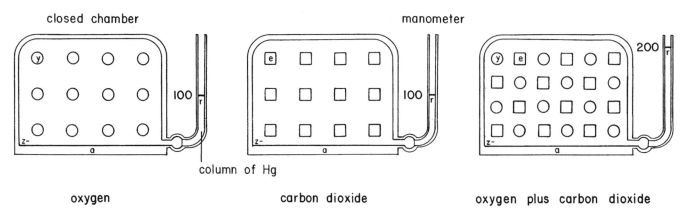

closed chamber

manometer

100 r

column of Hg

100 r

200 r

oxygen

carbon dioxide

oxygen plus carbon dioxide

Figure 6.6 Partial pressures. Color and count the O_2 molecules (circles) in the left panel. Color the chamber and the level of mercury in the schematic manometer (actual manometers contain a U-tube), which indicates that the pressure exerted by this gas on the walls of the chamber happens to be 100 mmHg, i.e., $PO_2 = 100$ mmHg. Repeat the process for the CO_2 molecules (squares) in the middle panel, noting that the same number of molecules exerts the same pressure on the walls of the chamber, i.e., $PCO_2 = 100$ mmHg. Finish the picture by coloring the right panel, noting that the gas mixture in this chamber represents the O_2 molecules from the left chamber plus the CO_2 molecules from the middle chamber. In accordance with Dalton's law, the total pressure exerted by this mixture of gases ($P_{TOTAL} = 200$ mmHg) can be calculated from the sum of the partial pressures of each of its constituents (i.e., $P_{TOTAL} = PO_2 + PCO_2$).

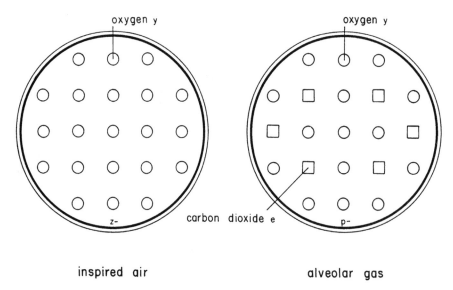

oxygen y

oxygen y

carbon dioxide e

z-

p-

inspired air

alveolar gas

Figure 6.7 Composition of inspired air and alveolar gas. Color and count the O_2 molecules (circles) and CO_2 molecules (squares) in inspired air (left panel) and alveolar gas (right panel). Observe that alveolar gas differs from inspired air in that it has fewer O_2 molecules and more CO_2 molecules. Compare these results with the partial pressures of O_2 and CO_2 in inspired air and alveolar gas (Table 6.1). Finish the picture by coloring the background areas.

Table 6.1   Partial pressures of oxygen and carbon dioxide

	Inspired Air	Alveolar Gas	Arterial Blood	Mixed Venous Blood
PO_2 (mmHg)	150	100	100	40
PCO_2 (mmHg)	0	40	40	46

Table 6.1, which itemizes the partial pressures of oxygen and carbon dioxide in inspired air, alveolar gas, arterial blood, and mixed venous blood, illustrates two points. First, in going from inspired air to mixed venous blood, PO_2 decreases and PCO_2 increases. Since gases diffuse from a region of higher partial pressure to one of lower partial pressure, the partial pressure gradients for oxygen steadily drive O_2 from the atmosphere into the mitochondria, where it is ultimately utilized, while the partial pressure gradients for carbon dioxide steadily drive CO_2 from the mitochondria into the atmosphere (Figure 6.8).

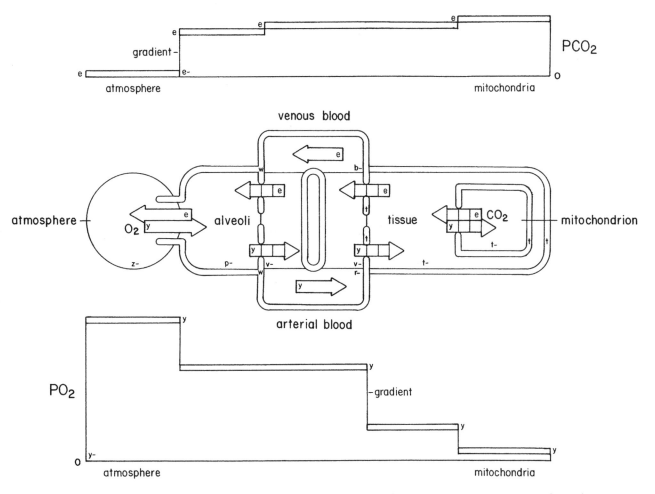

Figure 6.8   **Partial pressure gradients for oxygen and carbon dioxide.** Color the middle panel from left to right: beginning in the atmosphere, color the arrow labeled O_2 and follow the path of oxygen from the atmosphere to the mitochondrion, where it is ultimately utilized. Color the bar graph in the bottom panel, noting that the height of each level depicts the PO_2 in the structure just above it. Beginning in the mitochondrion, color the arrow labeled CO_2 and follow the path of carbon dioxide from the mitochondrion to the atmosphere, where it is ultimately expired. Color the bar graph in the top panel, noting that the height of each level depicts the PCO_2 in the structure just beneath it. Observe that the difference between the heights of steps indicates the partial pressure gradients between adjacent structures. Since gases diffuse from a region of higher partial pressure to one of lower partial pressure, these gradients enable O_2 to diffuse continuously from the atmosphere into the mitochondria and enable CO_2 to diffuse continuously from the mitochondria into the atmosphere. Also observe that the PO_2 of arterial blood is the same as that of alveolar gas and that the PCO_2 of venous blood is the same as that in the tissue. These latter findings demonstrate that blood spends enough time in the capillaries for equilibration of gases to occur. Compare this figure with Figure 6.1 and Table 6.1.

Dynamics of gas exchange in the lung

Second, the fact that the partial pressures of oxygen and carbon dioxide in alveolar gas and arterial blood are equal demonstrates that alveolar gas normally imposes its partial pressures on the blood. With respect to O_2, for example, mixed venous blood (having a PO_2 of 40 mmHg) coming in contact with an alveolus (having a PO_2 of 100 mmHg) creates a 60 mmHg partial pressure gradient that drives O_2 from the alveolus into the blood until equilibrium is reached (at a PO_2 of 100 mmHg) (Figure 6.9).

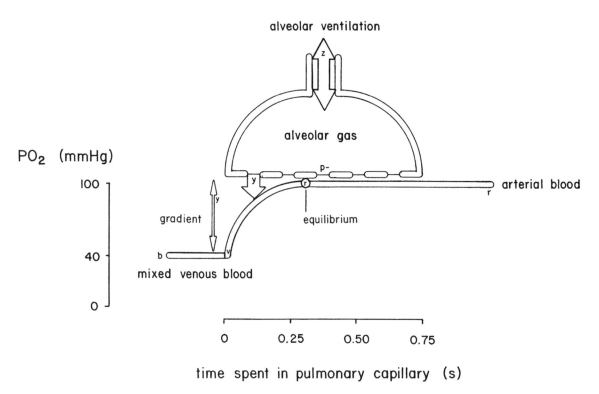

Figure 6.9   Dynamics of gas exchange in the lung. Color the alveolar gas and the arrow labelled alveolar ventilation. Color the horizontal segment at left that indicates the partial pressure of oxygen (PO_2) in mixed venous blood and the arrow labeled gradient. Observe that partial pressure gradient for oxygen is determined by the amount by which the PO_2 of alveolar gas exceeds the PO_2 of mixed venous blood. Color the downward arrow that indicates the diffusion of oxygen down its partial pressure gradient, from the alveolus into the blood. Finish the picture by coloring the remainder of the line, noting that the PO_2 of blood comes into equilibrium with the PO_2 of alveolar gas well before the blood leaves the lung. For this reason, the PO_2 of arterial blood is normally the same as the PO_2 of alveolar gas. Stated another way, the lung normally imposes its partial pressures on the blood, which, in turn, determines the concentrations of oxygen and carbon dioxide in arterial blood.

At rest, this process is normally completed in one-third of the time that the blood actually spends in the pulmonary capillary; the remaining two-thirds of the transit time provides sufficient reserve to allow equilibration to occur even when blood flows three times faster during maximal exercise. Another benefit of this reserve is that a mild to moderate diffusion impairment does not prevent the lung from providing a normal level of arterial PO_2 at rest (Figure 6.10, left panel). If a diffusion impairment and a high blood flow rate are both present, however, arterial PO_2 will be lower than alveolar PO_2 when the transit time is too short for equilibration to occur (Figure 6.10, right panel). These considerations explain why people with moderate diffusion impairments (due to lung disease) can oxygenate their blood adequately at rest but not during exercise.

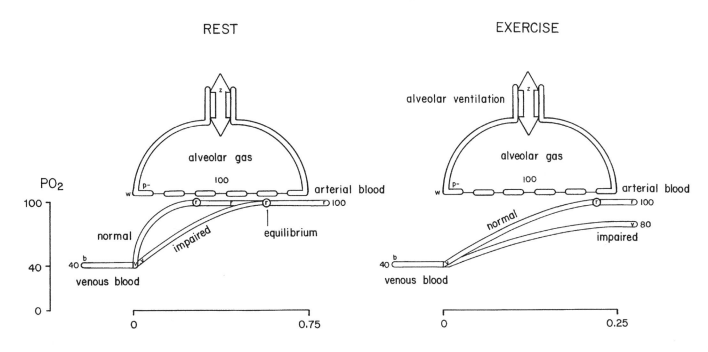

Figure 6.10 Dynamics of gas exchange in the lung during exercise. Color the left panel, noting that the line for the normal lung is identical to that shown in Figure 6.9 and that the line for the lung with a moderate diffusion impairment lies below the normal line, indicating correspondingly lower blood levels of PO_2. Also observe that the PO_2 of blood in the normal lung and the impaired lung come into equilibrium with the PO_2 of alveolar gas (points labeled equilibrium), and that the impaired lung requires more time to reach equilibrium. Thus, the arterial PO_2 of the normal and impaired lungs are both 100 mmHg (the normal value); this result explains why the resting levels of arterial blood gases are not a good indicator of a diffusion impairment. Color the right panel, noting that blood spends less time in the pulmonary capillary when blood flows faster during exercise. Note that the lines for the normal and impaired lungs are portions of those shown in the left panel. Observe that blood in the normal lung equilibrates with alveolar gas (circle) but blood in the impaired lung fails to equilibrate with alveolar gas. Also observe that the PO_2 of arterial blood is 100 mmHg (the normal value) in the normal lung and 80 mmHg (less than the normal value) in the impaired lung. These findings demonstrate that lungs with a moderate diffusion impairment can provide normal levels of arterial blood gases at rest but not during exercise. For this reason, diffusion tests should be performed during exercise.

Oxygen carriage by blood

Essentially all of the O_2 in arterial blood is carried by *hemoglobin* molecules that are contained in red blood cells. Because of its low solubility in plasma, only a negligible amount of O_2 is carried in dissolved form. For example, for every 20 mLO_2 in arterial blood, 19.7 mLO_2 are normally carried by hemoglobin and 0.3 mLO_2 are carried in dissolved form.

A hemoglobin molecule consists of two alpha and two beta polypeptide chains that each bond to a heme group, which is an iron-containing porphyrin, that is able to bond loosely

with an O_2 molecule. Each complete hemoglobin molecule (Hb_4) can combine reversibly with up to four O_2 molecules (Figure 6.11), i.e.,

$$Hb_4 + 4\,O_2 \rightleftarrows Hb_4O_8$$

The *oxygen saturation* of blood (SO_2) specifies the percentage of the total number of hemoglobin sites that are actually occupied by O_2 molecules. At 100% saturation, for example, all of the sites are filled with O_2, whereas at 50% saturation, only half of the sites are filled with O_2 (Fig 6.12).

153

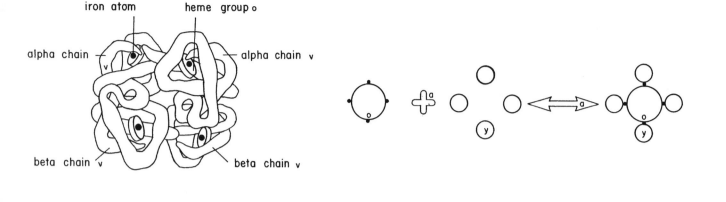

Figure 6.11   Carriage of oxygen by hemoglobin. Identify and color the chains of the hemoglobin molecule and the heme groups, which are the sites where O_2 molecules are carried. Color the reaction at the right, noting that each hemoglobin molecule (large circle) can combine reversibly with four O_2 molecules (small circles).

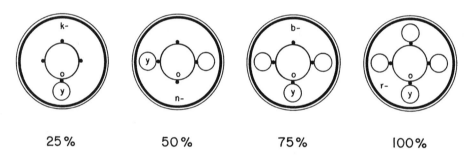

Figure 6.12   Oxygen saturation of hemoglobin. Color the hemoglobin (large circles) and O_2 molecules (small circles) in each condition, noting that the oxygen saturation represents the percentage of the total number of sites on hemoglobin that are actually filled with O_2. Color the background area in each condition, noting that the color of the blood reflects its oxygen saturation.

Oxyhemoglobin dissociation curve

The *oxyhemoglobin dissociation curve* describes the relationship between the oxygen saturation of hemoglobin, or SO_2, and the partial pressure of oxygen (PO_2), or oxygen tension, that is imposed on the blood. The oxyhemoglobin dissociation curve is characterized by a steep, S-shaped portion, and a flat, nearly horizontal portion (Figure 6.13).

The steep portion of the curve corresponds to the range of oxygen tensions over which SO_2 is dependent on PO_2, while the flat portion corresponds to the range of oxygen tensions in which SO_2 is essentially independent of PO_2. At the normal arterial PO_2 of 100 mmHg, which corresponds to a point on the flat portion of the curve, nearly 100% of the hemoglobin sites are occupied by oxygen molecules. At the normal mixed venous PO_2 of 40 mmHg, which corresponds to a point on the steep portion of the curve, approximately 75% of the hemoglobin sites are occupied by oxygen molecules (Figure 6.13).

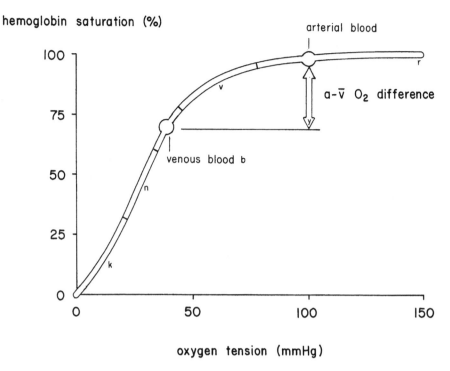

Figure 6.13 Oxyhemoglobin dissociation curve. Color the oxyhemoglobin dissociation curve, comparing the colors of its segments with the blood samples depicted in Figure 6.12. Identify the points that correspond to the partial pressures of oxygen in arterial and mixed venous blood and compare them with those listed in Table 6.1. Note that the hemoglobin saturation of arterial blood is nearly 100%, indicating that essentially all of the hemoglobin sites are filled by O_2 molecules. Note that the hemoglobin saturation of mixed venous blood is approximately 75%, indicating that only three-quarters of the hemoglobin sites are filled by O_2 molecules. Color the arrow that indicates the corresponding a-$\bar{v}$ O_2 difference, a measure of the amount of O_2 taken up by the tissues.

The a-$\bar{v}$ O_2 difference

The oxygen content of blood at 100% saturation is called the oxygen capacity and it reflects the maximal amount of O_2 that blood can carry. Given that the nominal hemoglobin concentration in blood is 15 g Hb per 100 mL of blood, and that each g of hemoglobin can carry 1.34 mL O_2, it follows that a normal value for oxygen capacity is 20 mL O_2 per 100 mL of blood. Similarly, the oxygen content of mixed venous blood, which is 75% saturated at rest, is 15 mL O_2 per 100 mL of blood. Thus, the oxygen content of blood depends on its oxygen capacity (determined by its hemoglobin concentration) and on its saturation (determined by its PO_2). For this reason, the oxygen capacity of blood decreases in anemia, a condition characterized by a deficiency of hemoglobin in the blood.

The difference between the oxygen content of arterial blood (C_aO_2, in mLO_2/100 mL blood) and that of mixed venous blood (C_vO_2, in mLO_2/100 mL blood) is normally 5 mL O_2 per 100 mL of blood at rest, and is called the a-$\bar{v}$ O_2 *difference;* it represents the oxygen that is taken up by the tissues (Figure 6.13). At rest, the tissues of the body normally deplete arterial blood of only one-quarter of the oxygen it carries. During exercise, however, the tissues extract more oxygen from arterial blood, the a-$\bar{v}$ O_2 difference widens, and the PO_2 of venous blood falls accordingly (Figure 6.14).

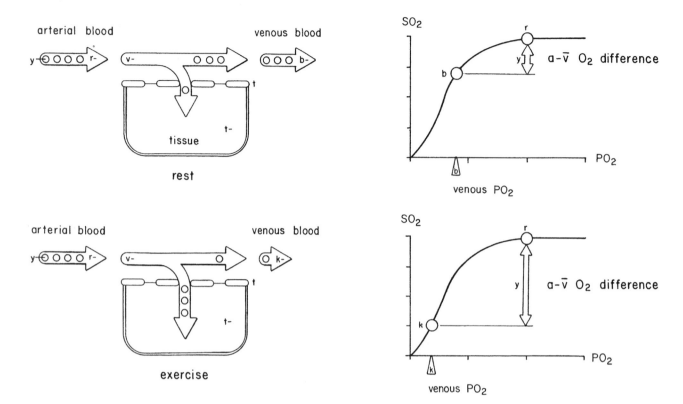

Figure 6.14   Effect of oxygen uptake on a-v̄ O₂ difference. For each condition, color the tissue and the membrane. Color and count the oxygen molecules (circles). Note that the difference between the number of oxygen molecules in arterial and venous blood represents the number of oxygen molecules that are taken up by the tissues. Color the arrows that indicate arterial blood, capillary blood, and venous blood. Color the points that correspond to arterial and venous blood on the oxyhemoglobin dissociation curve and the arrow that indicates the a-v̄ O₂ difference. Since the saturation of arterial blood is 100% in both conditions, note that a widened a-v̄ O₂ difference during exercise causes a corresponding reduction in the oxygen saturation of venous blood. These considerations explain why the oxygen content of venous blood falls when tissues take up more oxygen during exercise.

Fick equation

The a-v̄ O₂ difference is a factor in the *Fick equation,* which states that the rate of oxygen consumption ($\dot{V}O_2$, in L/min) is determined by the product of the cardiac output (CO, in L/min) and the a-v̄ O₂ difference (in mLO₂/100 mL blood), i.e.,

$$\dot{V}O_2 = CO \cdot (\text{a-}\bar{v}\ O_2\ \text{difference})$$

The Fick equation explains why the increase in oxygen uptake during exercise is achieved both by an increase in cardiac output and by an increase in oxygen extraction (a-v̄ O₂ difference) (Figure 6.15). Since the term a-v̄ O₂ difference in the Fick equation can be replaced by ($C_aO_2 - C_vO_2$), it also explains how cardiac output can be derived from simultaneous measurements of oxygen consumption [$\dot{V}O_2$, obtained from an analysis of expired air (Figure 3.19)] and the concentrations of oxygen in arterial (C_aO_2) and mixed venous (C_vO_2) blood (obtained from an analysis of arterial and venous blood samples), i.e., CO = $\dot{V}O_2/(C_aO_2 - C_vO_2)$.

Figure 6.15 Effect of blood flow and O_2 extraction on O_2 uptake. For each condition, color the tissue and color and count the O_2 molecules in arterial blood (arrow at left), O_2 uptake (downward arrow in middle) and venous blood (arrow at right). Note that the condition labeled rest (top panel) is identical to that shown in Figure 6.14 and that the O_2 uptake in this condition is one molecule of O_2. Note that the O_2 uptake in each condition is given by the difference between the O_2 contents of arterial and venous blood and that an increase in O_2 uptake (to two molecules) can be achieved by an increase in blood flow (wider arrow, second panel from top) or by an increase in O_2 extraction (third panel from top). Note that the tissues extract one-quarter of their O_2 supply in the panel labeled increased blood flow but one-half of their O_2 supply in the panel labeled increased O_2 extraction. Observe that the a-v̄ O_2 difference is unchanged by an increase in blood flow but widened by an increase in O_2 extraction. Also observe that the oxygen saturation of venous blood is unchanged by an increase in blood flow but decreased by an increase in O_2 extraction. Finally, observe that the increase in O_2 uptake during exercise (to four molecules of O_2, bottom panel) is mediated both by an increase in blood flow (wider arrow) and by an increase in O_2 extraction (widened a-v̄ O_2 difference). These examples illustrate the Fick principle, which states that the O_2 consumption ($\dot{V}O_2$) is given by the product of cardiac output (CO) and a-v̄ O_2 difference, i.e., $\dot{V}O_2 = CO \cdot (a\text{-}\bar{v} \, O_2 \text{ difference})$.

arterial blood   venous blood

rest

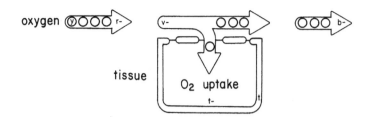

increased blood flow

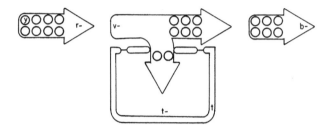

increased O_2 extraction

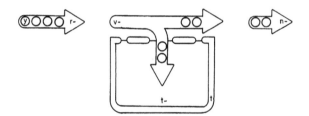

exercise

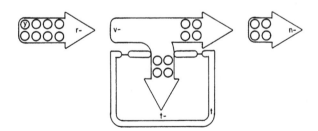

Factors affecting the oxyhemoglobin dissociation curve

The oxyhemoglobin dissociation curve is affected by the prevailing levels of carbon dioxide (PCO_2), acidity (pH), and temperature. Higher temperatures, elevated CO_2 levels, and decreased pH, as occur in exercising muscle, shift the oxyhemoglobin dissociation curve to the right (Figure 6.16), a phenomenon called the *Bohr effect*. The oxyhemoglobin dissociation curve is also shifted to the right by elevated concentrations of 2,3-diphosphoglycerate (2,3-DPG), a compound synthesized from glucose in the red blood cells. Higher concentrations of 2,3-DPG occur in healthy individuals exposed to high-altitude hypoxia (low PO_2 in alveolar gas).

This shift of the oxyhemoglobin dissociation curve to the right indicates a decreased affinity of hemoglobin for oxygen, which, in turn, enables hemoglobin to unload and therefore deliver an additional amount of oxygen to the tissues without requiring the tissues to lower their PO_2. For a given tissue PO_2, therefore, a shift to the right causes the a-$\bar{v}$ O_2 difference to widen, indicating an increased O_2 extraction by the tissues (Figure 6.16).

On the other hand, if temperature, PCO_2, and 2,3-DPG levels fall or pH rises, the oxyhemoglobin dissociation curve shifts to the left, indicating an increased affinity of hemoglobin for oxygen (Figure 6.16). A shift to the left occurs when CO_2 is removed from the blood in the lung; the resultant higher affinity of hemoglobin for oxygen facilitates the uptake of O_2 by the blood and thereby promotes gas exchange in the lung.

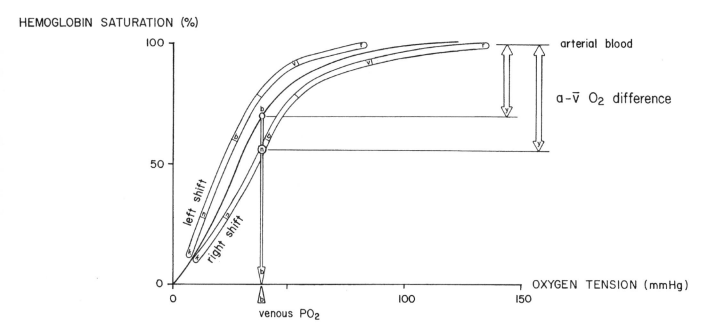

Figure 6.16   Factors affecting the oxyhemoglobin dissociation curve. Color the oxyhemoglobin dissociation curves labeled right shift and left shift, noting that the middle line depicts the oxyhemoglobin dissociation curve shown in Figure 6.13. A shift of the oxyhemoglobin curve to the right indicates a decreased affinity of hemoglobin for oxygen, whereas a shift to the left indicates an increased affinity. Color the arrowhead labeled venous PO_2, the vertical arrow associated with this particular PO_2, and the circles that mark the points at which the vertical line intersects the normal curve (solid line) and the right shift curve. Observe that the O_2 saturation of venous blood is lower in the right shift curve than in the normal curve; color the arrow that indicates the correspondingly wider a-$\bar{v}$ O_2 difference. These results demonstrate that a decreased affinity of hemoglobin for oxygen—as occurs when temperature and PCO_2 rise and pH falls during exercise—enables hemoglobin to unload and therefore deliver more O_2 to exercising muscles at any given PO_2.

Carbon dioxide carriage by blood

Carbon dioxide is carried by the blood in three different forms: (1) as bicarbonate ions (HCO_3^-) in plasma; (2) as carbamino compounds, which are formed when CO_2 molecules combine with NH_2 groups in proteins, such as hemoglobin; and (3) as dissolved molecules (Figure 6.17).

The *bicarbonate ion* is formed in a reaction between CO_2 and H_2O that is catalyzed by the enzyme carbonic anhydrase (CA), which is present in the red blood cell but is absent in blood plasma, i.e.,

$$[CA]$$

$$CO_2 + H_2O \rightleftarrows H_2CO_3 \rightleftarrows H^+ + HCO_3^-$$

Of the CO_2 that is picked up by the blood in the systemic capillaries, 60% is carried as bicarbonate ions, 30% is carried as *carbamino compounds,* and the remaining 10% is carried in dissolved form (Figure 6.17).

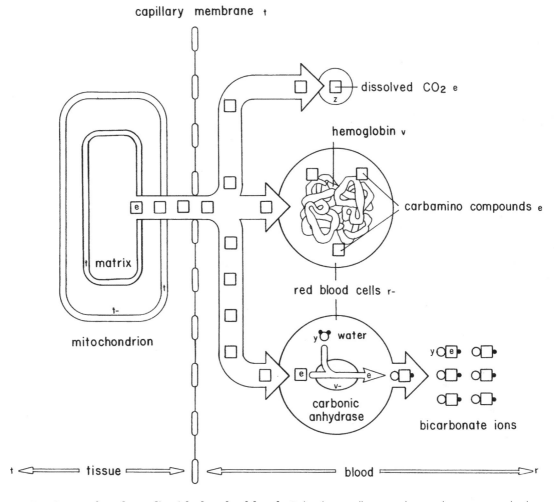

Figure 6.17 Carriage of carbon dioxide by the blood. Color the capillary membrane, the arrows at the bottom, the mitochondrion, and the CO_2 molecules (squares) that it produces. Color the CO_2 molecule that is in a dissolved state. Color the red blood cell just below, its hemoglobin molecule, and the CO_2 molecules that are carried in carbamino compounds. Finish the picture by coloring the red blood cell at the bottom, the enzyme (carbonic anhydrase), the water molecule, and the bicarbonate ions (HCO_3^-) that are formed by the reaction between carbon dioxide and water. Compare the relative numbers of CO_2 molecules that are carried in the different states.

Blood pH

The pH of arterial blood is maintained within normal limits by the buffering action of the HCO_3^-/CO_2 system and blood proteins, primarily hemoglobin. Reduced hemoglobin (Hb^-) buffers hydrogen ions that are generated in the red blood cell when carbonic acid (H_2CO_3) dissociates into H^+ and HCO_3^-, i.e.,

$$H^+ + Hb^- \rightleftarrows HHb$$

As for the HCO_3^-/CO_2 system, the *Henderson–Hasselbach equation* states that the pH of blood can be calculated by adding a constant term (6.1, the pK of the reaction) to a variable term given by the logarithm of the ratio of the HCO_3^- concentration to the CO_2 concentration, i.e.,

$$pH = 6.1 + \log([HCO_3^-]/[CO_2])$$

Since log (20) = 1.3, the pH of blood will be 7.4 whenever $[HCO_3^-]/[CO_2]$ is 20, i.e., $6.1 + \log 20 = 6.1 + 1.3 = 7.4$. One implication of the Henderson–Hasselbach equation is that the pH of blood can be maintained at its normal value of 7.4 by the balanced operation of the renal system, which regulates the HCO_3^- concentration, and the respiratory system, which regulates the CO_2 concentration (Figure 6.18). Because $[CO_2]$ is proportional to PCO_2 in the physiological range, it can be replaced in the Henderson–Hasselbach equation by the product of its solubility constant (0.03) and PCO_2, i.e., $[CO_2] = 0.03 \cdot PCO_2$.

Figure 6.18   Acid-base disturbances. For each condition, color the balance, the pointer, and the pH scale. Then color and count the carbon dioxide and bicarbonate rectangles on each side of the balance. Observe that an abnormal pH occurs whenever the levels of CO_2 and HCO_3^- do not exactly counterbalance one another. Observe also that respiratory acidosis is said to occur when arterial PCO_2 is greater than its normal value of 40 mmHg and respiratory alkalosis is said to occur when arterial PCO_2 is less than its normal value of 40 mmHg. Similarly, metabolic acidosis is said to occur when blood levels of bicarbonate fall below the normal value of 25 mEq/L and metabolic alkalosis is said to occur when blood levels of bicarbonate rise above the normal value of 25 mEq/L. These considerations explain why the formation of lactic acid during anaerobic glycolysis, which lowers blood levels of HCO_3^-, causes metabolic acidosis.

carbon dioxide   bicarbonate

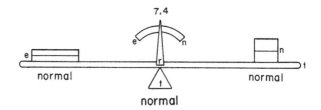
normal

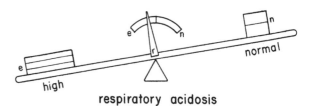
respiratory acidosis

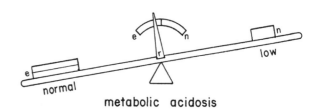
metabolic acidosis

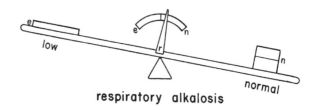
respiratory alkalosis

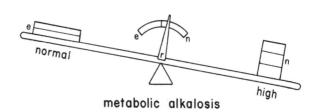
metabolic alkalosis

Acid-base disturbances

Another implication of the Henderson–Hasselbach equation is that the pH of blood will deviate from its normal value of 7.4 whenever the HCO_3^- : CO_2 ratio deviates from its normal value of 20:1. Alkalosis (pH > 7.4) occurs when $[HCO_3^-]$:$[CO_2]$ is greater than 20:1 and acidosis (pH < 7.4) occurs when $[HCO_3^-]$:$[CO_2]$ is less than 20:1.

It follows from these considerations that an abnormal pH could be due to an abnormal level of HCO_3^- (a metabolic component) and/or an abnormal level of CO_2 (a respiratory component) (Figure 6.18). It also follows that acidosis could be due to a high level of CO_2 (*respiratory acidosis*) and/or a low level of HCO_3^- (*metabolic acidosis*), and alkalosis could be due to a low level of CO_2 (*respiratory alkalosis*) and/or a high level of HCO_3^- (*metabolic alkalosis*). These considerations explain why the formation of lactic acid, which reduces the blood level of bicarbonate (Figure 3.25), causes metabolic acidosis.

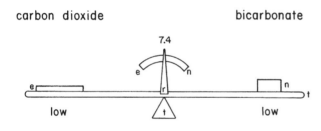
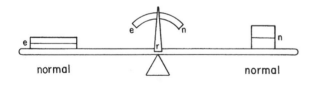
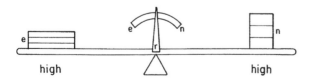

Figure 6.19   Compensated acid-base disturbances
For each condition, color the balance, the pointer, and the pH scale. Then color and count the carbon dioxide and bicarbonate rectangles on each side of the balance. Note that a normal pH results whenever the levels of CO_2 and HCO_3^- exactly counterbalance one another. Compare this figure with Figure 6.18.

Compensated acid-base disturbances

In reality, however, an abnormal pH that is due to a disturbance in one component is usually partially or fully compensated by an opposite adjustment in the other component (Figure 6.19). For example, respiratory acidosis due to chronically elevated CO_2 levels, as can occur in long-standing lung disease, is usually accompanied by a compensatory metabolic alkalosis due to the elevation of HCO_3^- levels by the kidney. As another example, respiratory compensation, which refers to an increase in ventilation at near maximal levels of exercise, causes blood levels of CO_2 to fall (respiratory alkalosis) and thereby offset the falling pH caused by high rates of lactic acid production (metabolic acidosis) (Figure 6.44).

Pulmonary ventilation

The ventilation of the lung is an important determinant of the oxygen and carbon dioxide tensions in alveolar gas and, thus, arterial blood (Figure 6.9). Two measures of pulmonary ventilation are minute ventilation and alveolar ventilation.

Minute ventilation refers to the rate at which air moves into and out of the trachea. Minute ventilation ($\dot{V}_E$, in L/min) is determined by the product of the tidal volume (V_T, the volume of air inspired per breath, in L) and the respiratory frequency (f, the number of breaths per minute). Thus,

$$\dot{V}_E = V_T \cdot f$$

Alveolar ventilation refers to the rate at which air moves into and out of the alveoli. Part of the inspired volume ventilates the dead space (V_D), where no gas exchange takes place, while the remaining part ventilates the alveoli, where gas exchange does take place (Figure 6.5). Alveolar ventilation ($\dot{V}_A$, in L/min) is determined by the product of the volume of air entering the alveoli per breath and the respiratory frequency (Figure 6.20). Since only that portion of the tidal volume that exceeds the dead space ($V_T - V_D$) actually enters and ventilates the alveoli, it follows that

$$\dot{V}_A = (V_T - V_D) \cdot f$$

The remaining portion of the tidal volume (V_D) is wasted ventilating dead space. Note that $\dot{V}_A$ becomes zero when V_T equals V_D; this shows that the alveoli are not ventilated when the tidal volume fails to exceed the dead space.

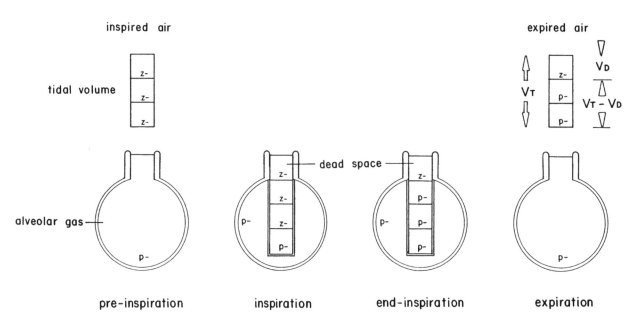

Figure 6.20   Pulmonary ventilation. Color the panels from left to right, noting the similarity between this schematic lung and that shown in Figure 6.5. Compare the composition of gases in the inspired and expired air, noting that only that fraction of the tidal volume (V_T) that exceeds the dead space volume (V_D) actually ventilates the alveoli, i.e., $V_T - V_D$. Since minute ventilation is determined by the product of V_T and f, it follows that a given minute ventilation can be achieved by a spectrum of V_T-f combinations, ranging from a rapid-shallow to a slow-deep breathing pattern. Because the respiratory frequency determines the number of times that the dead space will be ventilated per minute, a slow-deep breathing pattern provides more alveolar ventilation than does a rapid-shallow breathing pattern. Thus, the small tidal volumes used in rapid-shallow breathing are inefficient because an excessive amount of energy is wasted ventilating dead space where no gas exchange takes place. Compare this figure with Figure 3.18.

Effect of alveolar ventilation on arterial blood gases

The relationship between alveolar ventilation and arterial blood gases is governed by two alveolar gas laws.

The first alveolar gas law states that the level of CO_2 in alveolar gas (P_ACO_2) represents the balance between the rate of CO_2 production by metabolizing tissues ($\dot{V}CO_2$) and the rate of CO_2 removal by alveolar ventilation ($\dot{V}_A$), i.e.,

$$P_ACO_2 = K \cdot \dot{V}CO_2/\dot{V}_A$$

where K is a constant. It follows from this law that an increase in the rate of CO_2 production or a decrease in its rate of removal will increase P_ACO_2, but changing them both proportionally will not alter P_ACO_2 (Figure 6.21).

The second alveolar gas law states that the PO_2 of alveolar gas (P_AO_2) depends on the PCO_2 of alveolar gas (P_ACO_2), i.e.,

$$P_AO_2 = P_IO_2 - P_ACO_2/R$$

where P_IO_2 is the PO_2 of inspired air and R is the *respiratory exchange ratio*, defined as the ratio of the carbon dioxide production ($\dot{V}CO_2$) to the oxygen consumption ($\dot{V}O_2$), i.e., $R = \dot{V}CO_2/\dot{V}O_2$ (Figure 3.24). It follows from this law that any change in alveolar PCO_2 must be accompanied by an opposite change in alveolar PO_2. As a result, only certain combinations of PCO_2 and PO_2 can coexist in alveolar gas while breathing room air at sea level (Figure 6.22).

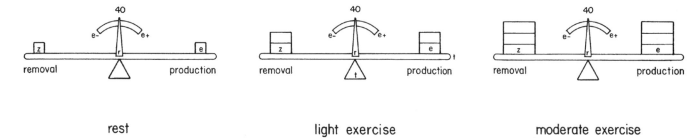

rest   light exercise   moderate exercise

Figure 6.21   Effect of alveolar ventilation on alveolar PCO$_2$. Color the balance, the pointer, and the PCO$_2$ scale (in mmHg). For each panel, color and compare the rectangles that depict the rate at which CO$_2$ is removed from the body by alveolar ventilation (left side of balance) and the rate at which CO$_2$ is produced by the body (right side of balance). Observe that CO$_2$ production increases with increasing exercise intensity and that these increases in CO$_2$ production are matched exactly by corresponding increases in CO$_2$ removal. These considerations explain why arterial PCO$_2$ remains constant at 40 mmHg over the range from rest (left panel) to moderate exercise (right panel).

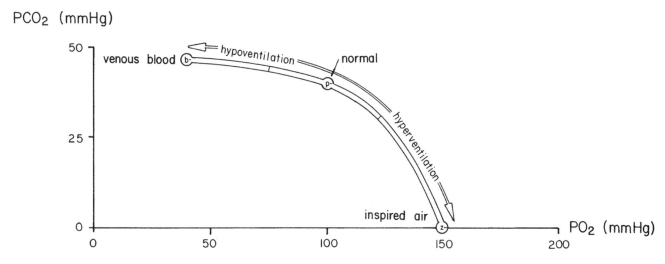

Figure 6.22   Possible PCO$_2$-PO$_2$ combinations in alveolar gas. Color the line that depicts the effect of alveolar ventilation on the composition of alveolar gas, noting that these results apply only to the breathing of room air (20.93% O$_2$, 0% CO$_2$) at sea level (P$_B$ = 760 mmHg). Identify the normal operating point (PO$_2$ = 100 mmHg, PCO$_2$ = 40 mmHg). Observe that a normal level of alveolar ventilation produces alveolar gas tensions that are intermediate between the two extremes of mixed venous blood (PO$_2$ = 40 mmHg, PCO$_2$ = 46 mmHg) and inspired air (PO$_2$ = 150 mmHg, PCO$_2$ = 0 mmHg). Since arterial blood normally equilibrates with alveolar gas in the lung (Figure 6.9), these findings show that hyperventilation causes the arterial blood gas tensions to more closely resemble those of inspired air, whereas hypoventilation causes the arterial blood gas tensions to more closely resemble those of mixed venous blood (Table 6.1). Because the oxyhemoglobin dissociation curve is essentially flat when PO$_2$ exceeds 100 mmHg (Figure 6.13), hyperventilation does not materially improve the O$_2$ content of arterial blood because the O$_2$ saturation is nearly 100% at a PO$_2$ of 100 mmHg. For these reasons, blood levels of PO$_2$ in excess of 100 mmHg can increase the concentration of dissolved O$_2$ but cannot increase the saturation beyond its maximal value of 100%.

Hypoventilation and hyperventilation

Hypoventilation is defined as a condition in which the rate of CO$_2$ production by the tissues exceeds the rate of CO$_2$ removal by the lung. In accordance with the alveolar gas laws described above, hypoventilation causes a high PCO$_2$ (hyper-capnia) and a low PO$_2$ (hypoxia) in alveolar gas (Figure 6.23). Since blood equilibrates with alveolar gas in the lung (Figure 6.9), hypoventilation also causes a high PCO$_2$ (hypercarbia) coupled with a low PO$_2$ (hypoxemia) in arterial blood. Hypoventilation therefore causes the PO$_2$ and PCO$_2$ levels of arterial blood to more closely resemble those of mixed venous blood (Figure 6.22).

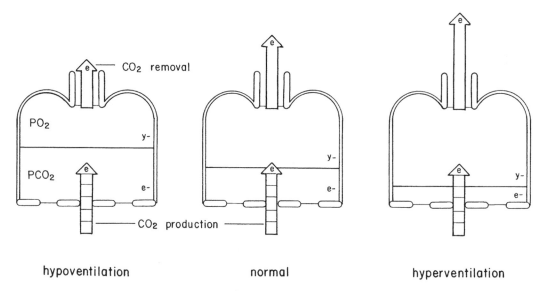

Figure 6.23   Effect of alveolar ventilation on alveolar PCO₂ and PO₂. Color the panels from left to right, noting that the length of the arrow at the bottom indicates the rate at which CO_2 enters the lung from tissues ($\dot{V}CO_2$). Note also that the length of the arrow at the top indicates the rate at which CO_2 is removed from the lung by alveolar ventilation ($\dot{V}_A$). Observe that hypoventilation (left panel) causes the alveolar gas to have a high level of CO_2 (hypercapnia) and a low level of O_2 (hypoxia). Observe also that hyperventilation (right panel) causes the alveolar gas to have a low level of CO_2 (hypocapnia) and a high level of O_2 (hyperoxia). Because alveolar gas and arterial blood normally equilibrate in the lung (Figure 6.9), hypoventilation causes arterial blood to have a high PCO₂ and a low PO₂). Similarly, hyperventilation causes arterial blood to have a low PCO₂ and a high PO₂. Compare this figure with Figure 6.22.

Conversely, *hyperventilation* is defined as a condition in which the rate of CO_2 removal by the lung exceeds the rate of CO_2 production by the tissues. Hyperventilation causes a low PCO₂ coupled with a high PO₂ in both alveolar gas (Figure 6.23) and arterial blood. Hyperventilation therefore causes the PO₂ and PCO₂ levels of arterial blood to more closely resemble those of inspired air (Figure 6.22).

Mechanics of breathing

Pulmonary ventilation depends on the balance between the pressures generated by the respiratory muscles and the mechanical properties of the respiratory system that oppose their contraction.

The outer surface of the lung and the inner surface of the thoracic cage are covered with slippery pleural membranes that slide easily over each other. This arrangement allows the lung to passively follow the movement of the *chest wall*, which is made up of the rib cage plus the diaphragm (Figure 6.24). Thus, the lung inflates when the vertical and/or lateral dimensions of the chest wall increase, and deflates when these dimensions decrease.

Figure 6.24 Lung and chest wall. Color the lung and chest wall, noting that the pleural cavity lies between them. Contraction of the respiratory muscles alters the pressure in the pleural cavity, which, in turn, provides the driving force to expand or collapse the lung. The actual change in lung volume depends on the magnitude of the change in pleural pressure and on the mechanical properties of the lung that oppose lung expansion.

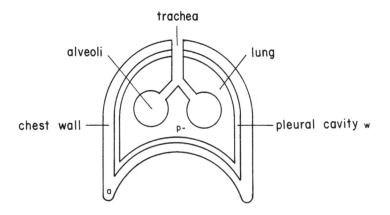

Respiratory muscles

The respiratory muscles are skeletal muscles that are divided into a group of *inspiratory muscles* and a group of *expiratory muscles* (Figure 6.25). Respiratory muscle contraction alters the pressure between the pleural membranes which, in turn,

creates a pressure gradient that expands or collapses the lung. The volume of the lung increases when the inspiratory muscles shorten and decreases when the expiratory muscles shorten.

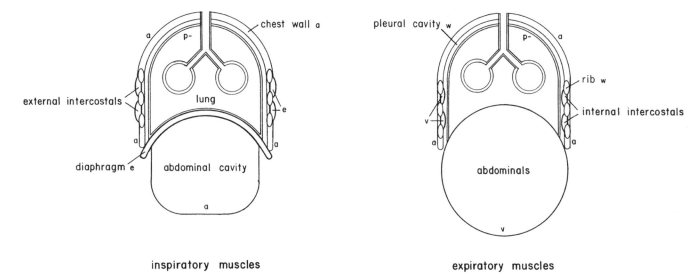

Figure 6.25 Respiratory muscles. Color the inspiratory muscles, which include the diaphragm and the external intercostal muscles, noting that the diaphragm and the rib cage collectively make up the chest wall (Figure 6.24). Color the expiratory muscles, which include the abdominal and the internal intercostal muscles, noting their relationship to the inspiratory muscles. Finish the picture by coloring the lung and the remainder of the chest wall in each panel.

Inspiratory muscles

The *diaphragm,* which is the most important inspiratory muscle, is a large, dome-shaped sheet of muscle that separates the thoracic cavity from the abdominal cavity. By pushing the abdominal contents down and out, diaphragmatic shortening increases lung volume by increasing the vertical dimension of the chest wall (Figure 6.26).

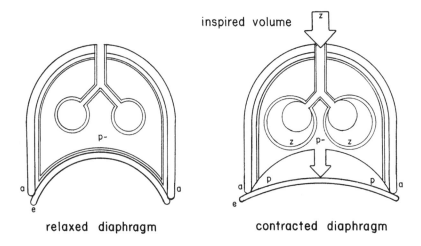

inspired volume

relaxed diaphragm   contracted diaphragm

Figure 6.26   Action of the diaphragm. Color the rib cage, lung, and diaphragm in the left panel, noting the domed configuration of the relaxed diaphragm. Color the same structures in the right panel, noting the flattened configuration of the contracted diaphragm. Observe that the length of the contracted diaphragm is shorter than that of the relaxed diaphragm; thus, diaphragmatic shortening increases the vertical dimension of the chest wall and thereby increases lung volume; this action is sometimes referred to as the "pump handle" effect. Color the arrow that indicates the volume of air that is inspired during diaphragmatic contraction and color the corresponding increase in alveolar volume. Color the rest of the picture, noting that the volume of inspired air is equal to the volume displaced by the descent of the diaphragm, i.e., the difference between the positions of the relaxed and contracted diaphragms.

The fibers of the *external intercostal muscles* connect adjacent ribs. By pulling the ribs upward and outward, contraction of the external intercostal muscles increases lung volume by increasing the anteroposterior (AP) and mediolateral (ML) diameters of the chest wall (Figure 6.27). Although the intercostal muscles usually exhibit minimal respiratory activity at rest, they contract vigorously during strenuous exercise.

The *accessory muscles* of inspiration include a group of neck muscles that attach to the upper part of the rib cage. The most important of the accessory muscles are the scalene muscles, which elevate the first two ribs, and the sternocleidomastoids, which elevate the sternum. Although these muscles usually exhibit no respiratory activity at rest, they also contract vigorously during strenuous exercise.

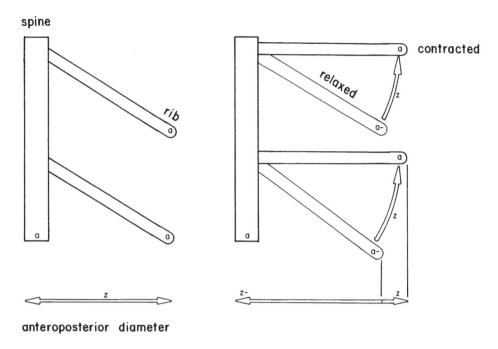

spine

rib

contracted

relaxed

anteroposterior diameter

Figure 6.27   Action of the external intercostal muscles. Color the ribs and spine for the condition at left, which corresponds to relaxed external intercostal muscles, and color the arrow that indicates the anteroposterior (AP) diameter of the rib cage. Color the ribs and spine for the condition at right, which corresponds to contracted external intercostal muscles. Color the arrow that indicates the new AP diameter of the rib cage, noting that it is longer than that in the left panel. Thus, contraction of the external intercostal muscle elevates the ribs, increases the AP and mediolateral (ML, not shown) diameters of the rib cage, and thereby increases lung volume; this action is sometimes referred to as the "bucket handle" effect.

Expiratory muscles

Expiratory muscles are not usually active during quiet breathing. The lung and chest wall are stretched during *inspiration,* the period in which air flows into the lung and the lung inflates. The elastic properties of the lung and chest wall cause them to recoil passively to their resting positions during *expiration,* the period in which air flows out of the lung and the lung deflates. Expiratory muscles contract vigorously during forced expirations, as occurs during strenuous exercise.

The muscles of the anterior abdominal wall are the most important expiratory muscles. Contraction of the *abdominal muscles* increases intra-abdominal pressure, compresses the abdominal contents, and actively forces the diaphragm upward, thereby reducing lung volume by decreasing the vertical dimension of the chest wall (Figure 6.26). Contraction of the *internal intercostal muscles* moves the ribs downward and inward. This action, which is the opposite of that produced by the external intercostal muscles, decreases lung volume by decreasing the AP and ML diameters of the chest wall (Figure 6.27).

Mechanical properties of the lung

The mechanical properties of the lung can be partitioned into an elastic component and a resistive component. The elastic component is due to the elastic fibers in the lung and chest wall and to the surface tension forces that occur at the air–liquid interface in the lung. The resistive component is due to the narrow airways that make up the tracheobronchial tree (Figure 6.5).

Elastic properties of the lung

Elasticity is that property of matter that enables it to return to its original shape after being deformed by an external force. The relationship between applied force and the resultant deformation can be expressed graphically. For example, an ideal spring for which stretch is proportional to force has a length–force relationship given by a straight line whose slope describes the compliance of the spring (stretch per unit of applied force) and whose y-intercept indicates its unstretched length (Figure 6.28).

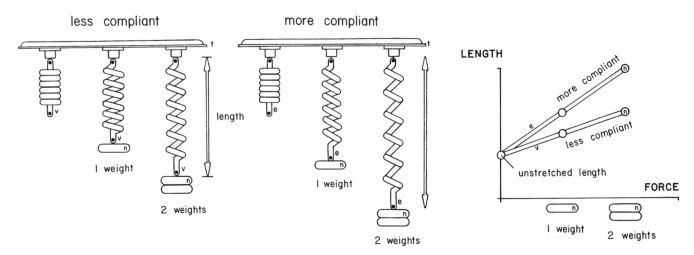

Figure 6.28   Elastic properties of springs. The elastic behavior of a spring can be expressed graphically by plotting its length (in cm) against the force (in g) that is applied to stretch the spring (left and middle panels). The length–force data obtained using a range of forces, or weights, determines a line in a length–force plane (right panel). The slope of the line thus formed represents the compliance of the spring (in cm/g), a measure of the ease with which the spring can be stretched, and the y-intercept represents its unstretched length. These considerations demonstrate that the compliance of a spring can be visualized from the steepness of the slope of its length–force curve, and the resting length of a spring can be visualized from its y-intercept.

In a similar manner, the elastic behavior of the lung can be expressed graphically by plotting the volume of the lung (in mL) against the magnitude of the pressure gradient (in cmH$_2$O) that is required to keep the lung inflated at that volume. The static volume–pressure data obtained using a range of inflation pressures determine a line whose slope describes the *compliance of the lung* (in mL/cmH$_2$O), a measure of the ease with which the lung can be inflated, and whose y-intercept indicates the minimum volume of the lung (Figure 6.29).

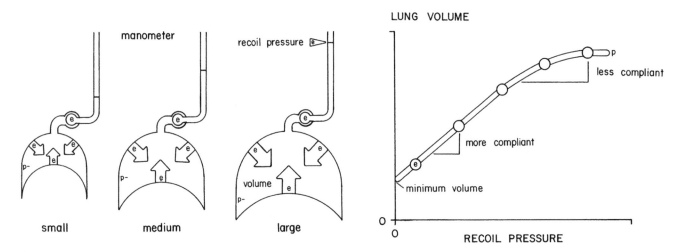

Figure 6.29   Elastic properties of the lung. Color the schematic lungs and water manometers in each of the conditions at left. Observe that the height of the water in the manometer is a measure (in cmH$_2$O) of the static (no movement) recoil pressure exerted by the lung at different lung volumes. Color and note the size of the lung recoil arrows (in the lung), which indicate that the recoil pressure increases with increasing lung volume. Color the graph at right, noting that the individual points on the line correspond to volume–pressure data obtained at different lung volumes. By analogy to the analysis shown in Figure 6.28, the y-intercept specifies the lung volume that would occur in the absence of external pressures (called the minimum volume) and the slope of the line specifies the compliance of the lung (C$_L$, in mL/cmH$_2$O). Observe that the volume–pressure curve for the lung is linear at low inflation pressures and nonlinear at high inflation pressures. Since compliance can be visualized from the steepness of a volume–pressure line, these results show that the compliance of the lung decreases, i.e., the lung becomes stiffer, when it is inflated to a large volume.

Resistive properties of the lung

Airway resistance (R_{aw}) specifies a relationship between the pressure gradient across the airways (ΔP, a measure of the driving force for airflow, in cmH_2O) and the corresponding airflow ($\dot{V}$, in L/s), i.e.,

$$R_{aw} = \Delta P / \dot{V}$$

where ΔP is determined by the amount by which the pressure at the mouth (atmospheric pressure) differs from the pressure in the alveoli (alveolar pressure) (Figure 6.30). Because air flows from a region of higher pressure to one of lower pressure (down a pressure gradient), atmospheric pressure is: (1) greater than alveolar pressure during inspiration (when air flows into the lung); (2) equal to alveolar pressure at end inspiration (when airflow ceases); and (3) less than alveolar pressure during expiration (when air flows out of the lung).

As expected from Poiseuille's law, airway resistance depends on the geometry of the airways, the viscosity of the gas being breathed, and the amount of energy that is dissipated in turbulent airflow. Since halving the diameter of an airway theoretically increases its resistance sixteen-fold (Figure 5.30), airway caliber is an important determinant of airway resistance.

In going from the trachea to the alveoli, the airways become narrower but more numerous with each succeeding division (Figure 6.5). These geometrical changes have opposite theoretical effects on airway resistance, i.e., narrower airways increase resistance but a greater number of airways decreases resistance. The magnitude of the airway resistance associated with any given generation, therefore, reflects a balance between these opposing factors. These considerations explain why the medium-sized bronchi are the major site of airway resistance in the tracheobronchial tree.

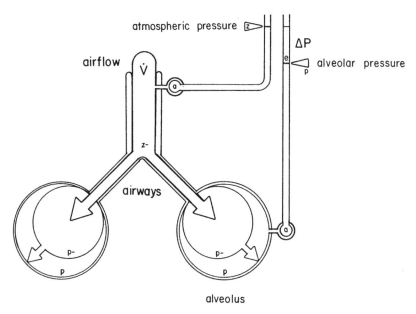

Figure 6.30 Airway resistance. Color the inspiratory airflow (arrow labeled $\dot{V}$, in L/s), the alveoli, and the manometers that measure the pressures (in cmH_2O) at the airway opening (atmospheric pressure) and in the alveoli (alveolar pressure). Identify the pressure gradient across the airways (ΔP), noting that it is determined by the amount by which atmospheric pressure exceeds alveolar pressure. Airway resistance (R_{aw}, in $cmH_2O \cdot s/L$) determines the relationship between ΔP and $\dot{V}$, i.e., $R_{aw} = \Delta P / \dot{V}$. As expected from Poiseuille's law, airway resistance depends on the geometry of the airways and on the amount of energy dissipated in turbulent airflow; turbulence increases the apparent resistance to airflow beyond that predicted by Poiseuille's law. Since halving the diameter of a cylindrical airway theoretically increases its resistance by a factor of sixteen (Figure 5.30), airway caliber is an important determinant of airway resistance.

Factors that affect airway resistance

Airway resistance varies in response to mechanical, neural, and humoral factors that influence the diameter of the airways.

A mechanical factor that alters the diameter of airways is the transmural pressure, which is determined by the amount by which the pressure inside the airway exceeds the pressure outside the airway. Because the action of the inspiratory muscles causes the pressure that surrounds the airways to become more negative during inspiration, transmural pressure and, therefore, airway caliber, increases during lung inflation and decreases during lung deflation. As a result, airway resistance varies inversely with lung volume (Figure 6.31).

AIRWAY RESISTANCE (cmH$_2$O·s/liter)

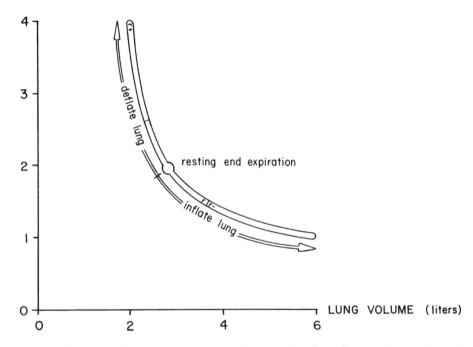

Figure 6.31 Effect of lung volume on airway resistance. Color the line depicting the effect of lung volume (in L) on airway resistance (in cmH$_2$O·s/L); identify the point that corresponds to resting end-expiration. Observe that increases in lung volume decrease airway resistance (segment labeled inflate lung) and that decreases in lung volume increase airway resistance (segment labeled deflate lung). These changes in airway resistance can be accounted for by changes in airway caliber, i.e., the airways become wider during lung inflation and narrower during lung deflation.

Neural and humoral factors alter the diameter of the airways by regulating the contraction of the smooth muscle fibers that reside in the walls of the airways. Bronchial smooth muscle cells contract when they are exposed to acetylcholine, which is the neurotransmitter released by the parasympathetic nerve fibers that innervate the airways. This process, called *bronchoconstriction*, narrows the airways and thereby increases airway resistance (Figure 6.32, middle panel). Conversely, bronchial smooth muscle cells relax when they are exposed to catecholamines, which are released by the sympathetic nerve fibers that innervate the airways and by the adrenal medulla (Figure 7.19). This process, called *bronchodilation*, widens the airways and thereby decreases airway resistance (Figure 6.32, right panel).

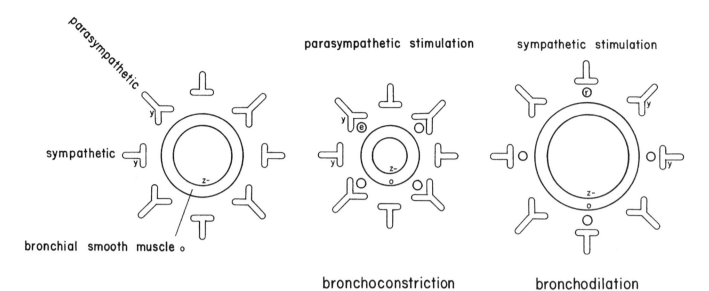

Figure 6.32   Effect of bronchial muscle tone on airway diameter. For each condition, color the bronchial smooth muscle, the airway opening (lumen), the parasympathetic (excitatory) and sympathetic (inhibitory) nerve fibers, and their neurotransmitters. Note that parasympathetic stimulation causes bronchial smooth muscle to contract, which constricts the airway and increases airway resistance. Note also that sympathetic stimulation causes bronchial smooth muscle to relax, which dilates the airway and decreases airway resistance. Compare this figure with Figure 5.31, noting the difference between the effects of acetylcholine and norepinephrine on vascular smooth muscle and bronchial smooth muscle.

Regulation of arterial blood gases

A relevant outcome of the alveolar gas laws is that the maintenance of normal values of carbon dioxide and oxygen in arterial blood requires that alveolar ventilation be matched precisely to the rate of CO_2 production by the tissues (Figure 6.21). This feat is accomplished through the operation of *respiratory reflexes* that adjust ventilation in accordance with the blood levels of carbon dioxide, oxygen, and acidity; these mechanisms are described in more detail below.

Respiratory reflexes

The respiratory control centers in the medulla and pons initiate and sustain a rhythmic breathing pattern. Respiratory reflexes modulate the rate and depth of the breathing pattern in response to chemical, mechanical, and other stimuli.

Respiratory reflexes represent the sequential operation of: (1) sensory receptors that transmit neural signals along afferent pathways to the CNS; (2) respiratory control centers in the CNS that transmit neural signals along efferent pathways to the respiratory muscles; (3) respiratory muscles, which convert their neural drive into respiratory muscle tension, which is the force that alters pleural pressure and thereby moves the lung; (4) the elastic and resistive properties of the lung, which determine the relationship between pleural pressure and lung volume (Figure 6.33).

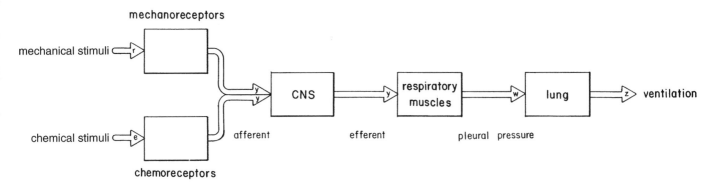

Figure 6.33   Block diagram of a respiratory reflex. Color the block diagram of a respiratory reflex. Observe that respiratory reflexes are mediated by the sequential operation of sensory receptors (chemoreceptors and mechanoreceptors), afferent pathways, a respiratory control (CNS), efferent pathways, and effector organs (respiratory muscles and lung). Compare this figure with Figure 4.9.

Chemoreceptor reflexes

The arterial blood levels of PCO_2, PO_2 and pH (collectively referred to as arterial blood gases) are continuously monitored by *chemoreceptors* that sense the chemical composition of the fluid that surrounds them. The most potent chemoreceptors are the central chemoreceptors, which are located on the surface of the medulla: these chemoreceptors respond to the level of PCO_2 in arterial blood. Peripheral chemoreceptors, which are located in the carotid bodies and in the aortic bodies, detect the PCO_2, PO_2, and pH of their arterial blood supply (Figure 6.34).

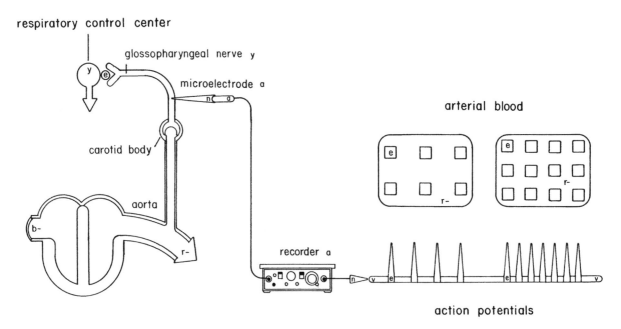

Figure 6.34   Transduction characteristics of arterial chemoreceptors. Color the blood in the heart, noting that the carotid body chemoreceptors are exposed to arterial blood. Color the glossopharyngeal nerve, its excitatory neurotransmitter, and the respiratory control center. Color the microelectrode, the recorder, and the arterial blood samples. Compare the concentration of CO_2 molecules (indicated by the density of squares), and the corresponding recordings of the action potentials generated by chemoreceptors exposed to this blood. Observe that the frequency of action potentials increases when blood levels of CO_2 rise. This feature of chemoreceptor function enables them to transmit information related to blood gases to the respiratory control centers. Compare this figure with Figure 5.34.

Any deviation from the normal values of PCO$_2$, PO$_2$, or pH in the arterial blood stimulates *chemoreceptor reflexes* that alter ventilation in such a way as to restore the normal levels of blood gases. The neural output from chemoreceptors stimulates the respiratory control centers in the brain stem, which, in turn, adjust ventilation by regulating the intensity and the timing of respiratory muscle contraction (Figure 6.35). The operation of chemoreceptor reflexes can be observed by measuring the changes in minute ventilation that occur when the blood levels of carbon dioxide and oxygen are varied.

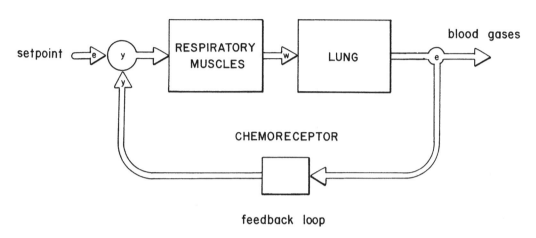

Figure 6.35 Block diagram of a blood gas control system. Color the block diagram. Observe that the setpoint (generated by a neural network in the respiratory control center) provides neural information related to the desired levels of blood gases to a comparator, which also consists of a neural network in the respiratory control center. Note that the comparator also receives neural information related to the actual levels of blood gases from the chemoreceptors (feedback loop). The difference between the two neural signals produces an error signal that drives the respiratory system (respiratory muscles plus lung) to alter its ventilation in such a way as to restore the normal levels of blood gases. Thus, the operation of this system can be regarded as a negative feedback control system that maintains normal levels of blood gases in the face of naturally occurring disturbances in homeostasis. Compare this figure with Figure 5.35.

Ventilatory responses to carbon dioxide and oxygen

The ventilatory response to carbon dioxide can be measured when a subject breathes a gas mixture that increases the level of CO$_2$, but does not change the level of O$_2$, in alveolar gas. Under conditions in which arterial blood levels of CO$_2$ gradually rise, central and peripheral chemoreceptor reflexes are stimulated, which, in turn, increase ventilation. As ventilation increases, more CO$_2$ is blown off in an attempt to restore the normal level of PCO$_2$ in arterial blood (Figure 6.21). The relationship between ventilation and arterial PCO$_2$ that emerges from such studies shows that ventilation increases when arterial PCO$_2$ rises above its normal value of 40 mmHg and decreases when arterial PCO$_2$ falls below its normal value (Figure 6.36, top panel). These findings demonstrate that arterial blood levels of CO$_2$ strongly influence ventilation.

Similarly, the ventilatory response to oxygen can be measured when a subject breathes a gas mixture that changes the level of O$_2$, but not the level of CO$_2$, in alveolar gas. Under conditions in which arterial blood levels of O$_2$ gradually fall, peripheral chemoreceptor reflexes are stimulated, which, in turn, increase ventilation. In contrast to the potent stimulation of ventilation by small increases in carbon dioxide levels, ventilation does not change appreciably even when arterial PO$_2$ falls to moderately low levels. These observations demonstrate that mild hypoxemia (low O$_2$ in arterial blood) only weakly stimulates ventilation, but severe hypoxemia strongly stimulates ventilation (Figure 6.36, bottom panel).

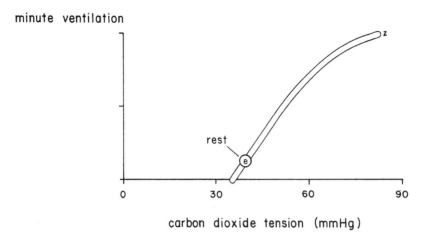

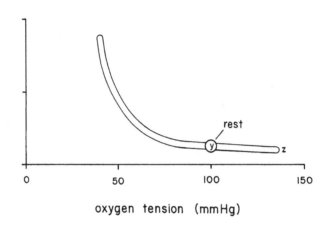

Figure 6.36   Ventilatory responses to carbon dioxide and oxygen. Color the top graph, identifying the point that corresponds to the normal resting condition (PCO_2 = 40 mmHg). Observe from the steepness of the line that minute ventilation increases markedly in response to small increases in arterial PCO_2. Then color the bottom graph, identifying the point that corresponds to the normal resting condition (PO_2 = 100 mmHg). Observe that minute ventilation does not change appreciably during mild hypoxemia, but increases markedly during severe hypoxemia. Observe that the breakpoint in the ventilatory response to O_2 (PO_2 ~ 60 mmHg) coincides with the breakpoint in the oxyhemoglobin dissociation curve (Figure 6.13). The ventilatory response to CO_2 is reduced by drugs that depress the respiratory centers in the central nervous system, by respiratory muscle weakness, or by pathological conditions that increase the stiffness of the lung or that narrow its airways. Compare this figure with Figure 6.33.

Phases of the ventilatory response to exercise

The ventilatory response to a fixed level of submaximal exercise can be divided into four distinct phases that have different time courses.

Phase I refers to a sudden increase in ventilation that occurs at the onset of exercise, Phase II describes a subsequent pe-

riod in which ventilation gradually increases to a higher steady-state level, and Phase III corresponds to the period in which the steady-state level of ventilation is maintained (Figure 6.37). Phase IV refers to the recovery period during which ventilation gradually returns to the resting level following the cessation of exercise. The higher than resting levels of ventilation during the recovery period coincide with the higher levels of O_2 consumption known as the excess postexercise oxygen consumption (EPOC, Figure 3.9).

VENTILATION (liters/min)

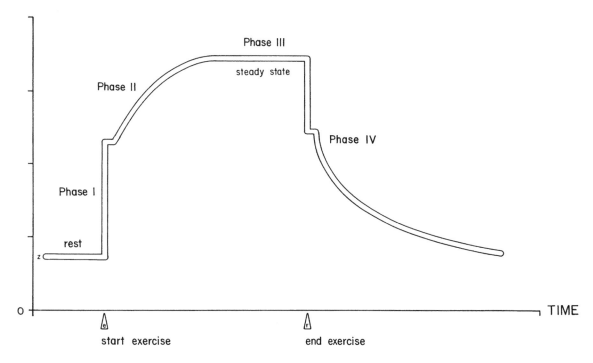

Figure 6.37   Phases of the ventilatory response to exercise. Color the line that depicts minute ventilation (in L/min) plotted against time. Identify the times at which a fixed intensity of continuous submaximal exercise begins and ends, and identify the four phases of the ventilatory response. The magnitudes of the Phase III (steady-state) and Phase IV (recovery) responses vary with the intensity of the exercise. Compare this figure with Figure 3.9.

Effect of exercise intensity on ventilation

The amount by which ventilation increases during exercise varies with the intensity of exercise. The relationship between ventilation and exercise intensity can be studied over a wide range of exercise intensities by plotting steady-state levels of ventilation (Phase III) against concomitant measurements of O_2 consumption (in L/min) or work rate (in watts). These data can be obtained from an analysis of expired air during a graded exercise test, which could be performed using a treadmill, cycle ergometer, or other exercise modality.

This analysis reveals that minute ventilation ($\dot{V}_E$) increases in proportion to oxygen consumption ($\dot{V}O_2$) over the range from rest to moderate exercise, but increases disproportionately to oxygen consumption over the range from moderate to strenuous exercise. The exercise intensity at which ventilation begins to deviate from its linear relationship with oxygen consumption is called the *ventilatory threshold* (VT) (Figure 6.38). Ventilatory thresholds occur at work rates that correspond to 50% to 60% $\dot{V}O_2$max in untrained persons and 70% to 80% $\dot{V}O_2$max in highly trained endurance athletes.

175

MINUTE VENTILATION (liters/min)   BLOOD LACTATE

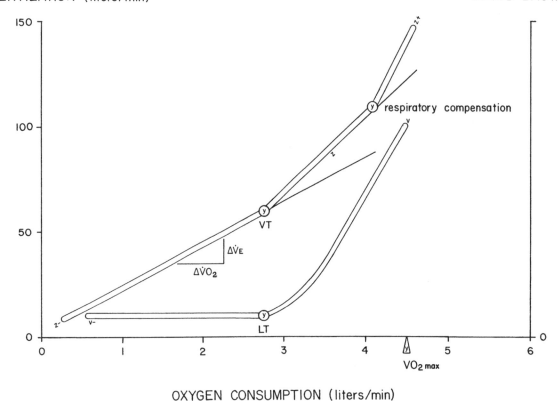

Figure 6.38   Ventilatory response to steady-state exercise. Color the lines depicting the steady-state values of minute ventilation (in L/min, y-axis on left) and blood lactate (in mmol/L, y-axis on right) plotted against oxygen consumption (in L/min), a measure of exercise intensity. Identify the points labeled VT (ventilatory threshold), LT (lactate threshold), and respiratory compensation. Observe that minute ventilation varies linearly with oxygen consumption over the range from rest to the ventilatory threshold and that ventilation increases disproportionately to oxygen consumption when the intensity of exercise exceeds the ventilatory threshold (line with steeper slope). Note that the ventilatory threshold is shown here to coincide with the lactate threshold, the exercise intensity beyond which lactate begins to accumulate in the blood (Figure 3.12). Finally, note that respiratory compensation refers to another point at which ventilation increases disproportionately to oxygen consumption at near maximal levels of exercise intensity.

Ventilatory and lactate thresholds

The ventilatory threshold and the *lactate threshold* (also called the anaerobic threshold) have been found to occur at approximately the same level of exercise intensity in many people. In these persons, the lactate threshold, defined as the point at which lactate begins to systematically accumulate in the blood, coincides with the point at which nonmetabolic CO_2 production begins to appear and with the point at which blood levels of bicarbonate begin to decline. These observations support the hypothesis that: (1) an observed increase in blood lactate is due to increased production of lactic acid by working muscle; and (2) the phenomenon of the ventilatory threshold is due to chemoreceptor reflexes that are stimulated by the nonmetabolic CO_2 that is produced when the hydrogen ions that dissociate from this lactic acid are buffered by bicarbonate ions in the blood (Figure 3.23). This hypothesis is

also supported by the observation that arterial PCO_2 remains essentially constant in the face of this disproportionate increase in ventilation. This result indicates that the higher rate of alveolar ventilation precisely matches the higher rate of CO_2 production; this behavior is referred to as *isocapnic buffering*. The above considerations provide a reasonable explanation of those cases in which ventilatory threshold and lactate threshold occur at the same exercise intensity (Figure 6.38). Under these conditions, therefore, ventilatory threshold can serve as an indicator of lactate threshold. In other words, the exercise intensity for which blood levels of lactate begin to rise can be inferred from noninvasive measurements of gas exchange at the mouth.

However, this mechanism does not account for the observation that the ventilatory threshold occurs at a higher exercise intensity than the lactate threshold in highly trained en-

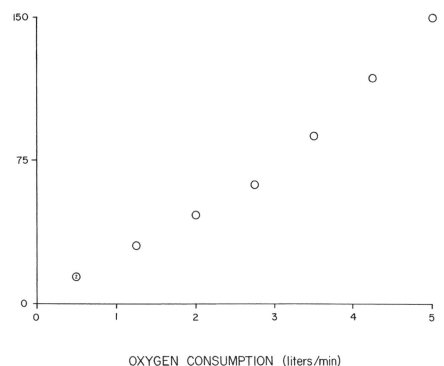

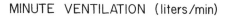

MINUTE VENTILATION (liters/min)

OXYGEN CONSUMPTION (liters/min)

Figure 6.39   Determination of VT from $\dot{V}_E$ and $\dot{V}O_2$ data. This figure illustrates a graphical method that can be used to determine the ventilatory threshold from gas exchange data obtained during a graded exercise test (stress test) in which work rate is progressively incremented. Color the points that represent measured values of minute ventilation (in L/min) plotted against concomitant values of oxygen consumption (in L/min). Fit two straight lines to these data and use the point at which they intersect to identify the ventilatory threshold (VT), the exercise intensity at which $\dot{V}_E$ begins to increase nonlinearly with $\dot{V}O_2$. Compare this figure with Figure 6.38.

durance athletes, or for the observation that glycogen depletion causes the lactate threshold to occur at a higher exercise intensity than the ventilatory threshold. Furthermore, the production of nonmetabolic CO_2 cannot account for the observation that persons with McArdle's syndrome, who do not produce lactic acid during exercise because they lack the enzyme lactate dehydrogenase (LDH), also exhibit a disproportionate increase in ventilation with respect to oxygen consumption during graded exercise tests. In other words, persons with McArdle's syndrome exhibit a ventilatory threshold despite the fact that they do not produce nonmetabolic CO_2. In these people, therefore, the phenomenon of ventilatory threshold cannot be attributed to the stimulation of chemoreceptor reflexes by a higher rate of CO_2 production. These findings demonstrate that other factors, which are

presently unknown, play a role in stimulating ventilation during exercise.

Measurement of ventilatory threshold

Ventilatory threshold can be estimated from steady-state measurements of minute ventilation ($\dot{V}_E$) and oxygen consumption ($\dot{V}O_2$) obtained over a range of exercise intensities (Figure 6.38). Because it is sometimes difficult to judge the $\dot{V}O_2$ value at which $\dot{V}_E$ begins to rise more steeply (Figure 6.39), other methods have been proposed to assess ventilatory threshold; one method employs calculated parameters known as the *ventilatory equivalents.*

Ventilatory equivalents for oxygen and carbon dioxide

Analysis of the ventilatory equivalents for oxygen and carbon dioxide is the most specific gas exchange method for the detection of ventilatory threshold. The ventilatory equivalents for oxygen (V_EO_2) and carbon dioxide (V_ECO_2) are calculated from simultaneous measurements of minute ventilation ($\dot{V}_E$, in L/min), oxygen consumption ($\dot{V}O_2$, in L/min), and carbon dioxide production ($\dot{V}CO_2$, in L/min) obtained during a graded exercise test (Figure 6.40), i.e.,

$$V_EO_2 = \dot{V}_E / \dot{V}O_2$$
$$V_ECO_2 = \dot{V}_E / \dot{V}CO_2$$

In algebraic terms, V_EO_2 is a measure of the volume of air that is expired (23 to 28 L at rest) during the period in which 1 liter of oxygen is consumed. Similarly, V_ECO_2 is a measure of the volume of air that is expired during the period in which 1 liter of carbon dioxide is produced.

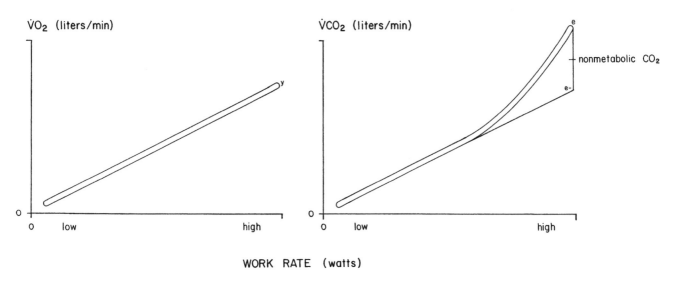

WORK RATE (watts)

Figure 6.40   Effect of exercise intensity on $\dot{V}O_2$ and $\dot{V}CO_2$. Color the lines depicting steady-state values of oxygen consumption ($\dot{V}O_2$, in L/min, left panel) and carbon dioxide production ($\dot{V}CO_2$, in L/min, right panel) plotted against work rate (in watts), a measure of exercise intensity. Observe that $\dot{V}O_2$ increases linearly with work rate over the range from low to high work rates. Observe also that $\dot{V}CO_2$ increases linearly with work rate over the range from low to moderate (~ lactate threshold) work rates, and disproportionately to work rate over the range from moderate to high work rates. Color the area labeled nonmetabolic CO_2; this production of extra CO_2 at high work intensities can be accounted for by the nonmetabolic production of CO_2 that occurs when hydrogen ions (generated during the formation of lactic acid) combine with bicarbonate ions in the blood and form CO_2 (Figure 3.23). The finding that the ventilatory threshold usually coincides with the lactate threshold supports this view. Compare this figure with Figure 3.24.

In graphical terms, V_EO_2 represents the slope of a line connecting the origin with a point on a graph of minute ventilation plotted against oxygen consumption. In other words, the numerical value of V_EO_2 associated with any given combination of $\dot{V}_E$ and $\dot{V}O_2$ can be visualized from the slope of a line from the origin to the data point (Figure 6.41). Thus, V_EO_2 remains constant over the range of exercise intensities for

which minute ventilation parallels oxygen consumption (data points on same line), but increases when minute ventilation increases disproportionately to oxygen consumption (data points on different line). These considerations explain why the point at which V_EO_2 begins to increase in a graded exercise test can serve as an indicator of ventilatory threshold (Figure 6.42).

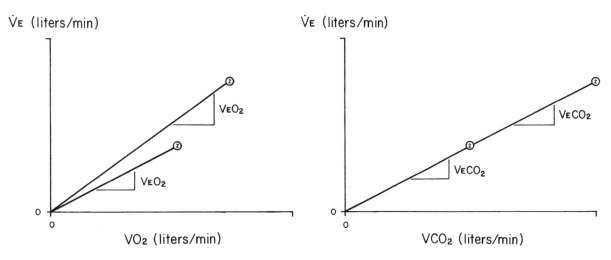

Figure 6.41   Ventilatory equivalents for oxygen and carbon dioxide. Color the data points that indicate measured values of minute ventilation (V_E, in L/min) plotted against the corresponding levels of oxygen consumption ($\dot{V}O_2$, in L/min, left panel) and carbon dioxide production ($\dot{V}CO_2$, in L/min, right panel). Note that the slope of a line from the origin to an individual data point in the left panel specifies a numerical value for the ventilatory equivalent for oxygen associated with the data point, i.e., $V_EO_2 = \dot{V}_E/\dot{V}O_2$. Observe that the V_EO_2 value for the data point at the lower exercise intensity (lower $\dot{V}O_2$) is smaller than the V_EO_2 value for the data point at the higher exercise intensity (higher $\dot{V}O_2$). These findings demonstrate that V_EO_2 increases when the exercise intensity exceeds the ventilatory threshold. Compare these results with those shown in Figure 6.38. Note also that the slope of a line from the origin to a data point in the right panel specifies a numerical value for the ventilatory equivalent for carbon dioxide associated with the data point, i.e., $V_ECO_2 = \dot{V}_E/\dot{V}CO_2$. Observe that the V_ECO_2 values for each data point are the same because they both fall on the same line. These results demonstrate that V_ECO_2 does not change when the intensity of exercise exceeds the ventilatory threshold because the increase in ventilation precisely matches the increase in CO_2 production. For these reasons, ventilatory threshold can be found by identifying the exercise intensity at which V_EO_2 increases but V_ECO_2 stays the same. This is the most specific method for identifying ventilatory threshold from gas exchange data.

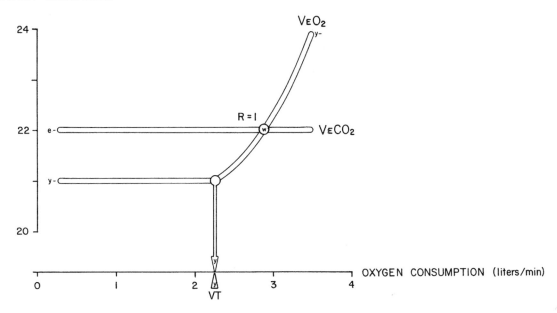

Figure 6.42   Determination of VT from V_EO_2 data. Color the lines that depict the ventilatory equivalents for oxygen (V_EO_2) and carbon dioxide (V_ECO_2) plotted against oxygen consumption ($\dot{V}O_2$, a measure of exercise intensity). Observe that the ventilatory threshold (VT) coincides with the point at which V_EO_2 increases, but V_ECO_2 remains the same (horizontal line indicating isocapnic buffering). Also observe that the respiratory exchange ratio (R= $\dot{V}CO_2/\dot{V}O_2$) equals unity at the point where the two lines intersect. R values that exceed 1 indicate that CO_2 production exceeds O_2 consumption, a finding that provides evidence of nonmetabolic CO_2 production (due to the formation of lactic acid). Compare this figure with Figures 3.24 and 6.41.

Similarly, V_ECO_2 defines the slope of a line connecting the origin with a point on the graph of minute ventilation plotted against carbon dioxide production (Figure 6.41). V_ECO_2 remains constant over the range of exercise intensities for which minute ventilation parallels carbon dioxide production. A relevant outcome of these considerations is that V_ECO_2 remains essentially constant at exercise intensities below and above the ventilatory threshold because the increase in ventilation matches the increased rate of CO_2 production during isocapnic buffering (Figure 6.42).

Blood levels of oxygen and carbon dioxide during exercise

The levels of oxygen and carbon dioxide in alveolar gas and therefore, arterial blood, remain essentially constant over a wide range of submaximal exercise (Figure 6.43). This constancy of arterial blood gases can be attributed to the operation of chemoreceptor reflexes that regulate alveolar ventilation in order to keep pace with the higher rates of oxy-

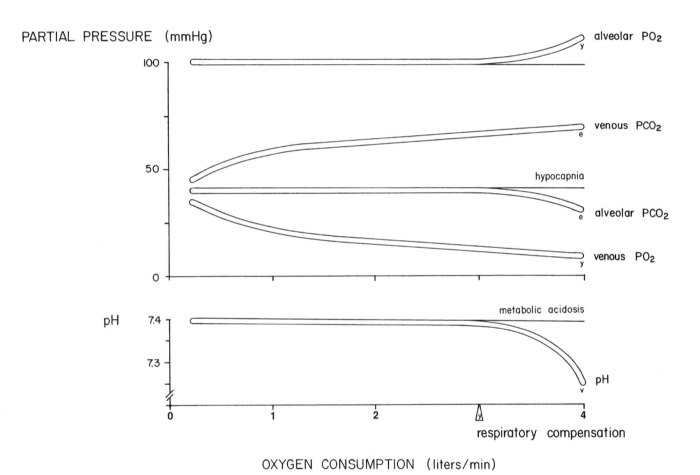

Figure 6.43   Effect of exercise intensity on PO₂ and PCO₂ levels. Color the lines that depict the partial pressures of oxygen (PO₂) and carbon dioxide (PCO₂) in alveolar gas and venous blood, and the pH of arterial blood, all plotted against oxygen consumption, a measure of exercise intensity. Note that the PO₂ of venous blood falls with increasing exercise intensity (indicating a widened a-v̄ O₂ difference, Figure 6.14), and that the PCO₂ of venous blood rises (indicating an increase in CO₂ content). Observe that alveolar PO₂, alveolar PCO₂, and arterial pH remain essentially constant (horizontal lines) over the range from rest (left endpoints of lines) to the exercise intensity labeled respiratory compensation (arrowhead). Observe also that beyond this point, alveolar PO₂ rises, alveolar PCO₂ falls, and pH falls (due to metabolic acidosis).

gen consumption and carbon dioxide production that occur during exercise (Figure 6.44).

In contrast, the levels of oxygen and carbon dioxide in mixed venous blood vary with exercise intensity (Figure 6.43). The oxygen content in mixed venous blood falls because the a-$\bar{v}$ O_2 difference widens when exercising muscles extract more oxygen from their arterial blood supply (Figure 6.14), and the carbon dioxide content rises because exercising muscles add more carbon dioxide to the blood.

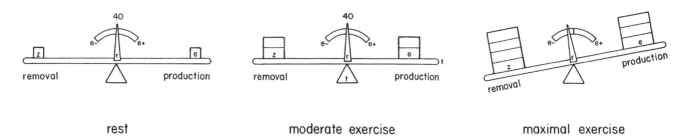

rest   moderate exercise   maximal exercise

Figure 6.44   Effect of exercise intensity on alveolar PCO$_2$. Color the balance, the pointer, and the PCO$_2$ scale (in mmHg). For each panel, color and compare the rectangles that depict the rate at which CO_2 is removed from the body by alveolar ventilation (left side of balance) and the rate at which CO_2 is produced by the body (right side of balance). Observe that CO_2 production increases with increasing exercise intensity and these increases are matched exactly by corresponding increases in CO_2 removal during rest (left panel) and moderate exercise (middle panel); thus, alveolar PCO$_2$ remains constant at its normal value of 40 mmHg. Observe also that CO_2 removal exceeds CO_2 production during maximal exercise (right panel). For this reason, alveolar PCO$_2$ falls below its normal value of 40 mmHg during maximal exercise. Compare this figure with Figure 6.21.

Respiratory compensation

Respiratory compensation, which refers to a further increase in ventilation that occurs at near maximal levels of exercise (Figure 6.38), causes alveolar PCO$_2$ to fall and alveolar PO$_2$ to rise (Figure 6.43); these changes in alveolar gas composition are similar to those observed during hyperventilation (Figure 6.23). The operation of chemoreceptors, which normally stimulates ventilation in response to rising CO_2 levels in arterial blood, is an unlikely candidate to explain why arterial blood levels of CO_2 fall at near-maximal levels of exercise. The resultant respiratory alkalosis (lowering of arterial PCO$_2$) offsets the falling pH due to the high rates of lactic acid production (metabolic acidosis) that accompanies high-intensity exercise (Figure 6.19).

A reduction in arterial PCO$_2$ indicates that alveolar ventilation increases disproportionately to carbon dioxide production at near-maximal levels of exercise (Figure 6.44). Since such changes in ventilation cannot be attributed entirely to the operation of chemoreceptor reflexes that regulate the blood levels of carbon dioxide and oxygen, it has been proposed that respiratory compensation is due to the combined effects of a number of factors that could also stimulate the respiratory control centers (Figure 6.45). Possible factors include the direct effects of increased temperature, the effects of lowered blood pH (mediated by carotid body chemoreceptors), as well as the effects of neural signals from higher brain centers, skeletal muscle mechanoreceptors, and respiratory mechanoreceptors (Figure 6.46).

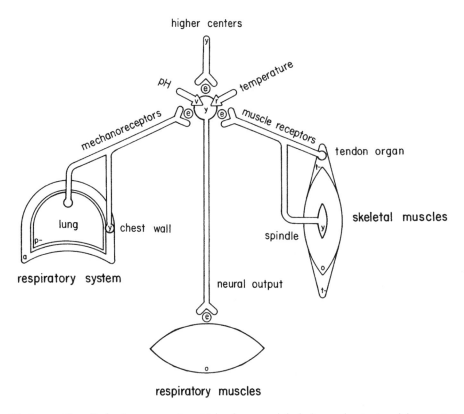

Figure 6.45   Ventilatory stimuli during exercise. Color the nerve labeled neural output and the respiratory muscle that it innervates. Observe that the neural output to the respiratory muscles is modulated by a variety of inputs. Identify and color the afferent nerve fibers from respiratory mechanoreceptors, skeletal muscle receptors, and higher centers, as well as the arrows labeled pH and temperature. Finish the picture by coloring the respiratory system and skeletal muscles.

Figure 6.46   Respiratory mechanoreceptors. Color the afferent nerve pathways from the respiratory mechanoreceptors, noting that they transmit neural signals from the airways, lung, chest wall, and diaphragm to the respiratory control center in the brain stem. Finish the picture by coloring the respiratory control center, the lung, and the chest wall.

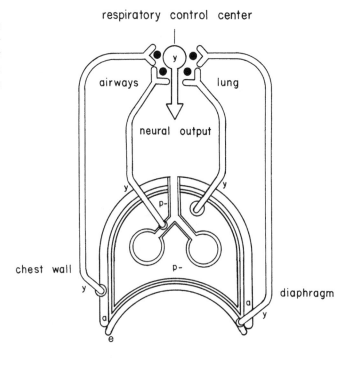

Pulmonary function tests

The standard tests of pulmonary function fall into three basic categories: (1) measurements of lung volume under static conditions; (2) measurements of airflow under dynamic conditions; and (3) measurements of gas exchange, which include diffusion capacity and determination of arterial blood gases (PO_2, PCO_2, and pH).

Lung volumes and capacities

Measurements of some lung volumes can be made with a *spirometer* (Figure 6.47), a device that can be used to record the changes in lung volume that occur when a maximal inspiration is followed by a maximal expiration. This procedure provides direct measurements of vital capacity (VC) and its subdivisions, inspiratory capacity (IC) and expiratory reserve volume (ERV) (Figure 6.48).

Since some air remains in the lung after a maximal expiration, other lung volumes cannot be measured directly by a spirometer. These volumes, which include total lung capacity (TLC), functional residual capacity (FRC), and residual volume (RV), must be measured by an indirect method, such as *helium dilution* (Figure 6.49).

Forced vital capacity and FEV₁

The forced vital capacity (FVC) is the volume of air that can be expired during a single maximal expiratory effort from TLC; the volume that is expired during the first second is called the FEV_1 (Figure 6.50). FEV_1 is usually reported on a pulmonary function test both as an absolute volume (in L) and as a percentage of the forced vital capacity, i.e., $FEV_1 \cdot 100\%/FVC$.

Maximum voluntary ventilation

The maximum voluntary ventilation (MVV) is the highest level of minute ventilation (in L/min) that a seated person can voluntarily achieve over a 15 s period (Figure 6.51). The fact that the observed values of MVV are somewhat higher than the actual values of ventilation attained during maximal exercise indicates that ventilation is not normally a limiting factor in exercise. This view is consistent with the observation that blood levels of PO_2 are usually maintained within the normal range during exercise (Figure 6.43).

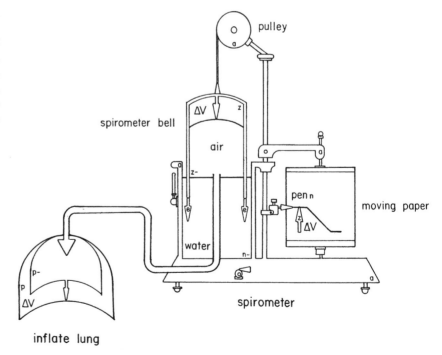

Figure 6.47 Spirometer. Color the spirometer; observe that the act of inspiring a given volume of air (ΔV) causes the descent of the spirometer bell to displace an equal volume of air. Note that the pen records this volume change on calibrated paper. Volumes can also be obtained from the electronic processing (integration) of airflow signals measured by a device called a pneumotachograph.

pulley

spirometer bell

air

ΔV

pen

moving paper

water

spirometer

inflate lung

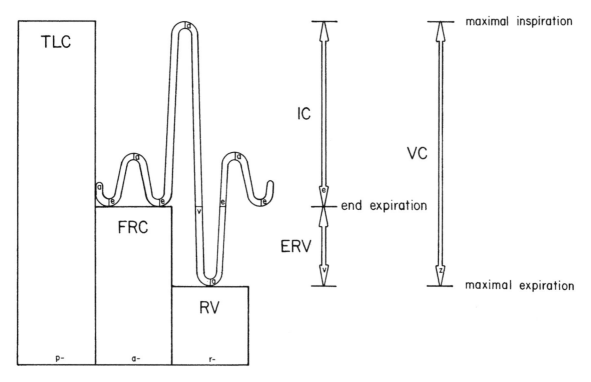

Figure 6.48   Lung volumes and capacities. Color the line depicting the lung volumes that are measured when a maximal inspiration is followed by a maximal expiration. Color the arrows labeled vital capacity (VC) and its subdivisions, inspiratory capacity (IC), and expiratory reserve volume (ERV); observe that VC is given by the sum of IC and ERV and that these lung volumes can be measured with a spirometer. IC is due to inspiratory muscle contraction and ERV is due to expiratory muscle contraction (Figure 6.25). Identify the total lung capacity (TLC), functional residual capacity (FRC) and residual volume (RV). FRC, also referred to as the resting end-expiratory position, is the lung volume associated with relaxed respiratory muscles. Because the lungs cannot be completely emptied voluntarily, TLC, FRC, and RV are measured by indirect techniques, such as helium dilution. Compare the colors in this figure with those in Figure 6.25, noting that volume changes due to inspiratory and expiratory muscle contraction are labeled e and v, respectively, and that volume changes that could be due to passive recoil of the respiratory apparatus are labeled a.

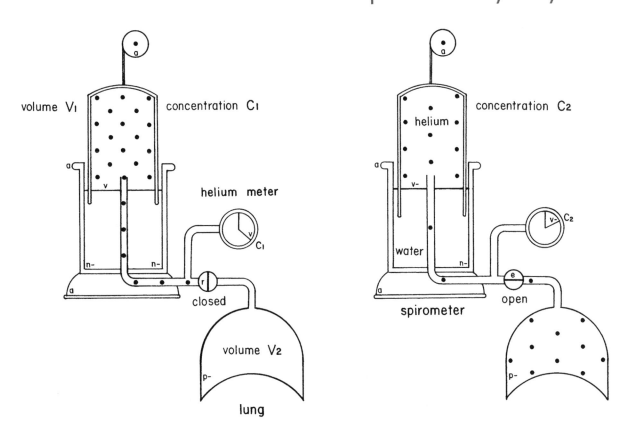

initial   final

Figure 6.49 Helium dilution. Color the spirometer in the left panel, noting that it contains a fixed number (N = 24) of helium molecules (dots). Note also that N is given by the product of the helium concentration (C_1) and the initial volume of gas in the spirometer (V_1), i.e., $N = C_1 \cdot V_1$. Observe the closed valve and the helium meter reading (C_1). Color the spirometer in the right panel, noting the open valve and helium meter reading (C_2, a lower concentration than C_1). Since helium does not cross the pulmonary membrane, observe that same number of helium molecules occupy a larger volume, given by the sum of V_1 (known spirometer volume) and V_2 (unknown lung volume), i.e., $N = C_2 \cdot (V_1 + V_2) = C_1 \cdot V_1$. This equation can be rearranged as $V_2 = [(C_1 - C_2)/C_2] \cdot V_1$. Thus, volume V_2 can be derived from C_1, C_2, and V_1. For example, if the volume of the lung happened to be the same as the volume of the spirometer ($V_1 = V_2$), the final concentration of helium (C_2) would be half the initial concentration (C_1) because the same number of molecules would occupy twice the volume, i.e., $C_2 = C_1/2$.

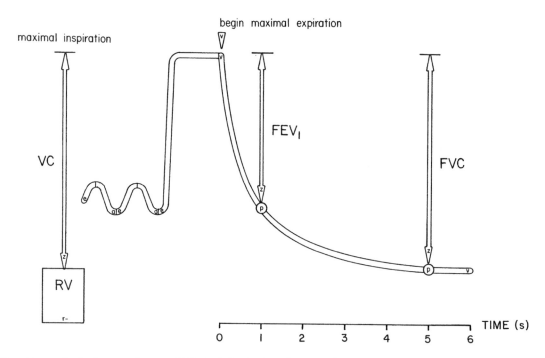

Figure 6.50   Forced vital capacity and FEV₁. Color the line depicting the spirometric tracing associated with a maximal expiratory effort from TLC (lung volume at maximal inspiration). Color the arrows labeled FEV₁ (forced expiratory volume in 1 s) and FVC (forced vital capacity). The FEV₁ /FVC ratio, calculated as $FEV_1 \cdot 100/FVC$, is ~80% in healthy subjects.

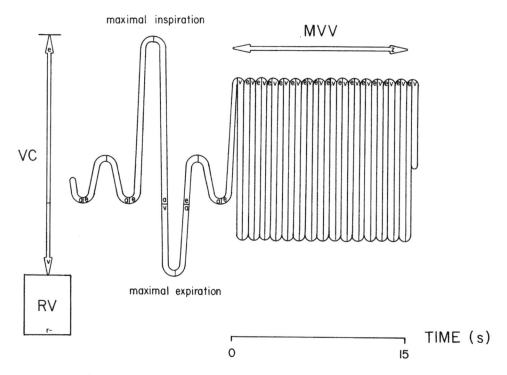

Figure 6.51   Maximum voluntary ventilation. Color the spirometric tracing, comparing the volumes associated with the MVV maneuver with those attained during the vital capacity maneuver.

chapter **seven**
endocrine

system

The greater energy demands of exercise are satisfied by increases in the activity of energy-yielding metabolic pathways and by increases in the delivery of fuels and oxygen to exercising muscles; these responses to exercise are modulated by the endocrine system.

Endocrine glands secrete hormones into the blood that regulate the activity of metabolic pathways to provide an adequate supply of ATP for muscle contraction and to maintain an adequate level of blood glucose for proper function of the nervous system. Hormones also enhance the capacity of the cardiovascular system to deliver fuels and oxygen to exercising muscle, and modulate the operation of the renal system to maintain normal concentrations of the constituents of body fluids.

Endocrine glands

The *endocrine system* consists of a number of glands, which are organs or tissues that secrete one or more chemical regulators, called *hormones* or *endocrines,* into the blood (Figure 7.1). The release of hormones by endocrine glands is regulated by a variety of stimuli, including neural signals from the autonomic nervous system (Figure 4.9), levels of other hormones in the blood, and concentrations of specific substances in the blood, such as glucose or sodium.

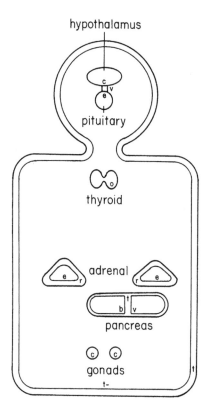

Figure 7.1 Schema of endocrine system. Color the endocrine glands, noting their locations relative to each other and within the body as a whole.

Hormones released by endocrine glands travel through the blood and act only on those cells that have specific receptor proteins for them in their cell membrane. These cells are referred to as their *target cells*, and they respond to their hormones in a predictable way. It is the response of the target cell that produces the biological effects of the hormone. The release of hormones is modulated by negative feedback loops that relay information related to the effects of the hormone back to the endocrine gland (Figure 7.2).

Figure 7.2 Schematic diagram of hormone action. Color the endocrine gland, hormone (triangles), blood, and target cell. Note that the hormone is released into venous blood, returns to the heart, passes through the lung, and reaches the target organ in the arterial blood supply. Observe that the target cell induces the biological effect of the hormone, and that the effect of the hormone modulates the activity of the endocrine gland by a negative feedback loop.

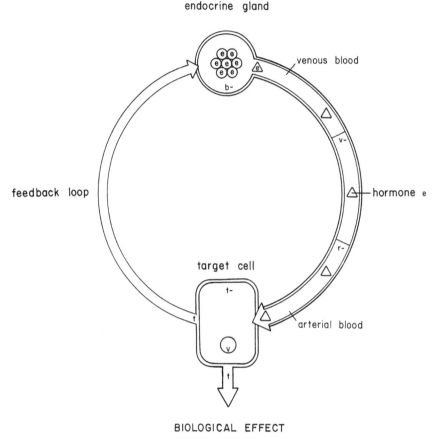

Classes of hormones

Hormones belong to different classes of chemical compounds, which include proteins, modified amino acids, and steroids (lipids with cyclic structures formed from cholesterol). Examples of protein hormones are insulin and glucagon, secreted by the pancreas; examples of modified amino acids are the catecholamines (epinephrine and norepinephrine, Figure 7.3), secreted by the adrenal medulla; and examples of steroid hormones (Figure 7.4) are the glucocorticoids (e.g., cortisol), secreted by the adrenal cortex.

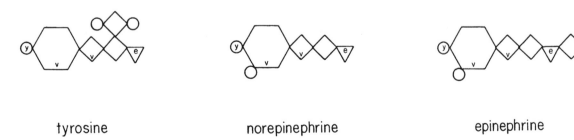

tyrosine　　　　norepinephrine　　　　epinephrine

Figure 7.3 Catecholamines. Color the carbon (diamonds), oxygen (circles), and nitrogen (triangles) atoms, and the benzene rings (hexagons), of the amino acid tyrosine (left panel) and the two catecholamines, norepinephrine (middle panel) and epinephrine (right panel), that are synthesized from it. Note that hydrogen atoms are not shown in this simplified diagram. Compare the structures of the three compounds, noting their similarities.

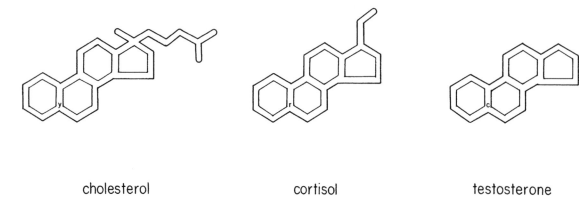

cholesterol   cortisol   testosterone

Figure 7.4 **Steroid hormones.** Color the molecule of cholesterol (left panel) and the two steroid hormones, cortisol (middle panel) and testosterone (right panel), noting their similarities and differences. These hormones and the other steroid hormones, such as progesterone, aldosterone, and estradiol, are synthesized from cholesterol and are structurally similar to it.

Mechanisms of hormone action

Hormones regulate the activity of their target organs through two different mechanisms; one mechanism produces effects that have a rapid onset and a short duration, while the other produces effects that have a slow onset and a long duration. The short-duration effect, which involves the activation of existing enzymes, is called the *second messenger mechanism*. The long-duration effect, which involves the synthesis of proteins, mediates its effects through the *control of gene transcription*.

Second messenger mechanism

In the second messenger mechanism (employed by insulin, glucagon, and catecholamines), the hormone, which is regarded as the "first messenger," binds to a specific receptor protein on the target cell membrane and changes the shape of the receptor, thereby transmitting a signal to the interior of the cell without having to enter the cell. This leads to the production of an intracellular substance (the "second messenger") which activates existing enzymes within the cell. It is the activation of these intracellular enzymes that is responsible for the biological effects of the hormone.

A ubiquitous example of a second messenger mechanism involves the synthesis of the compound, cyclic AMP (cAMP)

(Figure 7.5). The occupation of a receptor on a cell membrane by the hormone stimulates a membrane-bound enzyme, adenylate cyclase, to catalyze the reaction in which ATP is converted to cAMP plus pyrophosphate (two phosphate groups linked together). The newly formed cAMP (the second messenger) stimulates another enzyme (a protein kinase) that ultimately activates intracellular enzymes that regulate the rates of metabolic pathways. The effects of the second messenger mechanism are immediate (because it activates enzymes that are already present in the cell) but temporary (because cAMP is rapidly degraded in the cell).

A specific example of a second messenger system is the way in which glucagon stimulates the breakdown of glycogen into glucose in the liver (hepatic glycogenolysis). Glucagon binds to a receptor on the liver cell membrane and stimulates the enzyme, adenylate cyclase, to catalyze the reaction that converts ATP to cAMP plus pyrophosphate (Figure 7.5). Then cAMP, acting as the second messenger, initiates a series of intracellular events that ultimately activate glycogen phosphorylase, the rate-limiting enzyme in the pathway of glycogenolysis (Figure 2.12), thereby increasing the rate of glycogen breakdown. Because cAMP is rapidly degraded, its effect on glycogenolysis ends quickly unless another molecule of glucagon reinitiates the process by occupying its receptor in the cell membrane.

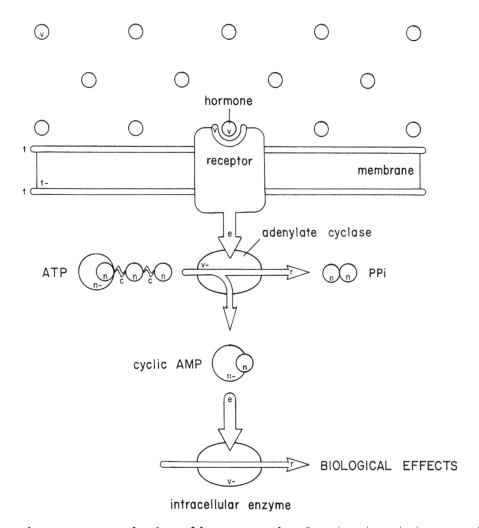

Figure 7.5   Second messenger mechanism of hormone action. Begin by coloring the hormone molecules in the blood (above the cell membrane), including the hormone that binds to its receptor on the cell membrane; color the receptor and the membrane that the receptor spans. Observe that the hormone does not enter the cell to exert its effect. Color the enzyme (adenylate cyclase) that is stimulated by the hormone-receptor complex, its substrate ATP, its products cyclic AMP (cAMP) and pyrophosphate (PPi), and the arrow that represents the reaction. Color the vertical arrow that represents a cascade of reactions that amplify the effect of an increase in cAMP and the intracellular enzyme whose activity is ultimately affected. Color the arrow indicating the biological effects that result from the activation of this intracellular enzyme. The effects of these changes in enzyme activity occur rapidly but are short-lived because cAMP is rapidly degraded in the cell.

Control of gene transcription

The slow-onset, long-duration mechanism of hormone action (employed by steroid hormones and thyroid hormone) is one in which hormones exert their effects on target cells through the synthesis of intracellular proteins. In this mechanism, the hormone actually enters the cell and ultimately binds to its specific protein receptor inside the nucleus; the hormone-receptor complex then directs the transcription of a specific portion of DNA into a strand of messenger RNA (mRNA). The mRNA thus formed leaves the nucleus and is decoded by the ribosomes to synthesize a protein having the sequence of amino acids specified by the mRNA; this process is referred to as *translation*. It is the production of more of the particular protein, which could be an enzyme, that is responsible for the biological effects of the hormone (Figure 7.6).

An example of this mechanism of hormone action involves cortisol, a steroid hormone released by the adrenal cortex. Cortisol causes liver cells to synthesize more molecules of a key enzyme in the pathway of gluconeogenesis (Figure 2.26). Thus, cortisol stimulates gluconeogenesis by making a greater amount of a particular enzyme available to catalyze a reaction in the pathway. For this reason, the effects of cortisol persist as long as the enzyme level remains elevated (hours).

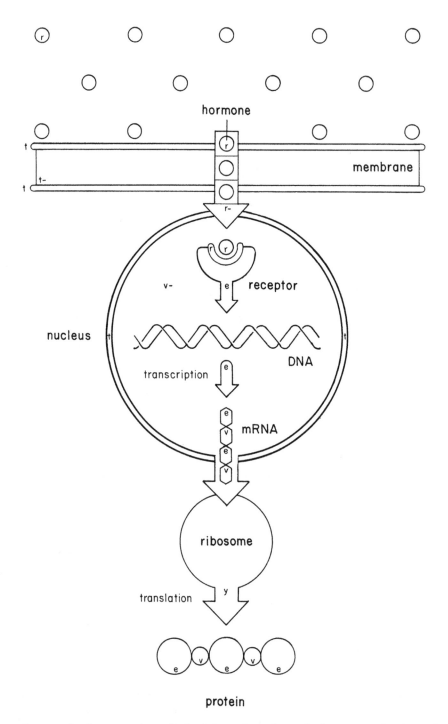

Figure 7.6 Hormonal control of gene transcription. Begin by coloring the hormone molecules in the blood (above the cell membrane) and the arrow that indicates their passage through the cell membrane and nuclear membrane to enter the nucleus. Color the hormone–receptor complex, noting the section of DNA to be transcribed to messenger RNA (mRNA). Color the mRNA strand, the ribosome, and the protein formed by the translation of mRNA into a sequence of amino acids (circles). Steroid hormones and thyroid hormone mediate their effects through the mechanism of gene transcription.

Effect of exercise on hormone release

Release of some hormones is stimulated at the onset of exercise, whereas for others it may not be stimulated until the exercise attains a sufficient intensity or duration. Exercise stimulates the secretion of fuel-mobilizing hormones (catecholamines, glucagon, growth hormone, and cortisol), result-

ing in higher blood levels of these hormones (Figure 7.7). Exercise can also increase blood levels of hormones that regulate body fluid composition (aldosterone and antidiuretic hormone) and blood levels of hormones that affect growth (growth hormone) and metabolic rate (thyroid hormone). In contrast, exercise suppresses the release of the fuel-storing hormone insulin, resulting in a lower blood level of this hormone. Each of these hormones is discussed below.

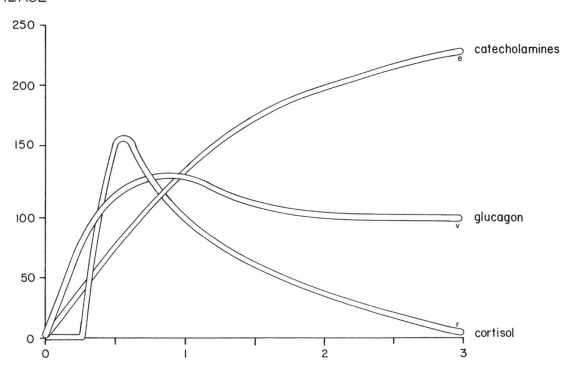

Figure 7.7 Time course of endocrine secretions during exercise. Color and compare the lines that plot blood levels of representative fuel-mobilizing hormones (percent increase above baseline levels) against time (in hr) during a fixed-intensity, long-duration exercise. Observe that blood levels of catecholamines and glucagon, but not cortisol, begin to rise at the onset of exercise. Note that catecholamines and glucagon mediate their effects through a second messenger mechanism, whereas cortisol mediates its effect through the synthesis of enzymes that regulate metabolic pathways.

chapter **seven**

Pituitary gland

The *pituitary gland,* which is also called the *hypophysis,* is located beneath the brain and functions as an intermediary between the hypothalamus and a number of endocrine glands. The hypothalamus is a region of the brain that coordinates processes involved in homeostasis (maintenance of a constant internal environment).

The pituitary gland is comprised of an anterior (front) portion, which is also called the adenohypophysis, and a posterior (back) portion, which is also called the neurohypophysis; the two regions of the pituitary gland differ anatomically and functionally (Figure 7.8).

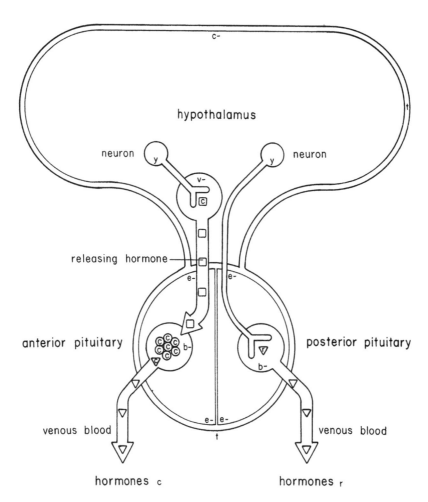

Figure 7.8   Pituitary gland. Color the neuron at left in the hypothalamus, the portal blood system that transports releasing and inhibiting hormones (squares) from the hypothalamus to the anterior pituitary gland, and the subsequent release of anterior pituitary hormones (triangles) into the blood. Color the neuron at right in the hypothalamus, its nerve ending in the posterior pituitary gland and the subsequent release of posterior pituitary hormones (triangles) into the blood. Observe that the release of anterior pituitary hormones is regulated by chemical signals that originate in the hypothalamus, and that the release of posterior pituitary hormones is regulated by neural signals that originate in the hypothalamus.

gr**a**y **b**lue **c**anary gr**ee**n blac**k** **n**avy **o**range **p**ink **r**ed **t**an **v**iolet **w**hite **y**ellow a**z**ure   [+] and [−] mean use heavy and light pressure, respectively

Anterior pituitary hormones

The anterior pituitary gland receives chemical signals, which are called *releasing hormones* (RH) and *inhibiting hormones* (IH), that travel from the hypothalamus to the anterior pituitary gland through a system of local blood vessels known as the *hypothalamic-pituitary portal system.* Each of the releasing hormones and inhibiting hormones regulates the secretion of a particular hormone by the anterior pituitary gland (Figure 7.9).

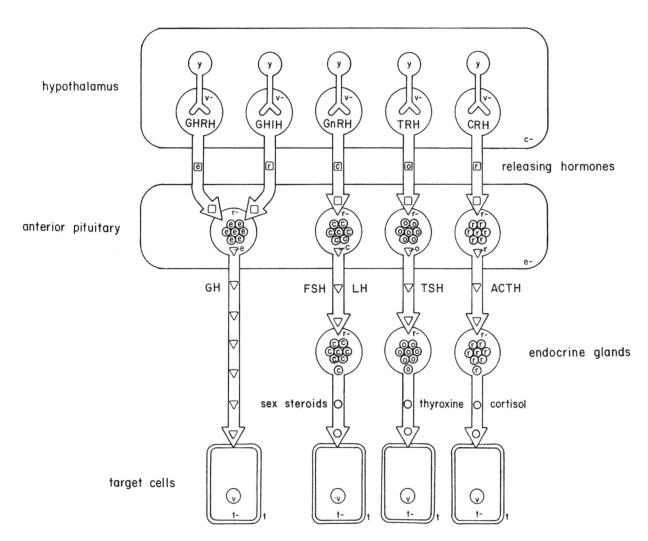

Figure 7.9   Anterior pituitary hormones. Color the hypothalamus and, for each hypothalamic neuron shown, color it and the path of the releasing (RH) or inhibiting (IH) hormone through the portal blood vessels to the anterior pituitary gland. For growth hormone releasing (GHRH) and inhibiting (GHIH) hormones, color the cells that secrete growth hormone (GH) and its path through the blood to its many target cells, which include liver and muscle. For gonadotropin-releasing hormone (GnRH), color the cells that secrete either follicle-stimulating hormone (FSH) or luteinizing hormone (LH), and their path through the blood to the ovary or testes. In the ovaries LH and FSH stimulate secretion of progesterone and estrogens that act on the uterus and mammary glands; in the testes LH increases the release of testosterone, which promotes growth and the development of sexual characteristics. For thyrotropin-releasing hormone (TRH), color its path to the pituitary cells that secrete thyroid-stimulating hormone (TSH), the path of TSH to the thyroid gland, and then the path of thyroid hormone (e.g., thyroxine) to all cells of the body. Finally, for corticotropin-releasing hormone (CRH), color the cells that secrete adrenocorticotropic hormone (ACTH), its path in the blood to the adrenal cortex, the adrenal cells that secrete glucocorticoids (e.g., cortisol), and then the path of glucocorticoids to their many target organs, including the liver. Note which hormones are released in response to hypothalamic hormones and which are released in response to tropic, or stimulating, hormones from the anterior pituitary gland. Compare this figure with Figure 7.8.

Anterior pituitary hormones, which are initially released into venous blood, eventually enter the general circulation. Some anterior pituitary hormones stimulate the release of hormones from other endocrine glands; these include thyroid-stimulating hormone (TSH, which acts on the thyroid gland), adrenocorticotropic hormone (ACTH, which acts on the adrenal gland), and follicle-stimulating hormone and luteinizing hormone (FSH and LH, respectively, which act on the gonads). Other anterior pituitary hormones act directly on their target cells; these include growth hormone (GH, which acts on all cells) and prolactin (which acts on the mammary gland) (Figure 7.9).

The secretion of hypothalamic releasing factors and the subsequent release of anterior pituitary hormones are modulated by multiple feedback loops that relay information related to the effects of the particular hormone back to the hypothalamus and the pituitary gland (Figure 7.10). For example, high levels of thyroid hormone inhibit the release of TSH by the anterior pituitary gland, and high levels of either thyroid hormone or TSH inhibit the release of thyroid-releasing hormone (TRH) by the hypothalamus.

Figure 7.10 Regulation of anterior pituitary hormone secretion. Beginning at the top, color the neuron, the hypothalamic releasing hormone (squares), its path in the blood to the anterior pituitary gland, and then the release of the pituitary hormone (triangles) into the general circulation. Follow the delivery of the pituitary hormone to an endocrine gland that releases a hormone (circles) that travels through the blood to its target cell, which produces the biological effect initiated in the hypothalamus. Color the multiple feedback loops that regulate hormone release by relaying information related to the effects of the particular hormone back to both the hypothalamus and the pituitary gland.

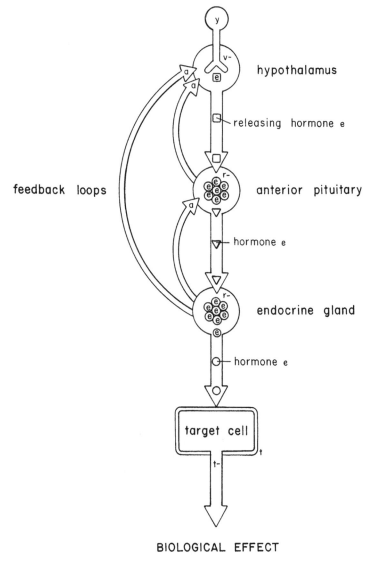

Growth hormone

The secretion of growth hormone into the blood by the anterior pitutitary gland is regulated by growth hormone–releasing (GHRH) and inhibiting (GHIH) hormones secreted by the hypothalamus (Figure 7.9). Continuous exercise stimulates the release of growth hormone; the amount by which blood levels of growth hormone rise under these conditions is directly related to the intensity and the duration of the exercise. Hypoglycemia (lower than normal blood glucose concentration), trauma, and sleep also stimulate the release of growth hormone. Growth hormone mobilizes fuels, promotes tissue growth, and is instrumental in the development of stature during childhood and adolescence.

The fuel-mobilizing effects of growth hormone include higher rates of lipolysis in adipose tissue (breakdown of stored triglyceride to glycerol plus three fatty acids, Figure 2.30) and higher rates of gluconeogenesis in liver (synthesis of glucose from noncarbohydrate sources, Figure 2.26). Thus, the release of growth hormone during exercise increases the availability of glucose and free fatty acids to serve as fuels for exercising muscles.

Growth hormone promotes tissue growth because it stimulates liver, muscle, and kidney cells to release substances called *somatomedins* (also called insulin-like growth factors, or IGFs) into the blood; somatomedins promote cell proliferation and protein synthesis. This mechanism of growth hormone action involves the control of gene transcription, which leads to the synthesis of proteins. For this reason, the effects of growth hormone on tissue development are slow in onset and long in duration.

Thyroid hormone

The thyroid gland produces triiodothyronine (T_3) and thyroxine (T_4), which are forms of thyroid hormone (Figure 7.11). They are small iodine-containing compounds derived from the amino acid tyrosine; T_3 contains three iodine atoms and T_4 contains four (Figure 7.12). Both forms of thyroid hormone are released into the blood. A fraction of each form is carried by the protein thyroid-binding globulin (TBG); the remaining unbound or "free" fraction can enter a cell. Once inside a target cell, T_4 is converted to the active form, which is T_3.

Figure 7.11 Thyroid gland. Color the cross sections of the follicles that comprise the thyroid gland and the capillaries that are outside of them. The lumen of each follicle contains a gel-like matrix (or colloid) into which the thyroid cells secrete iodine that was taken up from the blood. Note that thyroid hormone, which is formed in the matrix, passes through the thyroid cells, into the capillaries, and ultimately enters the general circulation to reach its target cells.

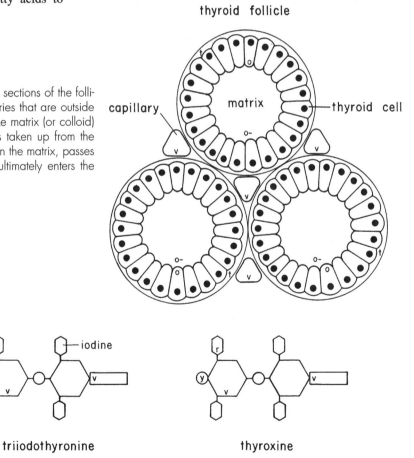

Figure 7.12 Thyroid hormone. Color the molecule of the amino acid tyrosine (left panel), noting that it is made up of a hydroxyl group (circle), a benzene ring (hexagon), and a rectangle that represents the rest of the amino acid. Note that hydrogen atoms are not shown in this simplified diagram. Color the molecules of triiodothyronine (T_3, middle panel) and thyroxine (T_4, right panel), which are forms of thyroid hormone. Color and count the iodine atoms (elongated hexagons) in each. Compare the structures of these thyroid hormones with that of tyrosine, from which they were synthesized.

chapter **seven**

The secretion of thyroid hormone is regulated by thyroid-stimulating hormone (TSH), released by the anterior pituitary gland (Figure 7.9). The secretion of TSH is controlled by thyroid-releasing hormone (TRH), which is released by the hypothalamus during exercise or in response to changes in the external environment. For example, chronic exposure to a cold environment can lead to increased secretion of thyroid hormone. Thyroid hormone increases resting metabolic rate (RMR), probably through its ability to increase the size and activity of mitochondria, and it can elevate resting heart rate and cardiac output.

The mechanism of thyroid hormone action involves the control of gene transcription, which leads to the synthesis of enzymes that regulate metabolic pathways. For this reason, the effects of thyroid hormone are slow in onset (at least six hours) and of very long duration (weeks), well beyond the period of physical activity during which its release was stimulated.

Adrenocorticotropic hormone

Adrenocorticotropic hormone (ACTH) is a protein secreted by the anterior pituitary gland into the blood in response to stimulation by its hypothalamic releasing hormone [corticotropin-releasing hormone (CRH), Figure 7.9]. CRH is secreted both in a diurnal (daily) pattern and in response to stress, as occurs during prolonged or intense physical activity. For this reason, blood levels of ACTH and the hormones whose release it stimulates do not rise during physical activity that does not attain a sufficient intensity or duration.

ACTH acts by way of the second messenger mechanism; its main target tissue is the adrenal cortex, which is the outer region of the adrenal gland (Figure 7.13). The adrenal cortex produces several types of steroid hormones from cholesterol (Figure 7.4), including glucocorticoids, mineralocorticoids, and androgens. Glucocorticoids promote fuel mobilization and suppress immune function; mineralocorticoids regulate body fluid composition.

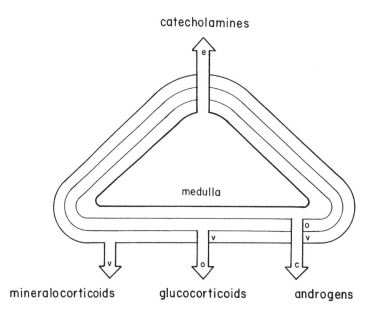

Figure 7.13   Adrenal gland. Color the inside portion, or medulla, and the arrow representing its secretion of catecholamines (~80% epinephrine and ~20% norepinephrine, Figure 7.3). Color the outer portion, or cortex, and the arrows that represent its secretion of mineralocorticoids (primarily aldosterone), glucocorticoids (primarily cortisol), and androgens.

Glucocorticoids

Cortisol is the major glucocorticoid in humans; its secretion is stimulated by ACTH (Figure 7.9). Increased secretion of cortisol causes: (1) skeletal muscle to break down its protein and release amino acids into the blood; (2) adipose tissue to break down its stored triglycerides and release fatty acids and glycerol into the blood; and (3) liver to increase its production of glucose by the pathway of gluconeogenesis, from lac-tate, glycerol, and amino acids that have been released into the blood. Thus, glucocorticoids promote fuel mobilization during periods of physical or emotional stress.

The mechanism of glucocorticoid action involves the control of gene transcription, which leads to the synthesis of enzymes that regulate metabolic pathways. For this reason, the effect of cortisol on gluconeogenesis, for example, is slow in onset and long in duration (hours).

gray blue canary green black navy orange pink red tan violet white yellow azure   [+] and [−] mean use heavy and light pressure, respectively

Mineralocorticoids

Mineralocorticoids maintain normal concentrations of sodium (Na^+) and potassium (K^+) ions in extracellular fluid. Aldosterone is the major mineralocorticoid in humans. Its release is stimulated by: (1) a high potassium concentration in extracellular fluid; (2) a low sodium concentration in extracellular fluid; or (3) a higher blood level of ACTH.

Aldosterone increases the activity of the sodium–potassium pump in the walls of the kidney tubules; this causes more sodium to be transported from the kidney tubules into the blood and more potassium to be transported in the opposite direction, from the blood into the kidney tubules (Figure 7.14). In this way, aldosterone causes the kidney to excrete less sodium and more potassium in urine.

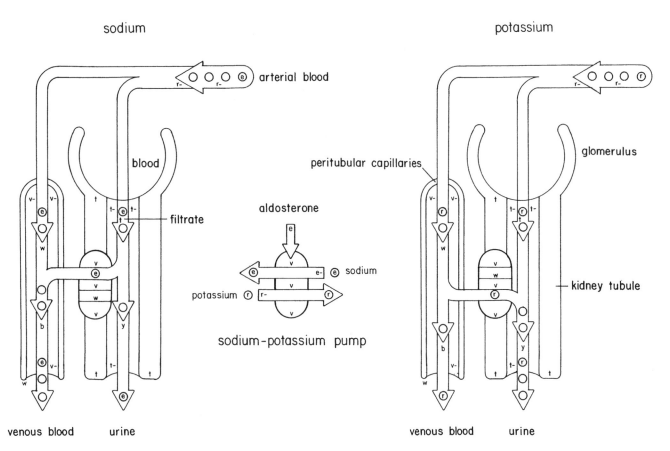

Figure 7.14 Mechanism of aldosterone action. Color the icon for the sodium–potassium pump, the arrows that depict the active transport of sodium and potassium in opposite directions, and the arrow that indicates that aldosterone increases the activity of the pump (middle panel). Color the arrow labeled arterial blood (left panel), noting that it contains four sodium ions (circles). Color the arrows that indicate the flow of blood to the kidney tubules and the peritubular capillaries; color these structures. Observe that two sodium ions enter the kidney tubules in the filtrate and two sodium ions enter the peritubular capillaries. Color the sodium–potassium pump in the wall of the kidney tubule and the transport of one sodium ion from the filtrate into the blood. Color the venous blood and urine, noting that three sodium ions are reabsorbed in venous blood and one sodium ion is excreted in urine. Repeat this process in the right panel, noting that the operation of the sodium–potassium pump results in the reabsorption of one potassium ion in venous blood and the excretion of three potassium ions in urine. These considerations explain how aldosterone causes the kidney to excrete less sodium (left panel) and more potassium (right panel) in urine.

The sodium–potassium pump in the initial portion of the kidney tubules (the proximal tubules and thick segment of the loop of Henle) actively reabsorb over 90% of the potassium that filters into the kidney tubules. Given that the dietary intake of potassium is normally more than sufficient to meet the needs of the body, the maintenance of the normal level of potassium in extracellular fluid (~4 mEq/L) requires that potassium be transported from the blood into the tubular fluid so that the kidney can excrete the excess potassium in the urine. The rate at which the cells that line the kidney tubules transport potassium from the blood into the tubular fluid is regulated by the concentration of aldosterone in the blood (Figure 7.14, right panel). High potassium concentrations in extracellular fluid stimulate the secretion of aldosterone, which, in turn, increases the activity of the sodium–potassium pump. As a result, more potassium is excreted in urine and the potassium concentration in extracellular fluid is reduced to the normal level. Thus, aldosterone plays an important role in the maintenance of normal concentrations of potassium in extracellular fluid (Figure 7.15).

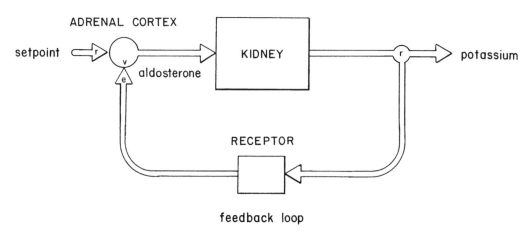

Figure 7.15   Block diagram of potassium control system. Color the block diagram of this negative feedback control system, identifying the setpoint (which signals the desired potassium concentration), the feedback loop (which signals the actual potassium concentration), and the comparator (which detects the difference between the desired and actual levels). Note that high concentrations of potassium stimulate aldosterone release so that more potassium is excreted, and the potassium concentration is restored to the normal level. Note also that low concentrations of potassium inhibit aldosterone release so that less potassium is excreted, and the potassium concentration is restored to the normal level. The operation of these mechanisms can be regarded as a negative feedback control system that maintains normal potassium concentrations in extracellular fluid.

Sweating during exercise causes a loss of both water and salts from the body, a condition that can lead to dehydration. Because sweat is a hypotonic solution, the loss of water is disproportionately greater than the concomitant loss of salt. Aldosterone released during exercise increases sodium reabsorption in the kidney tubules; this reduces the amount of sodium that is lost in urine (Figure 7.14, left panel). It also increases sodium reabsorption in the duct portions of the sweat glands (Figure 8.22); this reduces the amount of sodium that is lost in sweat. Thus, aldosterone conserves sodium by decreasing the amount of sodium that is lost in urine and sweat.

Antidiuretic hormone

The posterior pituitary gland contains the terminals of neurons whose cell bodies reside in the hypothalamus (Figure 7.8). These nerve terminals secrete antidiuretic hormone (ADH, also called arginine-vasopressin), which is classified as a neurohormone, into the blood. ADH release is regulated by neural signals from osmoreceptors, which reside in the hypothalamus and respond to intracellular dehydration.

The normal sodium concentration of ~142 mEq/L in extracellular fluid is maintained through a balance between the thirst mechanism, which regulates water intake, and the osmoreceptor-ADH system, which regulates water output by the kidney. The thirst mechanism and the osmoreceptor-ADH mechanism employ osmoreceptors in the hypothalamus that are stimulated by: (1) a high concentration of sodium in extracellular fluid; (2) a high concentration of potassium in intracellular fluid; or (3) a low blood volume. Under these conditions, the neural output from the osmoreceptors stimulates the posterior pituitary gland to secrete ADH, which, in turn, increases the permeability of the kidney tubules (distal tubules and collecting ducts) to water (Figure 7.16). As a result, more water is reabsorbed from the kidney tubules into the blood; this dilutes the extracellular fluid and reduces the sodium concentration to the normal level. Thus, ADH plays important roles in the maintenance of normal concentrations of sodium in extracellular fluid (Figure 7.17) and the maintenance of normal body fluid volumes.

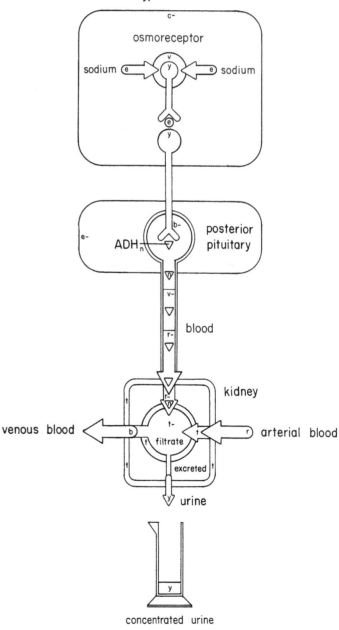

Figure 7.16 Mechanism of ADH action. Color the osmoreceptor, the arrows that indicate sodium concentration, and the hypothalamus. Color the hypothalamic neuron, the posterior pituitary gland, and the molecules of ADH (triangles) that are released into the blood. Observe that ADH is released in response to neural signals from hypothalamic osmoreceptors. Color the kidney and the arrows that depict arterial blood, venous blood, and urine. Color the circular icon, noting that ADH increases water reabsorption in the kidney. Finally, color the small volume of concentrated urine contained in the graduated cylinder.

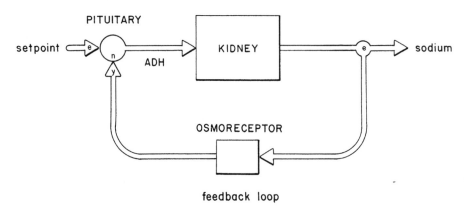

PITUITARY

setpoint — e / n / y — ADH → KIDNEY — e → sodium

OSMORECEPTOR

feedback loop

Figure 7.17   Block diagram of sodium control system. Color the block diagram of this negative feedback control system, identifying the setpoint (which specifies the desired sodium concentration), the feedback loop (which signals the actual sodium concentration), and the comparator (which detects the difference between the desired and actual levels). Note that high concentrations of sodium stimulate ADH release so that more water is reabsorbed, and the sodium concentration is restored to the normal level. Note also that low concentrations of sodium inhibit ADH release so that less water is reabsorbed, and the sodium concentration is restored to the normal level. The operation of these mechanisms can be regarded as a negative feedback control system that maintains normal concentrations of sodium in extracellular fluid.

Sweating during exercise causes loss of both salts and water from the body. Because sweat is a hypotonic solution, sweat loss can lead to a higher concentration of sodium in extracellular fluid (Figure 8.23) and a lower blood volume, conditions that stimulate osmoreceptors. The increased release of ADH during strenuous exercise (Figure 7.18) enables the kidney to reabsorb more water into the blood and therefore to excrete less water in urine; this increased fluid retention by the kidney results in a smaller volume of more concentrated urine (Figure 7.16). Thus, ADH release during exercise helps maintain normal levels of sodium in extracellular fluid and helps preserve blood volume; this latter factor plays a role in the regulation of cardiac output and the control of body temperature during exercise (Figure 8.24).

PERCENT INCREASE

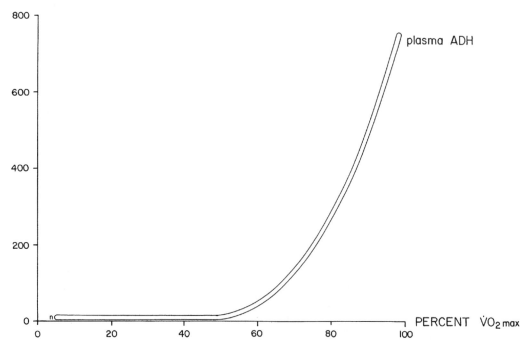

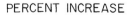

Figure 7.18   Effect of exercise intensity on ADH secretion. Color the line that plots plasma levels of ADH (percent increase above baseline) against oxygen consumption (percent $\dot{V}O_2max$), a measure of exercise intensity. Observe that blood levels of ADH remain low over the range from rest to moderate exercise and increase dramatically over the range from moderate to strenuous exercise. These findings demonstrate that ADH release varies with exercise intensity. Modified from V.A. Coventino et al. *J Appl Physiol* 54: 508, 1983.

Catecholamines

Catecholamines are a class of compounds that includes epinephrine and norepinephrine; they are produced by modification of the amino acid tyrosine (Figure 7.3). Catecholamines are released by the adrenal medulla, which is functionally part of the sympathetic nervous system (Figure 7.13). For this reason, increased activity of the sympathetic nervous system during exercise results in increased release of catecholamines. The adrenal medulla secretes epinephrine and, to a lesser extent, norepinephrine into the blood (~80% epinephrine, ~20% norepinephrine), whereas sympathetic adrenergic nerve fibers release norepinephrine at their axon terminals in cardiac muscle, smooth muscle, and glands (Figure 4.9). Because catecholamines act by way of the second messenger mechanism, their effects are immediate and persist only as long as catecholamine levels remain elevated.

Cardiac effects of catecholamines include increased heart rate (chronotropic effects) and myocardial contractility (inotropic effects), which improve the capability of the heart to pump blood. Systemic vascular effects of catecholamines include vasoconstriction, which helps redistribute cardiac output to exercising muscles, and venoconstriction, which promotes venous return by mobilizing blood contained in the veins (Figure 7.19, left panel). Respiratory effects of catecholamines include relaxation of bronchial smooth muscle in the airways of the lung (bronchodilation, Figure 6.32); this widens the airways, decreases airway resistance, and reduces the work of breathing (Figure 7.19, middle panel).

Metabolic effects of catecholamines include stimulation of glycogen breakdown (glycogenolysis) in both liver and muscle and stimulation of triglyceride breakdown (lipolysis) in adipose tissue. (Figure 7.19, right panel). Catecholamines also stimulate glucagon release by the α cells of the pancreas and inhibit insulin release by the β cells of the pancreas. Since the pathways of glycogenolysis in liver and lipolysis in adipose tissue are stimulated by glucagon but inhibited by insulin, the ability of catecholamines to increase glucagon release and decrease insulin release improves the efficacy with which catecholamines mobilize fuels.

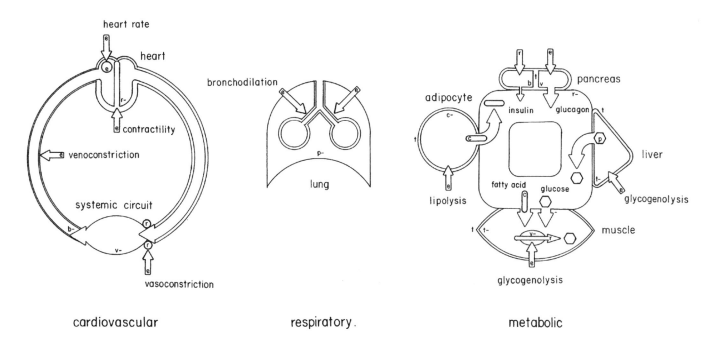

Figure 7.19   Effects of catecholamines. Color the panels from left to right. Note that cardiovascular effects of catecholamines include increased heart rate and myocardial contractility coupled with vasoconstriction and venoconstriction in the systemic circulation (left panel) (Figure 5.40). Observe that respiratory effects of catecholamines include bronchodilation (middle panel) (Figure 6.32). Observe also that metabolic effects of catecholamines include the breakdown of glycogen in liver and muscle, the breakdown of triglycerides in adipose tissue, and the modulation of pancreatic hormone release (right panel). These latter effects of catecholamines increase the availability of glucose and fatty acids to serve as fuels for exercising muscles.

Androgens and estrogens

Testosterone, which is the primary male sex hormone or androgen, is a steroid synthesized by the Leydig cells of the testis. In addition to its roles in the production of sperm and the development of secondary sexual characteristics, testosterone promotes protein synthesis in muscle and other tissues. Because testosterone increases muscle mass, men tend to have a larger muscle mass than do women.

Plasma levels of testosterone may increase during resistance exercise, such as weight lifting, and during moderate-intensity endurance exercise. Conversely, plasma levels of testosterone may decrease during prolonged exercise, such as marathon running.

Estrogens are a family of steroid hormones synthesized mainly in the ovaries and the placenta. Estrogens promote anabolism in bone and reproductive organs as well as storage of fat in certain depots of adipose tissue. Estradiol (17β-estradiol), which is the primary estrogen, is formed in adipose tissue from other steroids, including testosterone, in both men and women. Exercise does not appear to have any appreciable effect on the secretion of estrogens.

Pancreatic hormones

The pancreas is both an exocrine gland (secreting to the outside of the body) and an endocrine gland (secreting into the blood). The exocrine cells of the pancreas secrete digestive enzymes into the pancreatic duct, through which the enzymes enter the lumen of the intestine where they digest food. The endocrine cells of the pancreas make up a small portion of the gland (<5%). They consist of clusters of 100 to 1000 cells that form the islets of Langerhans, which are dispersed throughout the organ (Figure 7.20). Within the islets are the α cells, which secrete the hormone glucagon, and the β cells, which secrete the hormone insulin.

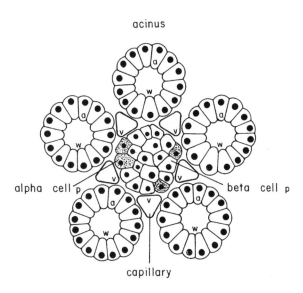

acinus

alpha cell p

beta cell p

capillary

Figure 7.20 Pancreatic islets. Color the cross sections of the clusters of exocrine cells, which are arranged as an acinus, and note the central lumen into which the cells secrete their digestive enzymes. Color the cluster of cells in the center of the figure; this represents an islet of Langerhans. The alpha cells (shaded) produce glucagon, and the beta cells (unshaded) produce insulin. Finally, color the cross-sections of capillaries through which insulin and glucagon ultimately enter the general circulation.

Insulin

Insulin is the primary anabolic hormone in the body; it promotes the storage of glucose and fat and the synthesis of protein. Insulin is secreted by the β cells of the pancreas in response to higher than normal blood levels of glucose (hyperglycemia), to gastrointestinal hormones involved in the regulation of digestion, and to parasympathetic stimulation, as occurs during eating.

Insulin removes glucose from the blood by increasing the rate at which glucose is taken up by skeletal muscle and adipose tissue. Insulin also increases the rate of glycogen synthesis (glycogenesis) in liver and muscle and decreases the rate of glycogen breakdown (glycogenolysis) in liver and muscle (Figure 7.21). All of these actions lower plasma glucose concentration, and thereby remove the stimulus for insulin secretion (Figure 7.22). Glucose uptake in muscle is accomplished by facilitated diffusion through the action of a glucose transport protein called *GLUT4* in the muscle cell membrane. Insulin stimulates the transfer of more of this transport protein to the cell membrane (Figure 7.23, middle panel), resulting in the uptake of more glucose by muscle when blood levels of insulin are high, as occurs in the fed state.

Insulin also stimulates the activity of the enzyme *lipoprotein lipase,* which increases the uptake of fatty acids from lipoprotein particles into adipocytes (Figure 2.32). Since glycerol is produced in adipocytes from glucose, and since glucose uptake by adipocytes is stimulated by insulin, insulin increases the availability of both components (fatty acids and glycerol) that are needed for the synthesis of triglycerides (Figure 2.30).

Figure 7.21 Effects of hormones on blood glucose levels. For each panel, color the cell membrane and the molecules of glycogen, glucose, and pyruvate within each liver cell, and the molecule of glucose outside the cell. Color the arrows within the cell, noting which reactions are catabolic and which reactions are anabolic. Color the arrows that show glucose entering or leaving each liver cell. Examine each panel, noting that insulin causes the liver to remove glucose from the blood while glucagon, epinephrine, and cortisol cause the liver to add glucose to the blood. For these reasons, insulin can be regarded as a fuel-storing hormone, whereas glucagon, epinephrine, and cortisol can be regarded as fuel-mobilizing hormones.

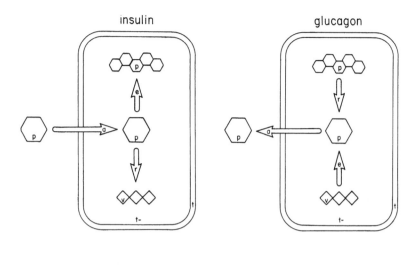

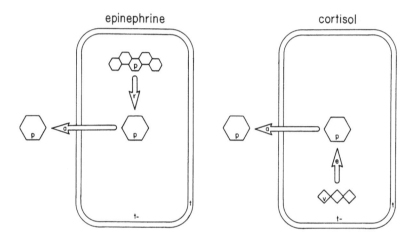

Figure 7.22 Block diagram of glucose control system. Beginning at the left, color the alpha cells that release glucagon, and the beta cells that release insulin. Color the arrows representing their effects on blood glucose concentration; glucagon stimulates the liver to release glucose into the blood, and insulin stimulates muscle, liver and adipose tissue to remove glucose from the blood. Color the feedback loops to the alpha and beta cells and the glucose setpoint, to which actual blood glucose levels are compared. When actual blood glucose levels are higher than the setpoint, more insulin is secreted in order to restore the normal concentration of blood glucose. When actual blood glucose levels are lower than the setpoint, more glucagon is secreted in order to restore the normal concentration of blood glucose. The operation of these mechanisms can be regarded as a negative feedback control system that maintains normal concentrations of glucose in blood.

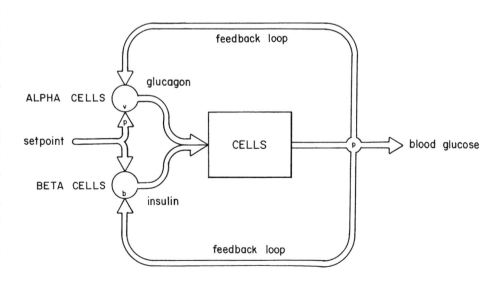

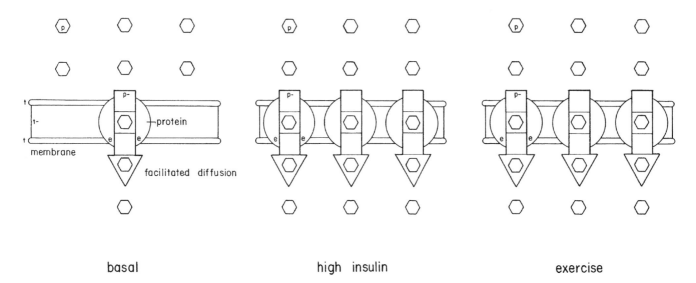

basal   high insulin   exercise

Figure 7.23   Glucose uptake by skeletal muscle. Color the molecules of glucose outside of the muscle cells (in the blood). Color the membrane, the arrow that indicates the basal uptake of glucose by facilitated diffusion, and the transport protein (GLUT4) that spans the muscle membrane (left panel). Color and compare these structures under high insulin conditions (middle panel), noting that insulin causes more molecules of GLUT4 to appear in the membrane and more glucose to enter the cell. Color and compare these structures under exercise conditions (right panel), noting that exercise also causes more molecules of GLUT4 to appear in the membrane and more glucose to enter the cell; this migration of glucose transporters to the cell membrane during exercise is stimulated by Ca^{2+} released during excitation–contraction coupling (Figure 4.14). Thus, exercise itself stimulates the uptake of glucose by muscle cells.

Insulin also inhibits lipolysis in adipose tissue. Thus, insulin promotes the storage of triglyceride in adipose tissue.

Insulin increases the transport of amino acids into tissues, as well as their incorporation into protein. Insulin is also necessary for other hormones, such as growth hormone, to exert their anabolic effects. Thus, insulin not only promotes the uptake and storage of fuels, but also inhibits the mobilization of stored fuels. These actions of insulin decrease the blood levels of glucose, fatty acids, and amino acids.

Glucagon

Glucagon is considered to be a catabolic hormone because it promotes the mobilization of fuels and increases the blood levels of glucose and free fatty acids (Figure 7.21). Glucagon is secreted by the α cells in response to lower than normal blood levels of glucose (hypoglycemia) or by sympathetic stimulation, as occurs during exercise.

Glucagon stimulates the liver to break down its glycogen into glucose (glycogenolysis), and to synthesize new glucose from noncarbohydrate sources (gluconeogenesis). These effects of glucagon enable the liver to release more glucose into the blood, thereby raising the blood level of glucose; this restoration of normal levels of blood glucose inhibits release of glucagon (Figure 7.22). Glucagon also stimulates lipolysis in adipose tissue; this increases the availability of fatty acids and glycerol to serve as fuels.

Effect of exercise on secretion of metabolic hormones

Given that the fuel needs of cardiac and skeletal muscle increase markedly during exercise, it is appropriate that the endocrine system stimulates the mobilization of fuels and inhibits the storage of fuels during exercise. The endocrine response to exercise is characterized by increased secretion of the fuel-mobilizing hormones, including glucagon, epinephrine, cortisol, and growth hormone (Figure 7.7), and decreased secretion of the fuel-storing hormone, insulin. The suppression of insulin release during exercise also inhibits the reincorporation of breakdown products of catabolic reactions into their stored forms; this results in greater availability of glucose and fatty acids to serve as fuels for exercising muscles.

Endocrine regulation of glycogenolysis and gluconeogenesis

Catecholamines released during exercise stimulate glycogenolysis in both liver and muscle, whereas glucagon stimulates glycogenolysis in liver but not muscle. Glucose derived from glycogen breakdown in liver can serve as a source of blood glucose, because it can leave the cell and enter the blood. In contrast, glucose derived from glycogen breakdown in muscle can serve as a substrate for glycolysis in muscle but not as a source of blood glucose, because it cannot leave the muscle cell (Figure 2.13). The breakdown of muscle glycogen is also stimulated by calcium ions released during the process of excitation–contraction coupling (Figure 4.14). In other words, muscle contraction itself also stimulates glycogenolysis.

Glucagon and growth hormone released during exercise stimulate gluconeogenesis in liver. Gluconeogenesis is also stimulated by cortisol if the exercise is sufficiently intense or prolonged to elicit its release (Figure 7.21). The pathways of glycogenolysis and gluconeogenesis represent two different mechanisms whereby the liver can supply glucose to the blood during exercise. The relative contribution of each pathway to the total amount of glucose formed by the liver varies with the duration of exercise. Glycogenolysis is more important in short-duration exercise, whereas gluconeogenesis becomes progressively more important during long-duration exercise and during the recovery period.

Endocrine regulation of lipolysis

Catecholamines, glucagon, and growth hormone released during exercise stimulate lipolysis in adipose tissue. Lipolysis is also stimulated by cortisol when the exercise is sufficiently stressful or prolonged. The breakdown of stored triglyceride and the subsequent release of glycerol and free fatty acids into the blood occurs early in exercise and becomes greater as the

duration of exercise increases. For this reason, long-duration exercises promote fat utilization (Figure 3.22).

Catecholamines increase the availability of fatty acids to serve as fuel for muscle by three different mechanisms: (1) they stimulate lipolysis in adipose tissue, causing the release of free fatty acids into the blood (Figure 7.19); (2) they promote the uptake of circulating triglycerides by muscle; the fatty acids obtained from the breakdown of triglyceride in lipoprotein particles enter the muscle fiber where they can serve as fuel for muscle contraction (Figure 2.33); and (3) they stimulate lipolysis of the triglyceride stored in muscle, also making fatty acids available to serve as fuel for muscle contraction.

Maintenance of plasma glucose levels during exercise

The concentration of glucose in the blood is maintained at a reasonably constant level of ~ 80 ± 20 mg/dL in the non-fed state. A transient rise in blood glucose occurs during the period in which carbohydrate from a meal is absorbed; this normally returns to the baseline level after about an hour (Figure 7.24). Because the central nervous system (CNS) normally uses only glucose as a fuel, hypoglycemia (plasma glucose

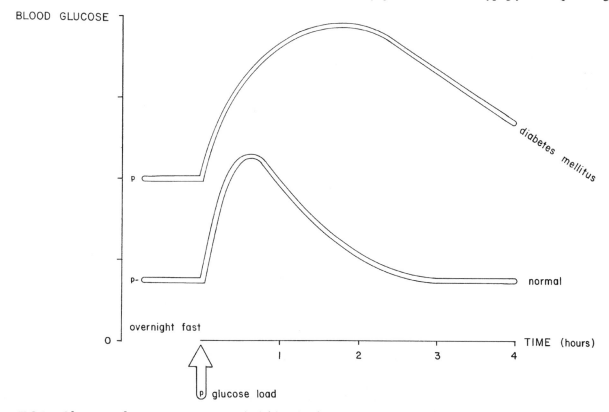

Figure 7.24 Glucose tolerance test. Begin at the left by identifying the baseline level of blood glucose for both conditions; color the arrow labeled glucose load that indicates the oral administration of a concentrated solution of glucose. Color the two lines that show the changes in blood glucose concentration over time (in hr). Note that individuals with diabetes mellitus show a higher baseline level of glucose (fasting hyperglycemia), a higher peak level of glucose, and a slower return to baseline values than individuals with normal control of blood glucose.

concentration <60 mg/dL) is a condition that can impair CNS function, resulting in fatigue, disorientation, and even coma. Therefore, the maintenance of normal levels of blood glucose is crucial to the proper function of the nervous system.

During exercise, muscle increases its utilization of glucose, both by breaking down its own stores of glycogen and by taking up more glucose from the blood. Because the prevail-

ing level of blood glucose reflects the balance between the rate at which glucose is added to the blood and the rate at which glucose is removed from the blood, the maintenance of normal levels of blood glucose during exercise requires that the higher rates of glucose uptake by exercising muscles be matched by correspondingly higher rates of glucose replenishment by the liver (Figure 7.25).

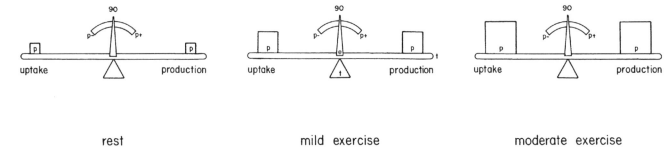

Figure 7.25   Maintenance of plasma glucose levels during exercise. Color the balance, the pointer, and the glucose scale (in mg/dL). For each panel, color and compare the rectangles that depict the rate at which glucose is removed from the blood (left side of balance) and the rate at which glucose is added to the blood (right side of balance). Observe that glucose removal increases with increasing exercise intensity and that these increases in glucose removal are matched exactly by corresponding increases in glucose production by the liver. These considerations explain why blood glucose levels remain essentially constant over the range from rest (left panel) to moderate exercise (right panel). However, glucose production may fail to keep pace with glucose removal during prolonged, strenuous exercise; this would result in a decline in plasma glucose levels.

Overview of endocrine regulation of fuel flux during exercise

Sources of blood glucose during exercise include glucose supplied by the liver (due to the action of its metabolic pathways) and glucose supplied by the gastrointestinal system (due to the ingestion of carbohydrates). The two metabolic pathways used by the liver to replenish blood glucose during exercise are glycogenolysis (the breakdown of liver glycogen) and gluconeogenesis (the synthesis of new glucose from noncarbohydrate sources) (Figure 7.26). The activity of these glucose-producing pathways are stimulated by catabolic hormones (catecholamines, glucagon, and cortisol) that are released during exercise (Figures 7.7 and 7.21).

The higher blood levels of glycerol (released during the breakdown of triglyceride in adipose tissue) and lactate (released mainly by skeletal muscle) during exercise provide more substrate for the pathway of gluconeogenesis in the liver (Figure 2.24). Catabolic hormones also stimulate the breakdown of triglyceride in adipose tissue and increase the quantity of free fatty acids and glycerol in the blood. Because increased utilization of fatty acids results in decreased utilization of glucose, higher blood levels of fatty acids have a glucose-sparing effect that helps preserve normal levels of blood glucose during exercise.

Therefore, both through provision of more glucose via glycogenolysis and gluconeogenesis, and through provision of fatty acids as an alternative fuel to glucose, plasma glucose levels are maintained within normal limits in the face of increased glucose uptake by exercising muscles; this enables individuals to sustain their physical performance and mental clarity during exercise.

Insulin-independent uptake of glucose by skeletal muscle

The uptake of glucose by muscle is dependent on insulin at rest but not during exercise. Although the suppression of insulin release during exercise reduces the uptake of glucose by most tissues, low blood levels of insulin do not limit glucose uptake in exercising muscles. The explanation for this phenomenon is that the higher intracellular Ca^{2+} concentration that occurs during muscle contraction causes more GLUT4 to be transferred to the muscle cell membrane; this mechanism does not involve insulin (Figure 7.23, right panel). Therefore, exercise itself stimulates the transport of glucose into muscle cells.

Exercise and diabetes mellitus

People with *diabetes mellitus,* a disease in which blood levels of glucose are higher than normal (hyperglycemia, Figure 7.24), can take advantage of the insulin-independent uptake

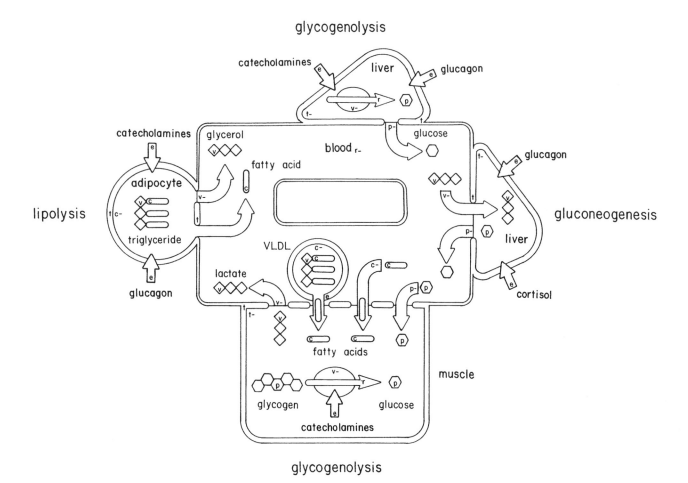

glycogenolysis

Figure 7.26   Endocrine regulation of fuel flux during exercise. Color the liver icon labeled glycogenolysis (at top), the arrows and enzyme of the reaction, and the arrows that indicate that glycogen breakdown in liver is stimulated by catecholamines and glucagon. Color the glucose molecule that is released into the blood. Color the liver icon labeled gluconeogenesis (at right), the arrow that indicates the uptake of 3-carbon substrates, and the arrows that indicate that the synthesis of glucose in liver is stimulated by glucagon and cortisol. Color the glucose molecule that is released into the blood. Color the adipocyte icon (at left), its internal triglyceride molecule, and the arrows that indicate that triglyceride breakdown (lipolysis) is stimulated by catecholamines and glucagon. Color the glycerol and fatty acid molecules that are released into the blood. Color the muscle cell (at bottom), the fuels that enter it from the blood (fatty acids from triglyceride in VLDL particles, free fatty acids, and glucose), and the lactate that leaves the muscle cell and enters the blood. Color the reaction in which catecholamines stimulate the breakdown of muscle glycogen, noting that the glucose produced remains in the muscle cell. Observe that these fuel-mobilizing hormones regulate the rates of metabolic pathways to provide an adequate supply of fuels for muscle contraction and to maintain adequate levels of blood glucose for proper function of the nervous system.

of glucose by muscle by using exercise as a means to lower their blood glucose levels. In these persons, moderate physical activity can increase glucose uptake by muscle and thereby lower plasma glucose to a more normal level. However, exercise also stimulates the release of fuel-mobilizing hormones that increase glucose output from the liver, an effect that could worsen hyperglycemia in individuals whose diabetes is not well-controlled. For these reasons, it is prudent for people with diabetes to monitor their blood glucose levels before, during, and after physical activity. Another relevant consideration is that the normal drop in insulin levels brought about by exercise will not occur in persons who receive insulin by injection. In these persons, care must be taken to adjust the dose of insulin and intake of carbohydrate

before the activity in order to prevent plasma glucose from falling to lower than normal levels (hypoglycemia) during exercise.

Because skeletal muscle becomes more sensitive to insulin after exercise, muscles will take up and store more glucose at any given insulin level during the postexercise period. This property of muscle can be utilized in the prevention and treatment of type 2 diabetes mellitus, a form of the disease characterized by poor tissue response to insulin. Regular mild to moderate exercise improves muscle's ability to remove glucose from the blood. Since the effect on muscle may continue long after the activity period, daily exercise helps maintain post-meal levels of plasma glucose within the normal range.

Postexercise endocrine effects

The effects of catecholamines and glucagon diminish rapidly in the postexercise period (when the levels of these hormones decrease), because they exert their effects through a second messenger mechanism. The effects of cortisol, growth hormone, thyroid hormone, and testosterone may persist for hours after the cessation of exercise because the effects of these hormones are mediated by the synthesis of enzymes that regulate the rates of metabolic pathways.

Growth hormone and testosterone, if sufficiently increased by exercise, can build muscle by stimulating protein synthesis. The effects of these hormones on protein synthesis is potentiated by high blood levels of insulin that stimulate the transport of amino acids into muscle as well as their incorporation into protein. For these reasons, muscle anabolism is best served by consumption of a high carbohydrate and protein meal immediately after an exercise session; this will stimulate insulin production and increase the availability of amino acids while blood levels of growth hormone and testosterone are still elevated.

chapter **eight**
temperature regulation

The prevailing level of body temperature reflects a balance between the rate at which heat is added to the body and the rate at which heat is removed from the body (Figure 8.1); body temperature rises when heat gain exceeds heat loss and falls when heat loss exceeds heat gain (Figure 8.2).

Deep body (core) temperature is maintained at an essentially constant level ($37 \pm 1°C$) by neural and hormonal mechanisms that cause the body to gain heat when *core temperature* falls below $37°C$, as can occur in a cold environment, and to lose heat when core temperature rises above $37°C$, as can occur during vigorous exercise.

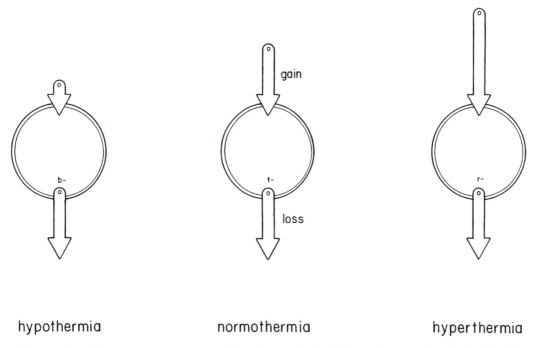

hypothermia   normothermia   hyperthermia

Figure 8.1   Effect of heat flux on temperature. Color the panels from left to right, noting that the length of the top arrow indicates the rate of heat gain and that the length of the bottom arrow indicates the concomitant rate of heat loss. Observe that hypothermia is a condition in which heat gain is smaller than heat loss (left panel), normothermia is condition in which heat gain equals heat loss (middle panel), and hyperthermia is a condition in which heat gain is larger than heat loss (right panel).

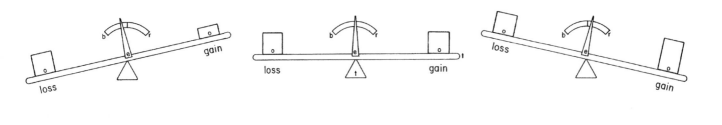

hypothermia   normothermia   hyperthermia

Figure 8.2   Principles of temperature regulation. Color the balance, the pointer, and the temperature scale. For each panel, color and compare the rectangles that depict the rate at which heat is lost from the body (left side of balance) and the rate at which heat is gained by the body (right side of balance). Observe that hypothermia occurs when heat loss exceeds heat gain (left panel), normothermia occurs when heat loss equals heat gain (middle panel), and hyperthermia occurs when heat gain exceeds heat loss (right panel). Body temperatures that range from 36.1 to 37.8°C are considered to be within normal limits. Compare this figure with Figure 8.1.

Heat production

Heat gain is due to the combined effects of heat production by the body (internal heat) and heat absorption from the environment (external heat) (Figure 8.3).

The heat produced by the body is a byproduct of chemical reactions that transform bond energy into work and heat (Figure 1.2). For example, because the efficiency of muscle contraction is 20% to 30%, approximately 70% to 80% of the energy released during the breakdown of ATP into ADP and Pi will be dissipated as heat (Figure 1.12). Heat production therefore varies with physical activity: involuntary physical activity (shivering) can increase heat production to three to five times the resting level, and voluntary physical activity (exercise) can increase heat production to twenty to twenty-five times the resting level (Figure 8.4).

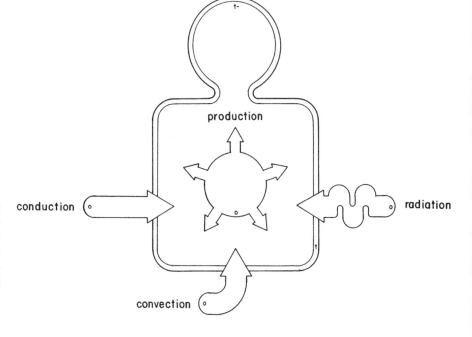

Figure 8.3 Mechanisms of heat gain. Color the diagram, noting that heat gain is due to the combined effects of heat production (internal heat) and heat absorption (external heat). Note also that heat absorption represents the combined effects of conduction (straight arrow), convection (curved arrow), and radiation (wavy arrow).

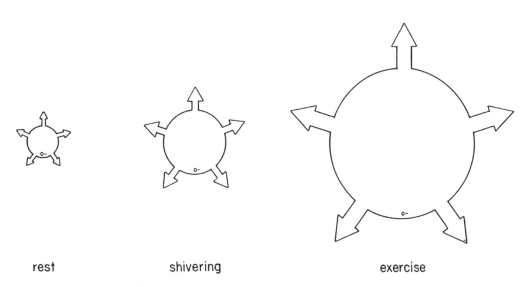

rest   shivering   exercise

Figure 8.4 Effect of physical activity on heat production. Color the panels from left to right, noting that the area of each symbol is a quantitative measure of heat production. Observe that shivering can increase metabolic heat production to three to five times the resting (basal) level and that exercise can increase metabolic heat production to twenty to twenty-five times the resting level.

Heat production also varies with blood levels of *thermogenic hormones* that generate heat by increasing metabolic rate (nonshivering thermogenesis). These hormones include catecholamines released by the adrenal gland in response to increased sympathetic stimulation and thyroid hormone released by the thyroid gland in response to prolonged or repeated exposure to a cold environment; high blood levels of thyroid hormone can double resting metabolic rate.

Heat exchange between the body and the environment

Heat exchange between the body and environment occurs by four different processes: radiation, conduction, convection, and evaporation (Figure 8.5).

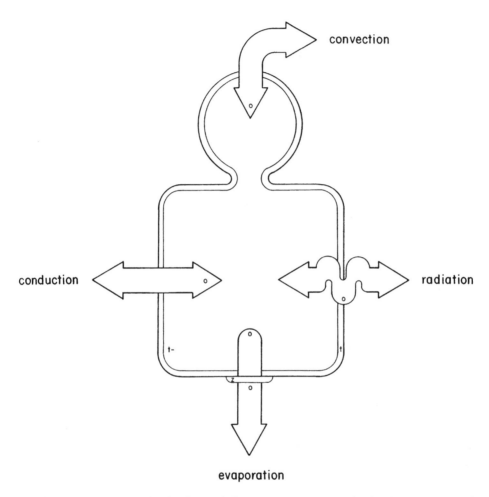

Figure 8.5 Heat exchange between the body and the environment. Color the diagram, noting that heat exchange between the body and environment occurs by four different processes, i.e., conduction, convection, radiation, and evaporation. Observe that conduction, convection, and radiation are mechanisms whereby the body can lose heat (arrowhead leaving body) or gain heat (arrowhead entering body), whereas evaporation is a mechanism whereby the body can lose heat (arrowhead leaving body).

Radiation

Radiation refers to a transfer of heat by infrared (a type of electromagnetic) waves that travel through the air from warmer to colder objects; radiation does not require molecular contact between objects.

Because radiant heat is transmitted from a region of higher temperature to one of lower temperature, radiation is said to occur down a temperature gradient (Figure 8.6). Radiation from the sun and from objects in the environment that are warmer than the skin causes the body to gain heat. Conversely, radiation from the skin to objects in the environment that are cooler than the skin causes the body to lose heat (Figure 8.7). Radiation is a major component of heat loss at rest, accounting for approximately 60% of the total heat loss at room temperature (21 to 25°C).

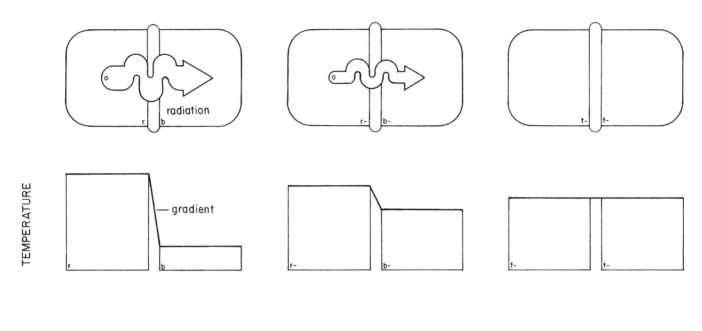

initial   intermediate   final

Figure 8.6   Effect of temperature gradient on radiation. Color the diagram from left to right, noting that the size of the arrow in each panel indicates the rate at which heat flows by radiation across the boundary between the left chamber and right chamber. Color the bar graphs below, noting that the height of each bar indicates the temperature in the chamber above it. Note that the magnitude of the temperature gradient can be visualized from the steepness of the line (labeled gradient) that connects the two bars. Observe that the flow of heat between the two chambers (size of arrow) is proportional to the temperature gradient (steepness of line connecting bars). Observe also that heat exchange ceases (no arrow) when the temperature gradient vanishes (horizontal line connecting bars), i.e., when the two chambers equilibrate at the same temperature (right panel). Because the flow of heat by radiation occurs from a region of higher temperature to one of lower temperature, radiation is a mechanism of heat loss when body temperature exceeds ambient temperature and a mechanism of heat gain when ambient temperature exceeds body temperature.

Figure 8.7   Radiation. Color the diagram, comparing the heat flow by radiation (size of arrow) with the temperatures of the objects. Note that heat flows by radiation from a region of higher temperature to one of lower temperature, and that the magnitude of heat flow between any two objects is directly related to the difference in temperature between them. At any given temperature gradient, black rough objects absorb a greater fraction of their radiation than do light shiny objects; over 90% of the radiant heat that strikes the skin is absorbed by the body.

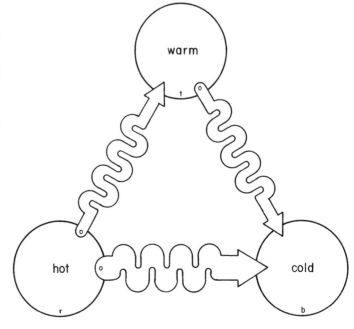

Conduction

Conduction refers to a direct transfer of heat from warmer to colder objects. In contrast to radiation, conduction requires molecular contact between objects.

Because conductive heat flows from a region of higher temperature to one of lower temperature, conduction is also said to occur down a temperature gradient (Figure 8.8). Temperature gradients, therefore, provide the driving force for heat transfer by both radiation and conduction. For this reason, ambient temperature influences the rate at which heat can be exchanged between the body and the environment by these processes.

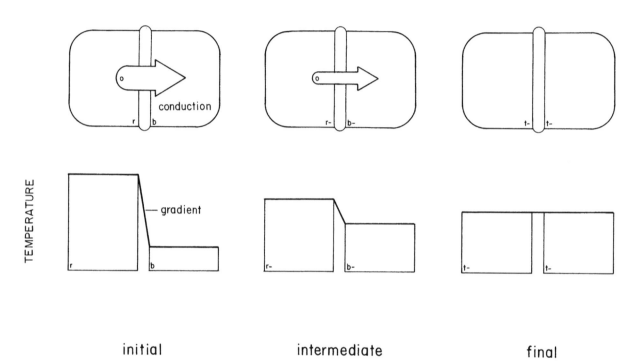

initial   intermediate   final

Figure 8.8   Effect of temperature gradient on conduction. Color the diagram from left to right, noting that the size of the arrow in each panel indicates the rate at which heat flows by conduction across the boundary between the left chamber and right chamber. Color the bar graphs below, noting that the height of each bar indicates the temperature in the chamber above it. Note that the magnitude of the temperature gradient can be visualized from the steepness of the line (labeled gradient) that connects the two bars. Observe that the flow of heat between the two chambers (size of arrow) is proportional to the temperature gradient (steepness of line connecting bars). Observe also that heat exchange ceases (no arrow) when the temperature gradient vanishes (horizontal line connecting bars), i.e., when the two chambers equilibrate at the same temperature (right panel). Because the flow of heat by conduction occurs from a region of higher temperature to one of lower temperature, conduction is a mechanism of heat loss when body temperature exceeds ambient temperature and a mechanism of heat gain when ambient temperature exceeds body temperature. Compare this figure with Fig-ure 8.6.

Conduction is a major component of heat transfer from the deep body tissues to the skin but a minor component of heat transfer from the skin to the environment. However, because the rate of conductive heat flow depends on both the magnitude of the temperature gradient and the thermal properties of the medium, conduction can become a significant component of heat loss in cold water because water is a better conductor of heat than is air (Figure 8.9).

Figure 8.9   Effect of medium on conduction. Color the panels from left to right, noting that the size of the arrow in each panel indicates the rate at which heat flows by conduction across the boundary between the left chamber and the right chamber. Color the bar graphs below, noting that the height of each bar indicates the temperature in the chamber above it. Observe that the rate of heat flow by conduction is greater in water (right panel) than in air (left panel) even though the magnitude of the temperature gradient (steepness of line labeled gradient) is the same in both conditions. Thus, heat flow by conduction depends on both the magnitude of the temperature gradient and the thermal properties of the medium. Because the thermal conductivity of water is approximately twenty-five times that of air, heat loss by conduction can be a significant factor in cold water.

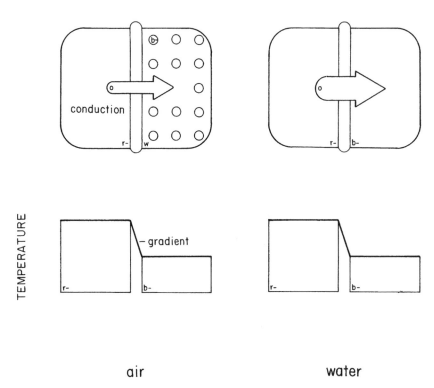

air   water

Convection

The effectiveness of heat loss by conduction depends on how rapidly warmed air or water molecules are removed from the body surface; this removal of warmed molecules helps main-

tain the temperature gradient. Thus, heat loss decreases when air movement *(convection)* is slow and increases when air movement is fast (Figure 8.10). For this reason, cycling at high speeds provides more convective cooling than does cycling at low speeds or running.

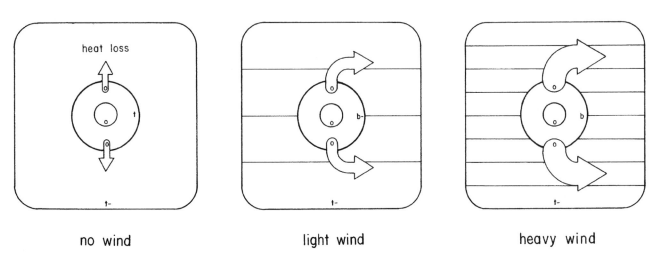

no wind   light wind   heavy wind

Figure 8.10   Convection. Color the panels from left to right, noting that the size of the arrows in each panel indicates the rate at which heat is lost by convection in each condition. Note also that the rate of heat production (size of small circle at center) and the prevailing environmental temperature are the same in all conditions. Observe that heat loss by convection increases with increasing wind velocity (indicated by density of horizontal lines).

The cooling effect of a particular wind speed is given by the *Wind Chill Index,* a measure of the temperature equivalent in the absence of convective heat loss (Figure 8.11). For exam-ple, because the body's rate of heat loss in 10°C in a 2.2 mph wind is the same as that in −10°C in still air, both conditions feel equally cold.

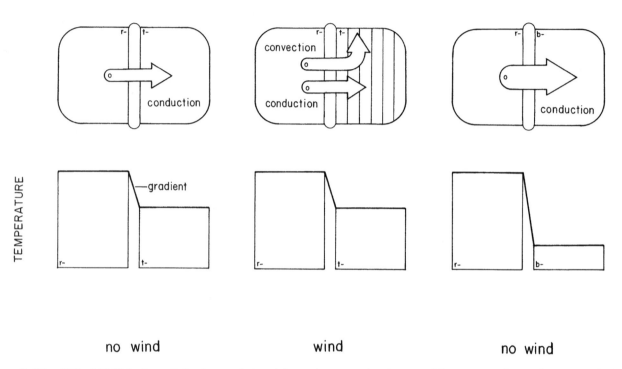

Figure 8.11   Wind Chill Index. Color the panels from left to right, noting that the size of the arrows indicates the rate at which heat flows across the boundary between the left chamber and right chamber. Color the bar graphs below, noting that the height of each bar indicates the temperature in the chamber above it. Note also that the magnitude of the temperature gradient can be visualized from the steepness of the line labeled gradient. Observe that the rate of heat loss is the same in the middle panel (small conduction arrow plus small convection arrow) and the right panel (large conduction arrow). For this reason, both conditions feel equally cold even though the tempera-ture gradient is smaller in the middle panel than in the right panel.

Evaporation

Evaporation occurs as a result of sweating and insensible water loss (which refers to water removed from the body in expired air and by diffusion through the skin).

The actual amount of heat removed from the body by evapo-ration (in kcal) is equal to the product of the amount of sweat that evaporates (in g) and the heat of vaporization of water, which specifies the amount of heat (in kcal) needed to change 1 g of water from the liquid phase to the vapor phase. Be-cause the *latent heat of vaporization* of water is 0.58 kcal/g,

580 kcal of heat are removed from the body for each liter of sweat that evaporates at the skin. Sweat that is wiped away or drips off the skin has no cooling effect on the body because it does not evaporate.

Evaporation is the major defense against overheating during exercise, and it is the only mechanism by which the body can lose heat when ambient temperature exceeds skin tempera-ture (Figure 8.5). Evaporation accounts for approximately 20% to 25% of the total heat loss at rest and approximately 80% of the total heat loss during strenuous exercise (Figure 8.12).

Figure 8.12 Evaporative heat loss. Color the diagram, noting that the areas of the rectangles are quantitative measures of heat loss. Observe that evaporation is a small portion of the total heat loss at rest (left panel) but a large component of total heat loss during exercise (right panel). Evaporation occurs as a result of sweating and insensible water loss, which refers to water lost in expired air (350 mL/day) and diffusion through the skin, but not to water lost in sweat, urine, and feces. Sweat evaporation becomes increasingly important with increasing exercise intensities.

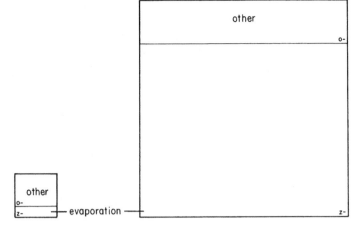

rest   exercise

Factors that influence evaporation

The driving force for evaporation of sweat is the amount by which the *vapor pressure* (PH$_2$O) at the body surface exceeds that of the surrounding air. Because vapor pressure is a function of both temperature and humidity, low ambient temperatures and relative humidities are factors that promote evaporation of sweat, whereas high ambient temperatures and relative humidi-

ties are factors that impede evaporation of sweat. For this reason, a vigorous exercise performed in a humid environment poses a greater risk of elevated core temperature (hyperthermia) than the same exercise performed in an arid environment at the same temperature. The *Heat Stress Index* provides a rating of the potential risk of heat injury associated with different combinations of temperature and humidity (Figure 8.13).

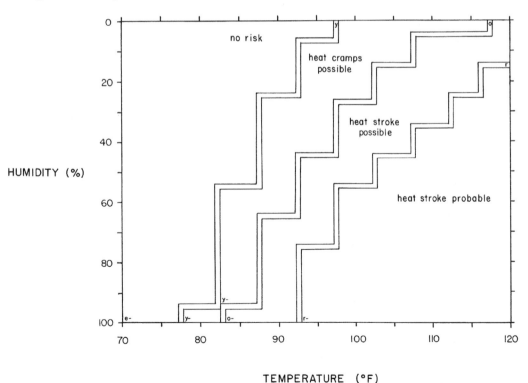

Figure 8.13 Heat Stress Index. Color the diagram, identifying the risks associated with different combinations of ambient temperature (°F, x-axis) and relative humidity (%, y-axis). Observe that higher levels of humidity increase the risk of heat injury at any given temperature. The relative humidity is determined by the ratio of the actual number of water molecules in ambient air compared with that carried if the air were fully saturated. In other words, the density of water molecules in air at 50% humidity is half that at 100% humidity.

Other factors that influence the rate at which sweat evaporates from the skin include the body surface area exposed to the environment (removal of clothing promotes evaporation) and the presence of convective air currents (air movement promotes evaporation).

Regulation of body temperature

Core temperature is maintained at an essentially constant level (37 ± 1°C) by the combined action of neural and hormonal mechanisms.

These mechanisms can be regarded as a negative feedback control system that causes the body to gain heat when core temperature falls below 37°C and, conversely, to lose heat when core temperature rises above 37°C. Heat gain is due to an increased rate of heat production coupled with a decreased rate of heat removal; heat loss is due to an increased rate of heat removal.

Room temperature control system

A common example of a negative feedback control system is a room temperature control system consisting of a thermostat, a furnace, and a thermometer (Figure 8.14). The thermostat compares the desired room temperature (indicated by the thermostat setting, or setpoint) with the actual room temperature (indicated by the thermometer) and uses the difference between the two readings (desired temperature minus actual temperature) to generate an error signal (Figure 8.15).

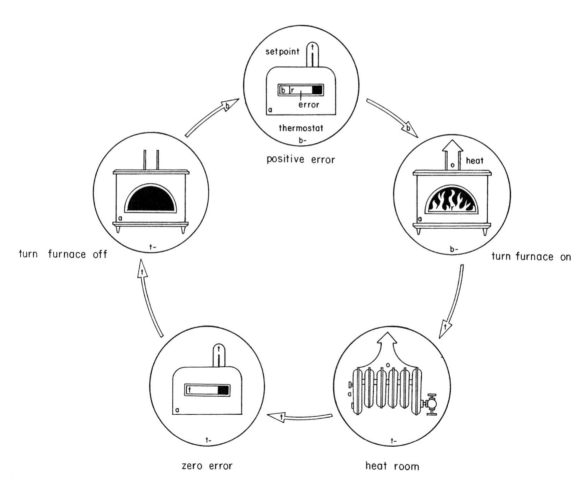

Figure 8.14   Room temperature control system. Begin by coloring the thermostat at the top. In this example, the cycle begins when the thermostat setpoint is suddenly moved to a higher setting. This generates a positive error signal that turns on the furnace and heats the room. When the room temperature rises to the point where it matches the new setpoint, the error signal becomes zero and the thermostat turns off the furnace. The cycle repeats whenever room temperature falls below the setpoint again.

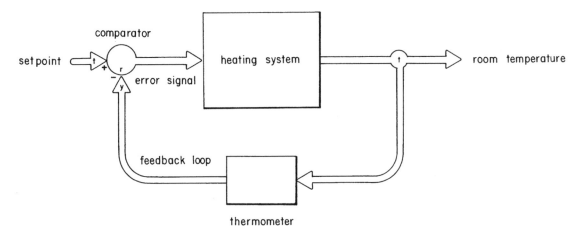

Figure 8.15 Block diagram of room temperature control system. Begin by coloring the arrow labeled setpoint and then work clockwise. By using the sign of the error signal to operate the furnace, this negative feedback control system automatically maintains room temperature at the level dictated by the setpoint. Compare this figure with Figure 8.14.

A salient feature of this configuration is that the sign (polarity) of the error signal is positive when the setpoint is higher than the actual temperature (the room is cooler than desired), and negative when the setpoint is lower than the actual temperature (the room is warmer than desired). In other words, a positive error signal means that room temperature should be raised and a negative error signal means that room temperature should be lowered. Thus, by using the sign of the error signal to operate the furnace switch, the system maintains room temperature at the desired level by automatically turning on the furnace when the room is too cold and turning it off when the room is too hot (Figure 8.14).

Body temperature control system

The body temperature control system works in a way that is similar to the room temperature control system described above. The components of the body temperature control system include thermoreceptors (analogous to the thermometer), a temperature regulatory center (the thermostat), and effector organs (the heating/cooling system) (Figure 8.16).

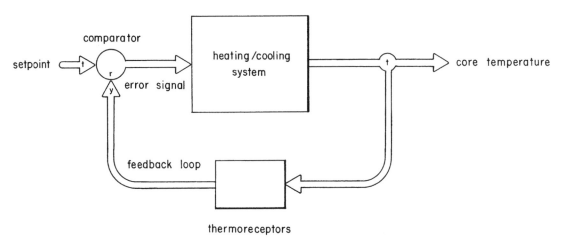

Figure 8.16 Block diagram of body temperature control system. Begin by coloring the arrow labeled setpoint and then work clockwise. By using the sign of the error signal to operate the heating/cooling system, this negative feedback control system automatically maintains body temperature at the level dictated by the setpoint. Compare this figure with Figure 8.15.

Thermoreceptors

Body temperature is monitored by *central thermoreceptors,* which detect core temperature, and *peripheral thermoreceptors,* which detect skin temperature.

Central thermoreceptors reside in the hypothalamus and detect the temperature of the blood perfusing the brain. Peripheral thermoreceptors are free nerve endings that detect the temperature of the skin. The two types of peripheral thermoreceptors are cold receptors and heat receptors: cold receptors are more abundant and more superficially located than heat receptors.

Temperature regulatory center

The *temperature regulatory center* is located in the hypothalamus. It receives afferent information related to core temperature from central thermoreceptors and afferent information related to environmental temperature from peripheral thermoreceptors (Figure 8.17). The cerebral cortex also receives afferent information from peripheral thermoreceptors, which allows for conscious perception of skin temperature; this allows for voluntary responses to these perceptions, such as putting on or taking off clothing.

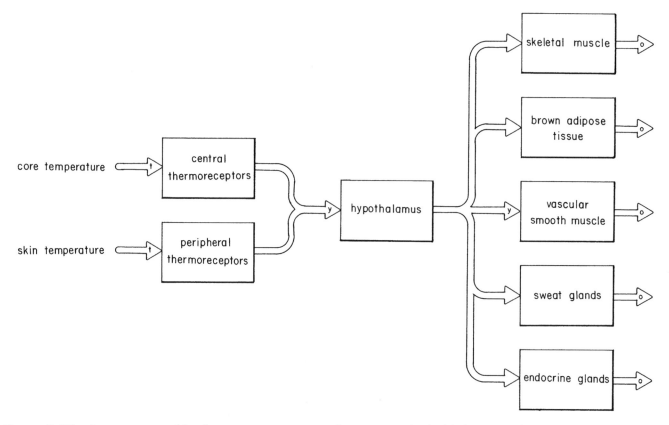

Figure 8.17 Components of body temperature control system. Color the block diagram from left to right. Note that the response to a change in temperature is mediated by the sequential action of central and peripheral thermoreceptors, afferent nerve pathways, the temperature regulatory center in the hypothalamus, efferent nerve pathways, and effector organs. Observe that effector organs include skeletal muscle, brown adipose tissue, vascular smooth muscle, sweat glands, and endocrine glands. Peripheral thermoreceptors also relay temperature information related to skin temperature to the cortex, which allows for conscious perception of skin temperature and therefore voluntary responses to these perceptions. Compare this figure with Figure 4.9.

Neurons in the posterior hypothalamus coordinate the mechanisms for heat gain, whereas neurons in the anterior hypothalamus coordinate the mechanisms for heat loss. The neural output from the hypothalamus controls the activity of the effector organs of the temperature regulating system, which include: (1) skeletal muscle; (2) brown adipose tissue; (3) vascular smooth muscle; (4) sweat glands; and (5) endocrine glands (Figure 8.17).

Thermoregulation in cold stress

During *hypothermia* (low core temperature), afferent signals from central and peripheral thermoreceptors stimulate the temperature regulatory center to increase the rate of heat production by the body and to decrease the rate of heat loss to the environment. These responses cause the body to gain heat in order to restore the normal level of core temperature (Figure 8.18).

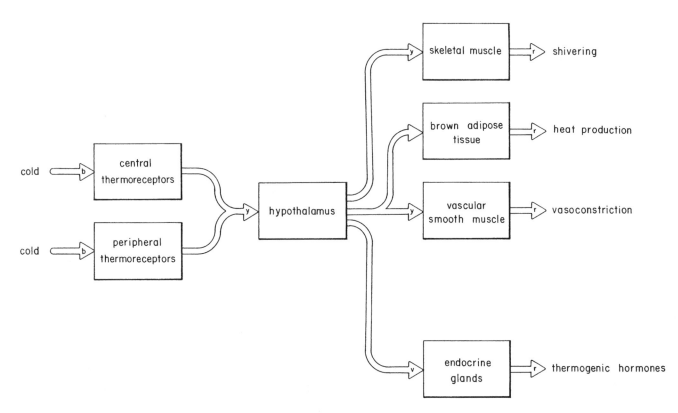

Figure 8.18   *Thermoregulation in cold stress.* Color the block diagram from left to right. Note that the response to hypothemia is mediated by the sequential action of central and peripheral thermoreceptors, afferent nerve pathways, the temperature regulatory center in the hypothalamus, efferent nerve pathways, and effector organs. Observe that effector organs for cold stress include skeletal muscle (which increases heat production by shivering), brown adipose tissue (which increases heat production by uncoupling the electron transport chain from ATP synthesis, a process called nonshivering thermogenesis), vascular smooth muscle (which constricts to decrease blood flow to the skin), and endocrine glands (which release thermogenic hormones). These mechanisms can sustain a normal level of core temperature in conditions of −30°C (−22°F). Compare this figure with Figure 8.17.

To increase heat production, the posterior hypothalamus: (1) stimulates the alpha and gamma motor neurons that innervate skeletal muscle; this causes shivering, a rapid involuntary cycle of skeletal muscle contraction and relaxation that increases metabolic rate (Figure 8.3); (2) stimulates the sympathetic nerve fibers to brown adipose tissue; this increases heat production; and (3) initiates the release of thermogenic hormones, such as thyroxine, which also increase metabolic rate.

To decrease heat loss, the posterior hypothalamus stimulates sympathetic nerve fibers that innervate the smooth muscle of peripheral blood vessels (Figure 5.31). The resultant vasoconstriction decreases blood flow to the skin, which, in turn, decreases the rate at which the body loses heat to the environment by radiation, conduction, and convection (Figure 8.19).

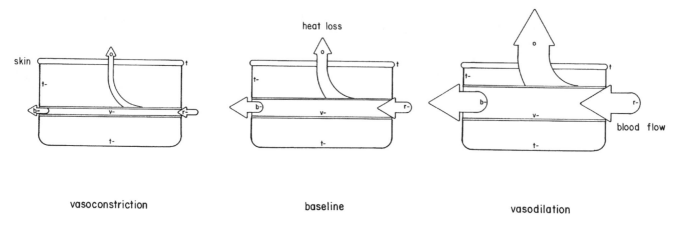

Figure 8.19 **Effect of vasomotor tone on heat loss.** Color the diagram from left to right, noting that the magnitudes of blood flow and heat loss through the skin can be visualized from the sizes of the arrows. Note that vasoconstriction decreases blood flow and heat loss (left panel) and that vasodilation increases blood flow and heat loss (right panel). Blood carries heat from deeper parts of the body to the skin where heat can be lost to the environment by radiation, conduction, and convection. Thus, stimulation of cold receptors constricts peripheral blood vessels and thereby enables the body to conserve heat whereas stimulation of heat receptors dilates peripheral blood vessels and thereby enables the body to lose heat. Cutaneous (skin) blood flow, which is nominally ~250 mL/min in a thermoneutral environment (baseline), can approach zero in a very cold environment and, at the opposite extreme, approach 15% to 25% of the cardiac output during vigorous exercise, as evidenced by flushed or reddened skin.

Thermoregulation in heat stress

During *hyperthermia* (high core temperature), afferent signals from central and peripheral thermoreceptors stimulate the temperature regulatory center to increase the rate of heat loss to the environment. This response causes the body to lose heat in order to restore the normal level of core temperature (Figure 8.20).

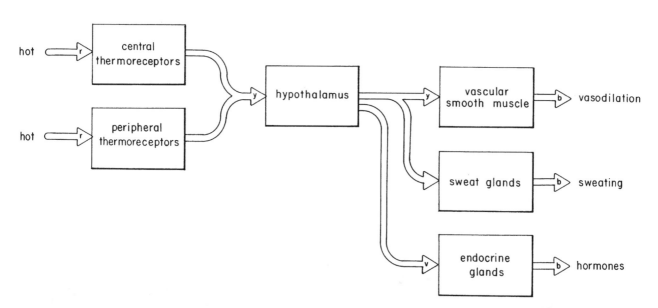

Figure 8.20 **Thermoregulation in heat stress.** Color the block diagram from left to right. Note that the response to hyperthemia is mediated by the sequential action of central and peripheral thermoreceptors, afferent nerve pathways, the temperature regulatory center in the hypothalamus, efferent nerve pathways, and effector organs. Observe that effector organs for heat stress include vascular smooth muscle (which dilates to increase blood flow to the skin), sweat glands (which increase heat loss by evaporation), and endocrine glands (which release ADH and aldosterone to conserve water and sodium). Compare this figure with Figure 8.17.

To increase heat loss, the anterior hypothalamus: (1) stimulates the sympathetic fibers that innervate sweat glands; the resultant secretion of sweat promotes heat loss by evaporation; and (2) inhibits the sympathetic fibers that innervate the smooth muscle of peripheral blood vessels. The resultant vasodilation increases blood flow to the skin which, in turn, causes more heat to be lost by radiation, convection, and conduction (Figure 8.19).

Blood flow to the skin increases dramatically during vigorous exercise in hot weather, as evidenced by flushed skin. Because the vascular beds of different organs are arranged in parallel (Figure 5.25), blood that is shunted to the skin does not perfuse exercising muscles. Thus, the need to dissipate heat and prevent hyperthermia is in conflict with the need to supply fuels and oxygen to exercising muscles. The resultant competition between skin and muscle for blood flow explains why maximal exercise performance, as indicated by $\dot{V}O_2$max, declines in hot/humid environments.

Effect of ambient temperature on mechanisms of heat loss

An increase in ambient temperature decreases the temperature gradient between the skin and environment so that less heat can be removed from the body by radiation, conduction, and convection (Figure 8.5). However, the total heat loss associated with a given level of submaximal exercise has been found to remain essentially constant over a wide range of ambient temperatures. This finding provides evidence that decrements in heat loss by the above mechanisms are counteracted by equal increments in heat loss by evaporation. Thus, evaporation becomes a progressively larger component of the total heat loss when ambient temperature rises (Figure 8.21).

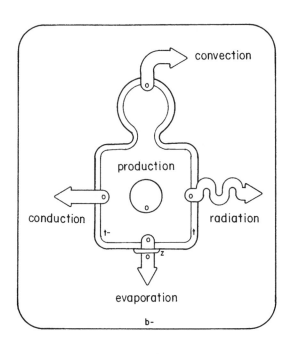

cool

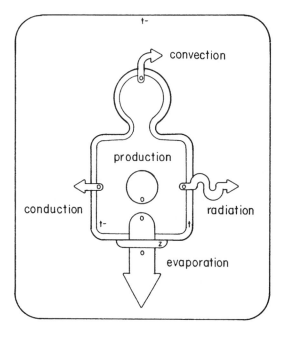

warm

Figure 8.21 Effect of ambient temperature on heat loss mechanisms. Color the panels, noting that heat production (area of circle) is the same in the cool (left panel) and warm (right panel) environments. Color and compare the components of heat loss in each condition, noting that arrow size indicates the magnitude of heat flow. Observe that warmer environments cause less heat to be lost by conduction, convection, and radiation, and correspondingly more heat to be lost by evaporation. Compare this figure with Figure 8.5.

Sweat glands

Stimulation of sympathetic nerve fibers causes sweat glands to secrete sweat, which is a hypotonic saline solution (0.2% to 0.4% NaCl) that they form by the filtration of plasma.

The two types of sweat glands are the *apocrine glands* and the *eccrine glands*. The apocrine glands are located in the axilla and genital area; their secretions contain a lipid substance responsible for body odor. The eccrine glands cover most of the body and are responsible for most of the evaporative heat loss. They consist of a deep coiled portion that secretes an essentially odorless sweat and a duct portion that allows sweat to pass outward through the layers of the skin (Figure 8.22).

Rates of sweat production vary among individuals in accordance with genetic factors and fitness level. They also vary with environmental conditions, exercise intensity, heat acclimatization, and degree of hydration.

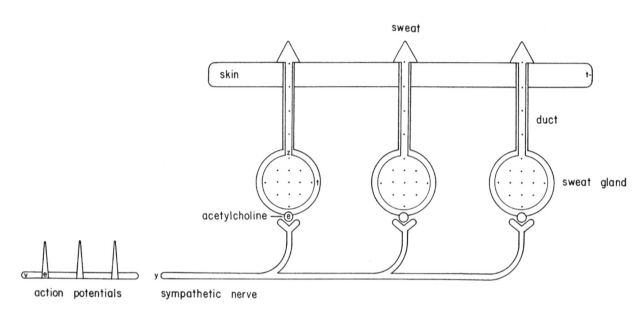

Figure 8.22   Sweat glands. Color the action potentials, sympathetic nerve fibers, molecules of acetylcholine, sweat glands, sweat, and skin. Observe that stimulation of sympathetic cholinergic fibers causes the secretion of sweat, a hypotonic saline solution (0.2% to 0.4% NaCl). Note that high sweat rates can increase the sodium and chloride concentrations in sweat because less time is available to reabsorb these ions in the duct portion of the sweat gland. The sweat rate of an acclimatized person can be three to four times that of an unacclimatized person; this adaptation increases the capacity for evaporative cooling.

Effect of sweat loss on body fluids

Sweating causes a loss of both water and salts from the body. Loss of fluid from the body is a condition referred to as *dehydration*. Because sweat is a hypotonic solution, the loss of water from the body is disproportionately greater than the concomitant loss of sodium and chloride (Figure 8.23). As a consequence, sweat loss decreases the blood volume and increases the sodium concentration in extracellular fluid.

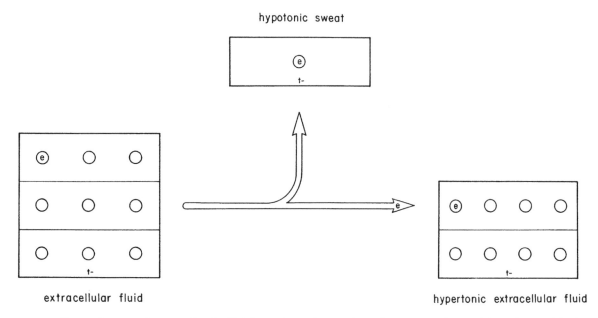

Figure 8.23 Effect of sweat loss on body fluids. Color and count the sodium ions (circles) and the volumes of fluid (rectangles) in the initial extracellular fluid (left panel), sweat (middle panel), and final extracellular fluid (right panel). Note that the concentration of sodium in each condition can be visualized from the space between the circles. Observe that the removal of one rectangle of hypotonic sweat (middle panel) from three rectangles of extracellular fluid (left panel) yields two rectangles of hypertonic extracellular fluid (right panel). Also observe that the total number of sodium ions and the total volume of fluid in the initial extracellular fluid are the same as that in sweat plus that in the final (hypertonic) extracellular fluid. These considerations explain why sweating causes the loss of water from the body to be disproportionately greater than the concomitant loss of sodium from the body. For this reason, sweating can lead to an increased sodium concentration in extracellular fluid coupled with a reduced blood volume.

Responses to sweat loss

Sweat loss activates the *thirst mechanism,* which is initiated by *osmoreceptors* in the hypothalamus that are stimulated by the higher sodium concentration in extracellular fluid (Figure 7.16). Because dehydration stimulates thirst, this mechanism, by itself, is activated too late to prevent dehydration due to fluid lost by sweating during exercise. For this reason, voluntary fluid intake is recommended before and during exercise to prevent dehydration.

Sweat loss also stimulates the release of hormones that conserve water and salt, including: (1) antidiuretic hormone

(ADH), which is released by the posterior pituitary gland in response to a high sodium concentration in extracellular fluid; and (2) aldosterone, which is released by the adrenal cortex in response to a high potassium concentration in extracellular fluid. ADH increases water reabsorption by the kidney tubules (Figure 7.16); this reduces the amount of water that is excreted in urine. Aldosterone increases Na^+ reabsorption by the kidney tubules (Figure 7.14) and the duct portions of the sweat glands (Figure 8.22); this reduces the amount of sodium that is excreted in urine and sweat.

Heat acclimatization

Heat acclimatization refers to adaptive responses to exercise in a hot environment, which include: (1) an expansion of blood volume; (2) an earlier onset of sweating and a higher sweat rate, which promotes evaporative heat loss; and (3) lower concentrations of sodium and chloride in sweat, which conserves electrolytes.

A thermoregulatory effect of an expanded blood volume is that a given increment in heat production causes a smaller rise in body temperature when more body fluid is available to absorb the added heat (Figure 8.24). A cardiovascular effect of an expanded blood volume is that a greater degree of filling of the venous circuit enhances stroke volume (Figure 5.16) and thereby reduces the heart rate associated with any given cardiac output (Figure 5.19).

The above adaptations explain why acclimatized individuals exhibit a lower heart rate and core temperature at any given level of submaximal exercise. They also explain why a reduction in blood volume due to excessive sweat loss causes a decline in maximal exercise performance.

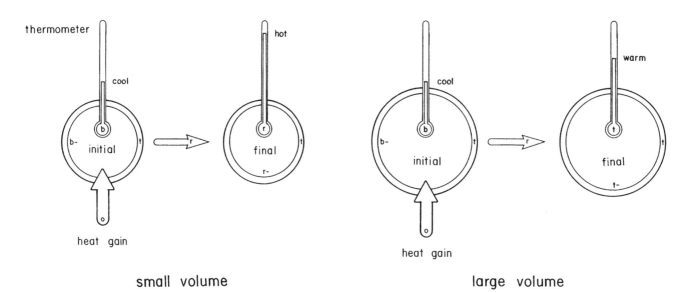

Figure 8.24 Effect of blood volume on thermoregulation. Color the panels from left to right, noting that the magnitude of the heat gain (size of arrow) and the initial temperature (indicated by the thermometer) are identical in the small volume (left panel) and large volume (right panel) conditions. Observe that the input of the same amount of heat causes the final temperature (indicated by the thermometer) to be higher in the small volume condition (left panel) than in the large volume condition (right panel). These results explain why a given increment in heat input causes a smaller rise in body temperature when more body fluid is available to absorb the added heat. For this reason, a low blood volume predisposes to hyperthemia during strenuous exercise.

Environmental factors that predispose to hyperthermia

Environmental factors that predispose to hyperthermia include: (1) high ambient temperature, which impairs heat loss by radiation and conduction; (2) low air movement, which impairs heat loss by convection; (3) high relative humidity, which impairs heat loss by evaporation; and (4) high levels of radiant heat from the sun, which increase heat gain (Figure 8.5).

In light of the above considerations, air temperature by itself is not an accurate index of environmental heat stress (Figure 8.13). The *wet bulb globe temperature* is an alternative index of environmental heat stress that takes into account the effects of air temperature, relative humidity, air movement, and radiant heat.

Wet bulb globe temperature

Wet bulb globe temperature (WBGT) is calculated from the weighted sum of three different temperature measurements: (1) dry-bulb temperature (DBT), obtained from a thermometer exposed to ambient air; (2) wet-bulb temperature (WBT), obtained from a thermometer surrounded by a wet wick exposed to rapid airflow (to detect evaporative cooling); and (3) globe temperature (GT), obtained from a thermometer placed in a black metal sphere (to detect radiant heat) (Figure 8.25), i.e.,

$$WBGT = 0.1\ DBT + 0.7\ WBT + 0.2\ GT$$

The difference between the dry bulb and wet bulb temperatures is due to the effects of evaporative cooling. For this rea-son, DBT exceeds WBT when humidity is low (a factor that promotes evaporation) but is similar to WBT when humidity is high (a factor that impedes evaporation). It is recommended that individuals exercise with caution when WBGT approaches 26.5°C (80°F) and avoid exercise when WBGT exceeds 31°C (88°F).

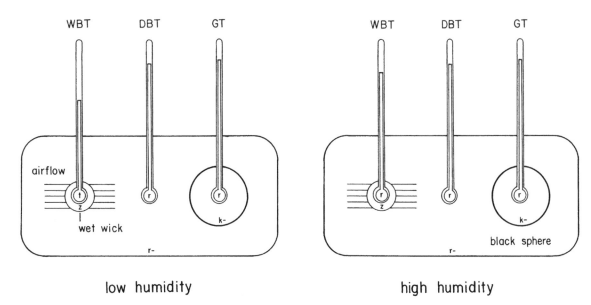

low humidity   high humidity

Figure 8.25   Wet bulb globe temperature (WBGT). Color the panels from left to right, comparing the temperatures measured by each thermometer in each condition. Note that the wet-bulb temperature (WBT) is lower in the low humidity condition (left panel) than in the high humidity condition (right panel), indicating corresponding differences in the rates of heat loss by evaporation. Note also that the dry-bulb temperature (DBT) and globe temperature (GT) are the same in the low and high humidity conditions.

Heat illness

Heat illnesses are complications of heat stress that include heat cramps, heat exhaustion, and heat stroke (Figure 8.13).

Heat cramps refer to involuntary muscle spasms that occur during or after intense exercise, probably as a result of electrolyte or body fluid imbalances. Heat exhaustion is a more serious condition characterized by pooling of blood in dilated peripheral vessels; its symptoms include a weak, rapid pulse, low arterial blood pressure in the upright position, general weakness, dizziness, and, in some cases, fainting. Heat stroke is a potentially lethal condition in which thermoregulation fails and body temperature rises to the point of tissue damage (> 41.5°C); its treatment can include alcohol rubs, application of ice packs, and whole-body immersion in cold water.

chapter **nine**
training for strength and endurance

chapter **nine**

Training to achieve measurable gains in physical performance requires exposure to physical stress of suitable intensity, duration, frequency, and mode (Figure 9.1).

This fundamental principle applies to the training of individual muscles to improve their strength (ability to generate more force), power (ability to perform more work in a given

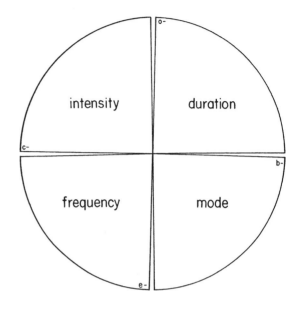

Figure 9.1 Components of an exercise prescription. Color each component of an exercise prescription. Note that intensity and duration are inversely related; high-intensity exercises can be sustained for only a short time, whereas low-intensity exercises can be sustained for a long time.

period of time), and endurance (ability to perform the same level of continuous work for a longer time) (Figure 9.2). It also applies to the training of individuals to increase their aerobic capacity. An increase in *aerobic capacity* is due to

improvements in the ability of the cardiovascular system to deliver oxygen and fuels to exercising muscles and in the ability of trained muscles to produce energy from the aerobic pathways of the oxidative system.

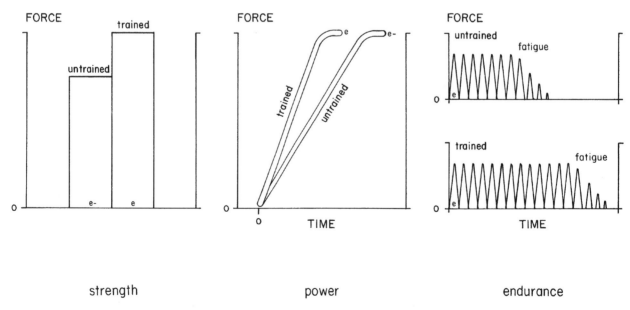

Figure 9.2 Components of muscle performance. Color each panel from left to right. Observe that an increase in the maximum force generated by a muscle (height of bar) provides evidence of increased strength (left panel). Observe also that an increase in the maximum rate of force development (slope of line in graph of force vs. time) provides evidence of increased power (middle panel). An increase in muscle power also manifests itself as a force–velocity curve in which a given muscle force is accompanied by a higher velocity of muscle shortening. Finally, observe that an increase in the number of repetitive stimuli that can be sustained before the muscle begins to exhibit signs of fatigue (decline in force in the face of same neural stimulation) provides evidence of increased endurance. Compare this panel with Figure 4.23.

Specificity of training

Specificity of training means that training effects in muscle are specific to the type of exercise utilized during training. In other words, training-induced improvements in one aspect of muscle performance may not carry over to other aspects. For example, training programs designed to increase muscle strength may not increase muscle endurance, and, conversely, training programs designed to increase muscle endurance may not increase muscle strength (Figure 9.3).

Specificity of training also means that training-induced improvements in one type of physical activity may not lead (carry over) to improvements in other types of physical activity. For example, running is a better exercise to train for a marathon than is cycling or swimming. For this reason, training programs ideally should employ the activity for which improved performance is desired.

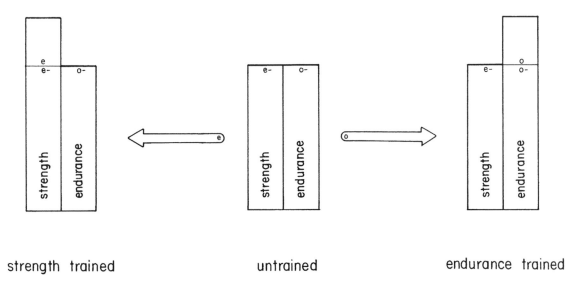

strength trained   untrained   endurance trained

Figure 9.3   Specificity of training. Color the bars in the middle panel, noting that their heights represent the untrained (pretraining) levels of muscle strength and endurance, respectively. Color the arrow at left, which indicates a period of strength training, and the bars that indicate the effects of strength training on strength and endurance. Compare the heights of these bars with those in the middle panel, noting that strength-trained muscles exhibit greater strength but not greater endurance. Color the arrow at right, which indicates a period of endurance training, and the bars that indicate the effects of endurance training on strength and endurance. Compare the heights of these bars with those in the middle panel, noting that endurance-trained muscles exhibit greater endurance but not greater strength. These hypothetical examples illustrate the principle of specificity of training. In actuality, muscles trained with weights often exhibit increases in both strength and endurance.

Cross-training

Cross-training refers to training for concurrent improvement in more than one type of physical activity (e.g., running and swimming) or more than one type of fitness (e.g., strength and endurance).

Because cardiovascular adaptations to endurance training are similar regardless of the physical activity used to stress the cardiovascular system, some carryover in cardiovascular improvement occurs across different types of endurance exercise. For this reason, cross-training is a useful technique to prevent cardiovascular deconditioning in injured athletes

who wish to abstain from activities that involve their injured body parts.

On the other hand, because muscular adaptations to training are specific to the muscles involved in the activity, little carryover in muscular improvement occurs across activities that employ different groups of muscles or different types of exercise. For these reasons, upper extremity exercises are not a useful technique to prevent deconditioning in lower extremity muscles, and anaerobic exercises are not a useful technique to prevent aerobic deconditioning. Adaptations to one type of exercise may even interfere with the training effects of another type of exercise. For example, strength training decreases capillary density in muscle, whereas endurance training increases capillary density in muscle.

The above considerations explain why swim training improves swimming performance more than it improves running performance and cycle training improves cycling performance more than it improves running performance (Figure 9.4).

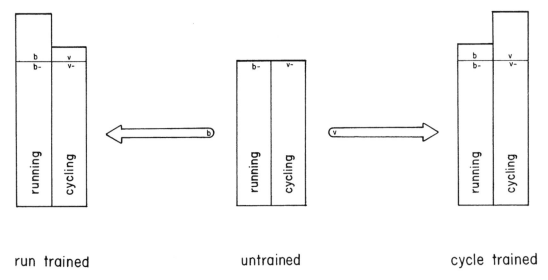

Figure 9.4   Effects of cross-training. Color the bars in the middle panel, noting that their heights represent the untrained levels of running and cycling performance. Color the arrow at left, which indicates a period of run training, and the bars that indicate the effects of run training on running and cycling performance. Compare these bars with those in the middle panel, noting that run training improves running more than it improves cycling. Color the arrow at right, which indicates a period of cycle training, and the bars that indicate the effects of cycle training on running and cycling performance. Compare these bars with those in the middle panel, noting that cycle training improves cycling more than it improves running. These hypothetical examples illustrate the principle of cross-training. Compare this figure with Figure 9.3.

Trainability and the overload principle

Individual differences in trainability (ability to improve performance with training) occur as a result of age, gender, and genetic endowment. An individual's initial level of fitness is another important determinant of trainability, because the *overload principle* states that, as the body adapts to a given level of stress, the workload must be incremented to achieve further improvement.

One consequence of the overload principle is that training proceeds safely and efficiently when exercise occurs at an appropriate fraction of an individual's maximal capacity—too low a workload may not be sufficiently intense to induce a training effect, and too high a workload may cause muscle or joint injury. Another consequence is that higher workloads are required to produce measurable gains in trained individuals than in untrained individuals (Figure 9.5). For example, a jogging protocol that improves $\dot{V}O_2$max in sedentary people may not be sufficiently rigorous to improve $\dot{V}O_2$max in elite marathon runners.

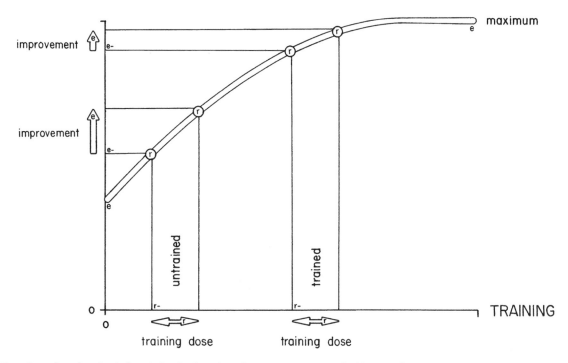

PERFORMANCE

Figure 9.5 Overload principle. Color the line that plots some measure of athletic performance against the duration of training (at a fixed intensity and frequency, Figure 9.1). Observe that performance increases nonlinearly with time from its initial level (y-intercept) to its final (maximum) level. Color the horizontal arrows labeled training dose, and the vertical and horizontal bands. Note that the same training dose (width of vertical band) yields more improvement in the untrained state [early in the training program (longer vertical arrow)] than in the trained state [later in the training program (shorter vertical arrow)].

Reversibility principle

The *reversibility principle* states that training-induced gains in physical performance quickly disappear when training stops; this process is referred to as *detraining*. Substantial reductions in exercise capacity occur within a few weeks of inactivity and many gains are completely lost within a few months.

To counteract the decline in physical performance associated with detraining, competitive athletes should initiate a reconditioning program several months prior to the start of their season or maintain a moderate level of sport-specific physical activity during the off-season.

Principles of muscle training programs

Muscle training programs are based on the premise that training sessions should employ the activity for which improved performance is desired (Figure 9.3). They are also based on the findings that: (1) weak contractions primarily recruit slow-twitch muscle fibers, whereas strong contractions recruit both slow-twitch and fast-twitch fibers (Figure 4.27); and (2) slow-twitch fibers rely heavily on aerobic sources of ATP (oxidative system), whereas fast-twitch fibers rely heavily on anaerobic sources of ATP (ATP-PCr and glycolytic systems) (Table 4.1).

As an example, muscle strength training programs are designed to exercise the fast-twitch muscle fibers that derive most of their energy from the ATP-PCr and glycolytic systems (Figure 3.1). Because these fibers are recruited during activities that require high-intensity, short-duration power surges, strength training protocols utilize high-resistance loads, such as heavy weights, to induce high-force, short-duration muscle contractions (Figure 9.6). For this reason, strength training is also called *resistance training*.

As another example, muscle endurance training programs are designed to exercise the slow-twitch, fatigue-resistant muscle fibers that derive most of their energy from the oxidative system. For this reason, endurance training protocols employ continuous submaximal activities, such as jogging, to induce low-force, repetitive contractions (Figure 9.6).

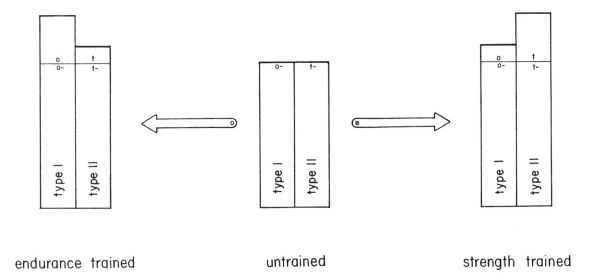

endurance trained   untrained   strength trained

Figure 9.6   Effects of strength and endurance training on muscle. Color the bars in the middle panel, noting that their heights represent the untrained levels of the type I (slow-twitch) and type II (fast-twitch) muscle fiber function. Color the arrow at left, which indicates a period of endurance training, and the bars that indicate the effects of endurance training on type I and type II muscle fiber function. Compare these bars with those in the middle panel, noting that endurance training causes more improvement in type I muscle fibers than in type II muscle fibers. Color the arrow at right, which indicates a period of strength training, and the bar graphs that indicate the effects of strength training on type I and type II muscle fiber function. Compare these bars with those in the middle panel, noting that strength training causes more improvement in type II muscle fibers than in type I muscle fibers. Compare this figure with Figure 9.4.

Assessment of muscle strength

Muscle strength is assessed from measurements of muscle force during maximal voluntary contractions. Some techniques assess muscle strength under static conditions, during which muscle length remains constant, whereas other techniques assess muscle strength under dynamic conditions, during which muscle length changes.

Dynamometry is a technique that employs a device called a dynamometer to measure maximum muscle force under static or dynamic conditions. In static dynamometry, the application of an external force to the dynamometer compresses an internal spring that, in turn, moves a pointer on a calibrated scale; the maximum value of recorded force is taken as a measure of strength (Figure 9.7).

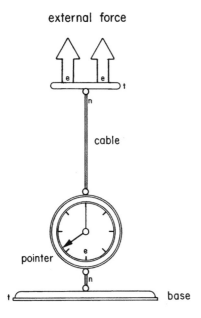

external force

cable

pointer

base

dynamometer

Figure 9.7 Static dynamometry. Color the components of the dynamometer and the arrows labeled external force, noting that the applied force moves a pointer on a calibrated scale. The maximum value of recorded force is taken as a measure of strength.

Weight lifting is a technique that employs fixed weights to measure maximum muscle force under dynamic conditions. Through the progressive addition of weight, the method determines the maximum weight that a person can lift throughout the full range of motion one time only: this maximum weight is referred to as the 1-RM load (one-repetition maximum load). According to this definition, a person whose 1-RM load is 100 kg has twice the strength of a person whose 1-RM load is 50 kg.

Isokinetic dynamometry is another technique that measures muscle force under dynamic conditions. The method employs an isokinetic dynamometer, which is a computer-assisted mechanical device that imposes a variable resistance (sometimes called an accommodating resistance) so that the speed of contraction can be held constant at a predetermined level (Figure 9.8). The resultant graphs of force (or torque) versus joint angle, obtained over a range of speeds, can be used to assess how muscle force varies with limb velocity and limb position (Figure 9.9); this information is not provided by the 1-RM test.

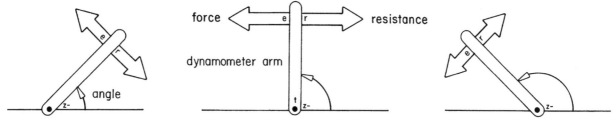

force   resistance

dynamometer arm

angle

isokinetic dynamometry

Figure 9.8 Isokinetic dynamometry. Color the diagram from left to right, noting that each panel depicts the dynamometer arm at a specific joint angle. For each joint angle, color the external force generated by the muscle at that angle (arrows labeled force), and the opposing force generated by the isokinetic dynamometer (arrows labeled resistance). In an isokinetic dynamometer, force is detected by an internal force transducer and joint angle is detected by an internal position sensor. Observe that muscle force (length of arrow labeled force) varies with joint angle. Observe also that the resistance imposed by the dynamometer (length of arrow labeled resistance) matches the muscle force at all joint angles. Under these conditions, net force and therefore limb acceleration is zero, and the resultant angular velocity of limb motion (in degrees/s) can be held constant at some predetermined level throughout the full range of motion. The ability of the isokinetic dynamometer to impose a high resistance when the muscle generates a strong force and a low resistance when the muscle generates a weak force enables the muscle to be maximally loaded throughout its full range of motion. Thus, isokinetic dynamometry makes it possible to activate the maximal number of motor units at every point in the range of motion.

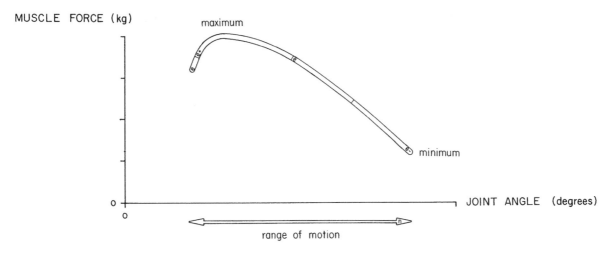

Figure 9.9   Effect of joint angle on maximal muscle force. Color the line depicting maximal muscle force plotted against joint angle. These data were obtained using an isokinetic dynamometer to measure the external force generated by a muscle during a maximal voluntary contraction at a fixed angular velocity of limb motion. Observe that muscle force varies with joint angle throughout the full range of motion, and identify the minimum and maximum values.

Muscle strength training programs

Gains in muscle strength can be achieved with different types of muscle contraction, including: (1) *concentric* (muscle length decreases during tension development); (2) *isometric* (muscle length remains constant during tension development); and (3) *eccentric* (muscle length increases during tension development) (Figure 4.16). Gains in strength can also be achieved with different types of exercise, including: (1) *isotonic exercise,* in which muscles contract against a fixed external load; (2) *isometric exercise,* in which muscles contract against an immovable load; and (3) *isokinetic exercise,* in which muscles contract against a variable external load.

Because the ability of skeletal muscle to generate tension decreases as the muscle shortens, the maximum tension that a given muscle can generate depends on the type of contraction; it is highest in an eccentric contraction, intermediate in an isometric contraction, and lowest in a concentric contraction. Despite differences in developed tension (a crucial factor in strength training) it remains unclear which type of contraction or which type of exercise is most effective in building muscle strength.

Dynamic strength training

One method of dynamic strength training employs fixed weights (sometimes referred to as *isotonic exercise*) to increase the tension developed by contracting muscles over a range of muscle lengths.

Progressive resistance exercise (PRE) is a method of weight training that is based on the overload principle. Programs typically utilize an "n-RM" load; that is, the number (n) of repetitions (R); maximum load (M). Stated another way, the n-RM load is the maximum weight (resistance) that can be successively lifted n times but is too heavy to be lifted (n + 1) times (Figure 9.10). For example, a 1-RM load is the maxi-

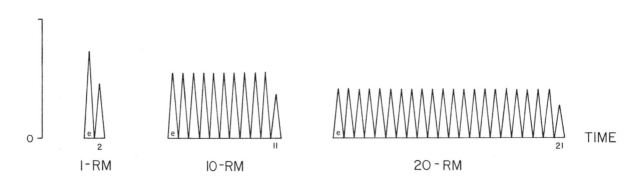

Figure 9.10   The n-RM load. Color the panels from left to right, noting that the height of the individual spikes indicates the force generated when a muscle attempts to lift a fixed weight in a series of sequential contractions. Observe that the 1-RM load is the maximum weight that can be lifted once but not twice, the 10-RM load can be lifted 10 but not 11 times, and the 20-RM load can be lifted 20 but not 21 times. Observe also that the 1-RM load is larger than the 10-RM load and that the 10-RM load is larger than the 20-RM load.

mum weight that can be lifted once but not twice and a 10-RM load is the maximum weight that can be lifted 10 times but not 11 times (a 10-RM load is typically 75% as heavy as a 1-RM load). Since muscles must generate near maximal levels of tension for gains in strength to occur, strength training programs utilize high resistance (3-RM to 12-RM loads), whereas endurance training programs utilize low resistance (20-RM loads, or lighter).

Although the optimal training program remains uncertain, two to three sets of ten repetitions (20–30 total repetitions per session) using weights that correspond to 60% to 80% of the 1-RM load are sufficient to build strength. Because the 1-RM load can be regarded as a quantitative measure of muscle strength, this method of specifying the training weight as a particular fraction of the 1-RM load allows training intensity to be incremented as gains in strength occur (overload principle). The optimal number of training days per week remains uncertain; improvements can be observed whether training occurs 1 day or 5 days per week. Too frequent training might prevent adequate recuperation between sessions; it is normally recommended that training occur 2–3 days per week.

Static strength training

Exercises employing static muscle contractions (also called *isometric exercises*) can increase muscle strength using short-duration, maximal contractions lasting only a few seconds when repeated 5 times per day, 3 days per week. A disadvantage of isometric training is that the maximal gains in strength occur at the limb position (joint angle) and therefore, muscle fiber length, at which training occurred. As a result, strength gains decrease as muscle fiber length (joint angle) deviates from its trained length. For this reason, isometric training should be implemented at several points throughout the range of motion of the joint.

Because of the specificity of muscle training, a statically-trained muscle is stronger when evaluated under static conditions, and a dynamically-trained muscle is stronger when evaluated under dynamic conditions.

Isokinetic strength training

Isokinetic strength training protocols utilize an isokinetic dynamometer to resist muscle contraction in such a way as to maintain a constant velocity of limb motion throughout the full range of motion (Figure 9.8). Because the maximal external force generated by a muscle varies with joint angle, the ability of the isokinetic dynamometer to adjust its resistance to match the force applied by the muscle enables the muscle to be maximally loaded throughout the full range of motion. In other words, the isokinetic dynamometer makes it possible to activate the maximal number of motor units at every point in the range of motion (Figure 9.11, left panel).

In contrast, the maximum weight that can be lifted during isotonic (fixed weight) exercise is determined by the force generated at the weakest point in the range of motion. For this reason, isotonic exercises do not allow a muscle to be maximally loaded throughout the full range of motion (Figure 9.11, right panel). However, since isokinetic exercises do not simulate natural movement, with the possible exception of swimming, the functional significance of isokinetic training remains uncertain.

Muscular adaptations to resistance training

Muscle strength is determined largely by muscle girth; a muscle with a larger cross-sectional area can generate more force and therefore lift more weight than one with a smaller cross-sectional area (Figure 9.12). Because the male hormone testosterone enlarges muscles, men tend to be stronger than women.

Strength training programs increase muscle strength and muscle cross-sectional area. The greater quantity of contractile protein results from an increase in the rate of protein synthesis and a decrease in the rate of protein degradation; these processes may involve compensatory responses to repeated muscle injury. Muscle biopsy data in humans reveal that training-induced muscle enlargement is due primarily to an enlargement of individual muscle fibers (*hypertrophy*) rather than an increase in the number of muscle fibers (*hyperplasia*) (Figure 9.13).

Measurements of myofibrillar ATPase activity also reveal that most strength training programs do not modify the relative percentages of slow-twitch and fast-twitch muscle fibers. These data indicate that resistance training does not usually cause appreciable conversion of slow-twitch fibers to fast-twitch fibers. However, some studies suggest that some resistance training protocols can result in a decrease in the percentage of fast-twitch, fatigable fibers (type IIb) and a corresponding increase in the percentage of fast-twitch, fatigue-resistant muscle fibers (type IIa) (Table 4.1).

Eccentric contractions have been found to be more effective in enlarging muscles than isometric or concentric contractions, probably because eccentric contractions create more tension and therefore cause more overload. However, the advantage of eccentric contractions in building muscle mass is offset by the fact that they also cause more muscle soreness than do isometric or concentric contractions, probably because they produce more structural damage to muscle fibers.

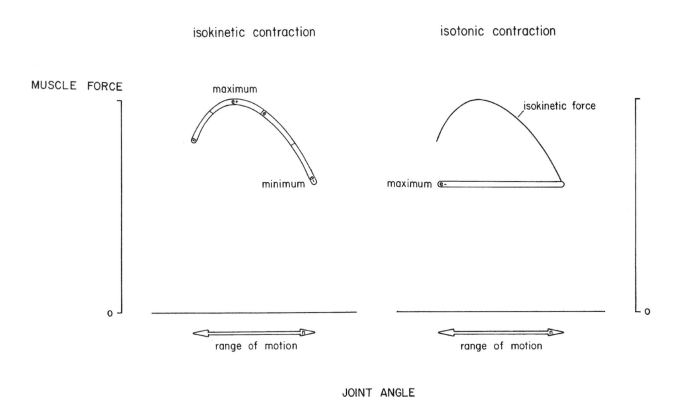

Figure 9.11 Maximal isokinetic and isotonic contractions. Color the line that depicts the maximal force generated by a muscle plotted against joint angle during a maximal isokinetic contraction (left panel); these data were obtained using the isokinetic dynamometer described in Figure 9.9. Note that the force generated by a muscle during an isokinetic contraction varies with joint angle and that the muscle is maximally loaded throughout its full range of motion. Color the line that depicts the maximal force generated by the same muscle plotted against joint angle during a maximal isotonic contraction; these data were obtained using a fixed external weight. Observe that the maximum fixed weight that a muscle can lift through its full range of motion is determined by force generated at the weakest point in the range of motion and that the muscle is not maximally loaded throughout its full range of motion.

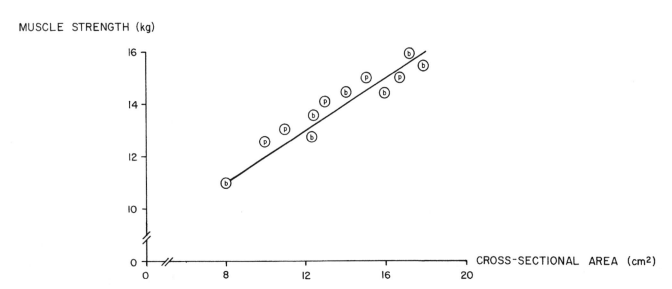

Figure 9.12 Effect of muscle cross-sectional area on strength. Color the plots of muscle strength (in kg) against muscle cross-sectional area (in cm²) obtained from different men and women, and identify the line that has been fitted to the data by linear regression analysis. Observe that the data from men (circles labeled b) and women (circles labeled p) fall on the same line. This linear relationship between muscle strength and cross-sectional area shows that strength of a muscle is determined largely by its cross-sectional area, with estimates ranging from 2.5 to 4.0 kg per cm² cross-sectional area.

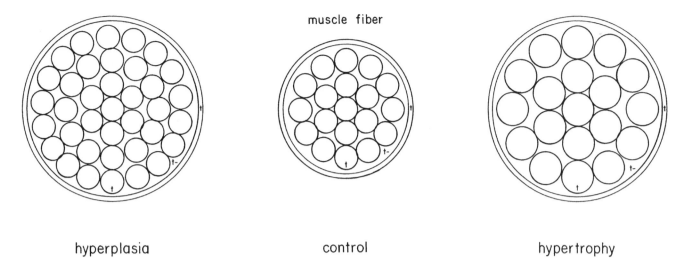

muscle fiber

hyperplasia   control   hypertrophy

Figure 9.13   Hypertrophy and hyperplasia. Color the cross sections of the individual muscle fibers in each of the conditions shown. Observe that the increase in muscle cross-sectional area in hyperplasia (left panel) compared to control (middle panel) is due to a greater number of the same size muscle fibers. Observe also that the increase in muscle cross-sectional area in hypertrophy (right panel) compared to control is due to the same number of larger muscle fibers. These results illustrate that hypertrophy and hyperplasia are two different mechanisms whereby a muscle can increase its girth. Hypertrophy due to resistance training occurs predominantly in fast-twitch fibers that are recruited during short-duration power surges that rely heavily on anaerobic sources of ATP (the ATP-PCr and glycolytic systems).

Metabolic adaptations to resistance training

Metabolic adaptations to strength training include higher resting levels of substrates for the ATP-PCr system (ATP, phosphocreatine, and free creatine) and the glycolytic system (intracellular glycogen). They also include increased activity of enzymes of the ATP-PCr system (creatine kinase, myokinase) and the glycolytic system (glycogen phosphorylase, phosphofructokinase) (Figure 9.15); these adaptations permit stronger and faster muscle contractions. In contrast, strength training does not increase the activity of oxidative enzymes; this result is compatible with the view that strength training does not improve muscle endurance (Figure 9.3).

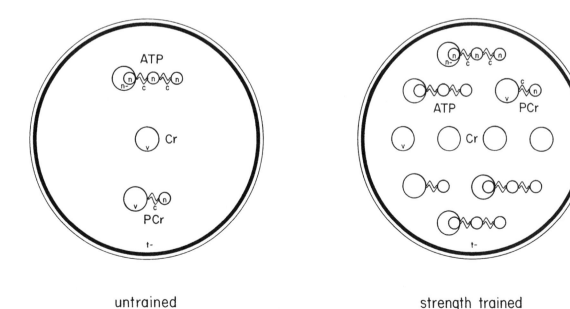

untrained   strength trained

Figure 9.14   Effects of resistance training on ATP-PCr system. Color and count the molecules of ATP, phosphocreatine (PCr), and free creatine (Cr) in the untrained (left panel) and strength-trained (right panel) conditions. Observe that strength training increases the concentrations of high-energy phosphate bonds (ATP and PCr) as well as free creatine (Cr) in muscle. These adaptations to strength training greatly enhance the capacity of the ATP-PCr system to supply ATP for muscle contraction. Compare this figure with Figure 3.2.

Higher substrate levels coupled with increased enzyme activity endow trained muscles with a greater immediate supply of ATP from the ATP-PCr system and a greater short-term supply of ATP from the glycolytic system (Figure 3.1). A greater ATP supply enables trained muscles to utilize ATP at a higher rate than untrained muscles, and an enhanced glycolytic capacity causes trained persons to produce higher levels of blood lactate during all-out exercise (Figure 9.15). Trained muscles also have a greater capacity to buffer the hydrogen ions that are released when lactic acid is formed; this delays the onset of fatigue during strenuous exercise.

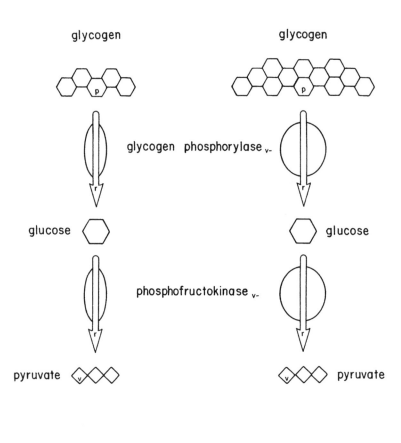

glycogen

glycogen

glycogen phosphorylase ᵥ₋

glucose

glucose

phosphofructokinase ᵥ₋

pyruvate

pyruvate

untrained

strength trained

Figure 9.15 Effects of resistance training on glycolytic system. For each condition, color and compare the molecules of glycogen, the arrows that indicate the pathway of glycogenolysis, the molecules of glucose, the arrows that indicate the pathway of glycolysis, and the final molecules of pyruvate. Observe that strength training (right panel) increases muscle glycogen (indicated by larger molecule). Observe also that strength training increases the activities of glycogen phosphorylase and phosphofructokinase (indicated by larger symbols for enzymes). These adaptations to strength training greatly enhance the capacity of the glycolytic system to supply ATP for muscle contraction. Compare this figure with Figure 3.4.

Neural adaptations to resistance training

Strength measurements obtained during maximal voluntary contractions represent the combined effects of neural drive to the muscle (neural factors) and the conversion of neural drive into muscle tension (muscle factors) (Figure 9.16). Gains in strength can therefore be partitioned into one component due to neural factors and one component due to muscle factors. Analysis of the time course of each of these factors reveals that gains in strength in the short term are due primarily to improvements in neural drive, whereas gains in strength in the long term are due primarily to hypertrophy of muscle fibers (Figure 9.17).

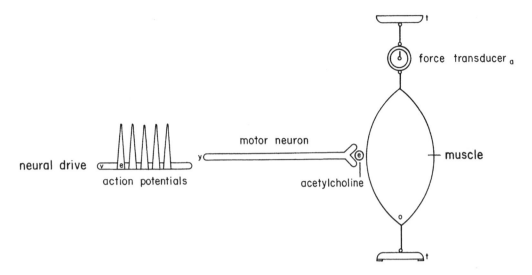

Figure 9.16 Components of muscle strength. Color the action potentials, motor neuron, molecule of acetylcholine, and the muscle. Color the force transducer, noting that it measures the isometric force generated by the muscle. Observe that the maximum force generated by the muscle under these conditions (a measure of strength) represents the combined effects of neural drive to the muscle (neural factors) and the conversion of this neural drive into force (muscle factors). For these reasons, training-induced gains in strength could be due to improvements in neural factors and/or to improvements in muscle factors. Compare this figure with Figure 4.15.

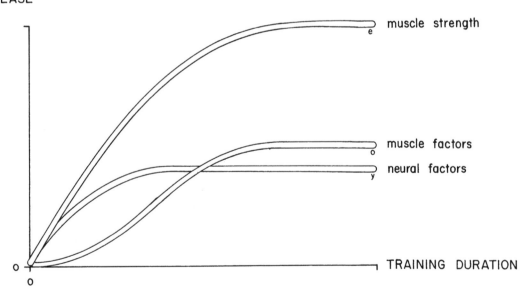

Figure 9.17 Longitudinal changes with strength training. Color the line that plots gains in muscle strength (% increase) against training duration (at a fixed intensity and frequency). Observe that strength increases in a nonlinear fashion from its initial level (y-intercept) to its final level. Color and compare the graphs that depict the concomitant improvements in neural factors and muscle factors. Observe from the different time courses of the two curves that gains in strength in the short term are due primarily to improvements in neural drive, whereas gains in strength in the long term are due primarily to hypertrophy of muscle fibers. Compare this figure with Figure 9.5. Modified from D. G. Sale *Med Sci Sports Exer* 20:S135, 1988.

The operation of neural factors explains why increased strength can be observed in the absence of visible hypertrophy, a phenomenon that has been attributed to: (1) increased neural drive to muscles; (2) enhanced synchrony of motor units; and (3) decreased neural drive to antagonistic muscles. Increased neural drive to muscles could be achieved by: (1) a greater number of stimulated motor units (spatial summation); (2) a higher frequency of stimulation of individual motor units (temporal summation); or (3) a reduced number of inhibitory impulses from nerve fibers originating in Golgi tendon organs, the reticular formation, or the cerebral cortex (Figure 9.18).

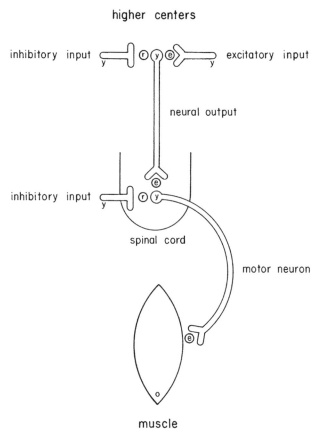

Figure 9.18 Neural factors that influence muscle strength. Color diagram from top to bottom, identifying the nerves and their neurotransmitters as you go. Observe that the activity of the alpha motor neuron that controls muscle contraction is modulated by excitatory neural output from higher centers and inhibitory neural input from peripheral sensory receptors (such as tendon organs, Figure 4.29). Observe also that the neural output from higher centers is modulated by excitatory and inhibitory inputs from other regions of the brain, such as the cerebral cortex. These inputs represent the effects of psychological factors, such as motivation, and physiological factors, such as pain, both of which can influence neural output. Thus, alpha motor neurons are controlled by nerve fibers that originate in different parts of the central nervous system, including the spinal cord, the lower regions of the brain, and the motor area of the cerebral cortex. Any factor that increases the alpha motor neuron output to a muscle, that enhances the synchrony of its motor units, or that decreases the neural drive to antagonistic muscles can be regarded as a neural factor that increases muscle strength. Compare this figure with Figure 4.25.

Aerobic training

Aerobic training programs employ continuous submaximal exercises, such as cross-country skiing, distance running, or cycling. These activities are classified as aerobic exercise because they derive their energy primarily from the oxidative system (Figure 3.6), which requires a continuous supply of oxygen to serve as the final electron acceptor in the electron transport chain (Figure 2.21). Oxygen consumption ($\dot{V}O_2$) can be regarded as an index of exercise intensity because it parallels the rate of aerobic ATP production.

For a given absolute workload, upper extremity exercises are associated with a higher heart rate, a greater perceived effort, and a higher level of ventilation than lower extremity exercises. These findings indicate that endurance training is more effective and less strenuous when a large muscle mass is exercised; cross-country skiing (which employs both upper and lower extremities) is therefore a preferable modality to arm ergometry (which employs only upper extremities) in developing aerobic fitness. Although the optimal duration and frequency of training sessions remain uncertain, programs employing 20 to 30-minute sessions per day, two to three days per week, have proven effective in increasing aerobic capacity.

Individual differences in aerobic trainability occur because of age, genetic endowment, and initial level of aerobic fitness. Although a training intensity of approximately 50% $\dot{V}O_2$max may be sufficient to achieve a training effect in deconditioned individuals, it is normally recommended that training occur at an oxygen consumption that corresponds to approximately 70% to 85% $\dot{V}O_2$max. Heart rate, rating of perceived exertion, or blood lactate levels are alternative measures of exercise intensity that can be used to guide training when measurements of oxygen consumption are not available.

Use of heart rate to guide training intensity

Heart rate can serve as an indicator of exercise intensity because heart rate varies nearly linearly with oxygen consumption and work rate. Training heart rates can be expressed as a percentage of maximal heart rate (% HR_{max}). HR_{max} can be measured directly during a maximal graded exercise test, or it can be estimated by subtracting an individual's age (in years) from 220, i.e.,

$$HR_{max} = (220 - age)$$

As a general guideline, aerobic conditioning should occur when the training heart rate is maintained at a level that falls between 55%–65% HR_{max} and 90% HR_{max}; this range is referred to as the *training-sensitive zone* (Figure 9.19).

HEART RATE (beats/min)

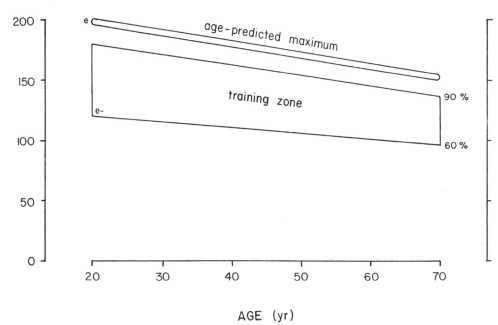

AGE (yr)

Figure 9.19   Use of heart rate to guide training intensity. Color the line labeled age-predicted maximum, which plots calculated values of heart rate (220 – age, in beats/min) against age (in yr). Observe that the age-predicted maximum heart rate (HR_{max}) decreases linearly with age, from 200 beats/min at age 20 to 150 beats/min at age 70. Color the band labeled training zone, noting that its lower and upper limits represent 60% and 90% HR_{max}, respectively. As a general guideline, aerobic conditioning should occur when the training heart rate is maintained at a level that falls within the training-sensitive zone.

Use of rating of perceived exertion to guide training intensity

Rating of perceived exertion (RPE) can be used to guide training intensity because RPE values have been shown to correlate well with other indices of exercise intensity, such as heart rate and oxygen consumption.

Perceived effort is rated by the exerciser on a numerical scale (Borg scale) that ranges from 6 to 20 (Figure 9.20). Although

RPE values of approximately 13–14 (somewhat hard) generally coincide with heart rate values of about 70% HR_{max}, this level of perceived effort could correspond to a lower heart rate in some individuals and a higher heart rate in other individuals. To account for individual differences in perceived effort, a personalized relationship between RPE and heart rate can be determined in an individual by using a graded exercise test to obtain RPE-HR data over a range of exercise intensities; this method allows training to occur at an RPE value that translates to the desired heart rate (Figure 9.21).

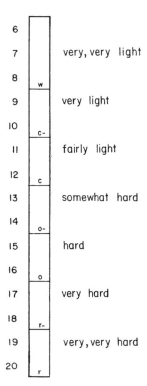

Figure 9.20   Rating of perceived exertion (RPE). Color the bar graph, comparing the numerical values of RPE, which range from 6 to 20, with their corresponding verbal descriptions, which range from very, very light to very, very hard. Values of RPE obtained over a range of exercise intensities have been found to correlate well with concomitant values of heart rate and oxygen consumption; RPE values can therefore serve as an index of exercise intensity under these conditions. The category–ratio RPE scale is another method in which perceived effort is rated by the exerciser on a scale that ranges from 0 (nothing at all) to 10 (very, very strong). The category–ratio PRE scale correlates well with exercise parameters that exhibit a nonlinear relationship with exercise intensity, such as blood lactate levels (Figure 3.12) and minute ventilation (Figure 6.38). Modified from G. A. Borg *Med Sci Sports Exer* 14:377, 1982.

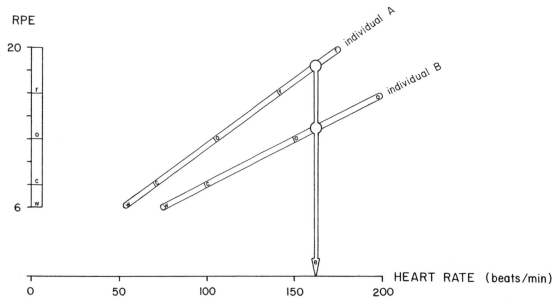

Figure 9.21   Individual differences in RPE. Color the lines that plot hypothetical RPE values of two different individuals against their concomitant heart rates (lines fitted to data obtained during a graded exercise test). Observe that the difference between the lines indicates corresponding differences in perceived effort at any given level of heart rate. Color the vertical line indicating a given heart rate; note that this heart rate corresponds to a higher RPE in individual A (upper line) than in individual B (lower line). Such individualized relationships between RPE and heart rate enable RPE values to be more accurate indicators of heart rate and therefore, more useful parameters to guide training intensity.

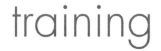

Use of blood lactate levels to guide training intensity

Blood lactate levels can be used to guide training intensity because effective training occurs when an individual trains at an exercise intensity that corresponds to the lactate threshold, i.e., the exercise intensity at which lactate begins to build up in the blood.

This method plots measured values of blood lactate against an index of exercise intensity, such as running speed or oxygen consumption, and determines the lactate threshold (LT) from the point at which lactate begins to systematically accumulate in the blood (Figure 3.12). This procedure enables a person to train at an intensity that coincides with the individual's lactate threshold. Because high levels of muscle and blood lactic acid are associated with fatigue, the functional significance of the lactate threshold is that it represents a high level of exercise intensity that can be sustained indefinitely.

Effects of aerobic training

Aerobic training effects include higher maximal levels of oxygen consumption ($\dot{V}O_2$max) and cardiac output and an improved capacity to perform continuous submaximal exercise (Figure 9.22). Other beneficial effects of aerobic training include a lower resting level of arterial blood pressure, a higher plasma level of high density lipoprotein particles (HDL), and an increase in lean body mass.

These improvements in physical performance are due largely to the combined effects of cardiovascular, respiratory, metabolic, and muscular adaptations to continuous submaximal exercise.

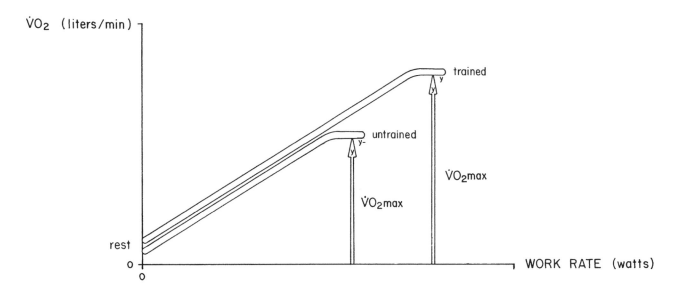

Figure 9.22   Effect of endurance training on $\dot{V}O_2$max. Color the lines that plot oxygen consumption ($\dot{V}O_2$, in liters/min) against work rate (WR, in watts); lines fitted to data obtained during a graded exercise test in same individual before (untrained) and after (trained) an endurance exercise (aerobic) training program. Observe that aerobic training increases $\dot{V}O_2$max, a quantitative measure of aerobic capacity. Increases in $\dot{V}O_2$max reflect increases in the ability of the cardiovascular system to supply fuels and oxygen to exercising muscles as well as increases in the capacity of trained muscles to oxidize fuels for energy. Compare this figure with Figure 3.11.

Effects of endurance training on $\dot{V}O_2$max

The Fick equation shows that training-induced increases in oxygen consumption ($\dot{V}O_2$) can be attributed to higher levels of cardiac output coupled with greater oxygen extraction by tissues, as evidenced by a widened a-$\bar{v}$ O_2 difference (Figure 6.15). Since cardiac output is equal to the product of heart rate and stroke volume, the Fick equation also shows that $\dot{V}O_2$max is determined by the maximal levels of heart rate (HR$_{max}$), stroke volume (SV$_{max}$), and oxygen extraction [(a-$\bar{v}$ O_2 difference)$_{max}$], i.e.,

$$\dot{V}O_2max = HR_{max} \cdot SV_{max} \cdot (\text{a-}\bar{v} \ O_2 \ difference)_{max}$$

Because maximum heart rates in highly trained endurance athletes are slightly lower than their untrained counterparts, their higher levels of $\dot{V}O_2$max can be attributed entirely to larger stroke volumes and greater O_2 extraction from arterial blood.

Cardiac adaptations to endurance training

Cardiac adaptations to endurance exercise training include larger cardiac muscle mass, higher maximal cardiac output, and lower heart rate at any given level of submaximal exercise.

Endurance training increases the maximal levels of cardiac output and oxygen consumption. However, cardiac output at any given level of submaximal exercise is the same before and after training, indicating that training does not alter the relationship between cardiac output and O$_2$ consumption (Figure 9.23, left panel). Because cardiac output is equal to the product of heart rate and stroke volume, the lower heart rates exhibited by trained individuals at any given level of submaximal exercise (middle panel) signify correspondingly larger stroke volumes (right panel). For this reason, the heart rate at a given exercise intensity can be regarded as an index of cardiovascular fitness, and a reduced heart rate at the same exercise intensity can be regarded as evidence of a cardiovascular training effect.

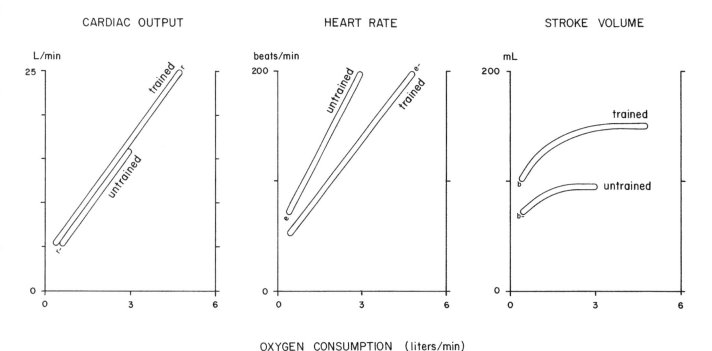

CARDIAC OUTPUT   HEART RATE   STROKE VOLUME

OXYGEN CONSUMPTION (liters/min)

Figure 9.23   Cardiac adaptations to endurance training. Color the panels from left to right, comparing the responses of the untrained individual with those of the highly trained endurance athlete. Note that the trained athlete exhibits significantly higher values of V̇O$_2$max and cardiac output than the untrained individual (right endpoints of lines in left panel) and that the relationship between cardiac output and oxygen consumption is the same in the untrained and trained persons (lines overlap in left panel). Note also that the trained individual exhibits a lower heart rate (middle panel) and a correspondingly larger stroke volume (right panel) than the untrained individual at any given level of cardiac output or oxygen consumption. These findings explain why the heart rate at any given level of exercise intensity can be regarded as an index of cardiovascular fitness, and a reduced heart rate at the same exercise intensity can be regarded as evidence of a cardiovascular training effect. Other cardiovascular benefits of physical fitness include a lower resting level of arterial blood pressure, an increase in the serum concentrations of high-density lipoprotein particles (HDL), and a reversal or retardation of other risk factors for cardiovascular disease. Psychological benefits of physical fitness include improvements in mood and self-esteem and reductions in stress and anxiety. Modified from B. Saltin et al. *Circulation* 38(suppl 7): 18, 1968.

Effect of endurance training on capillary density

Endurance training increases the *capillary density* in trained muscles; this refers to a greater number of capillaries per muscle fiber (Figure 9.24). The expanded interface between blood vessels and muscle fibers facilitates: (1) the delivery of O$_2$ and fuels to muscle; (2) the removal of CO$_2$ and waste products from muscle; and (3) the transfer of heat from muscle to blood. Stated another way, these features of a higher capillary-to-fiber ratio enhance the oxidative capacity of trained muscles and promote the removal of heat from exercising muscles.

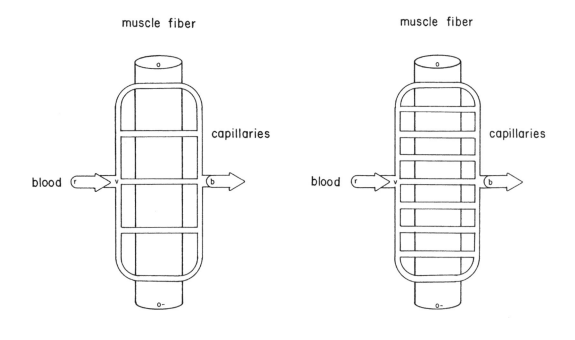

Figure 9.24   Effect of endurance training on capillary density. Color the schematic muscle fiber and its blood supply before (untrained, left panel) and after (trained, right panel) an endurance exercise training program. Observe that endurance training increases the number of capillaries per muscle fiber; this facilitates the delivery of fuels and oxygen to muscle, the removal of metabolic waste products from muscle, and the transfer of heat from muscle to blood.

Effect of endurance training on blood volume

Endurance training increases blood volume by expanding plasma volume and by increasing the number of red blood cells. The expansion of plasma volume is due both to changes in the levels of hormones that increase water reabsorption in kidney tubules and to a greater amount of plasma protein which increases water reabsorption in the capillaries.

Hormones that increase plasma volume include antidiuretic hormone (ADH), which is released by the posterior pituitary gland (Figure 7.16), and aldosterone, which is released by the adrenal cortex. The major plasma protein that increases plasma volume is albumin, which is a nondiffusible molecule that influences fluid balance at the capillaries through its effect on plasma osmotic pressure. A greater number of albumin molecules in the capillaries causes more water to be retained in the blood vessels; this increases plasma volume (Figure 5.36).

Endurance training also increases the absolute number of red blood cells by stimulating their production in bone marrow. However, because the increase in plasma volume is disproportionately greater than the increase in red blood cell volume, hematocrit falls and causes a condition referred to as hemodilution (Figure 9.25).

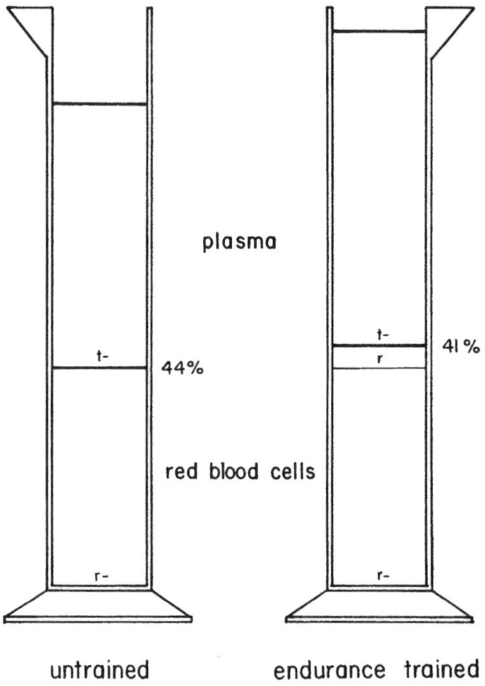

Figure 9.25 Effect of endurance training on blood volume. Color and compare the absolute volumes of red blood cells and plasma before (untrained, left panel) and after (trained, right panel) an endurance exercise training program. Observe that endurance training increases both the red blood cell volume and the plasma volume. Observe also that hematocrit (% red blood cell volume, Figure 5.29) falls slightly with endurance training because plasma volume increases disproportionately to red blood cell volume.

Circulatory and thermoregulatory effects of expanded blood volume

Expansion of blood volume improves cardiovascular function because a larger blood volume increases ventricular preload and therefore increases stroke volume (Figure 5.16). This mechanism helps elite endurance athletes to produce larger stroke volumes than do sedentary persons (Figure 9.23).

Expansion of blood volume also improves thermoregulatory function because a larger blood volume enables the body to absorb more heat for a given rise in body temperature. Stated another way, a larger blood volume blunts the rise in body temperature associated with a given increment in heat production. This mechanism helps trained persons to defend against hyperthermia during strenuous exercise (Figure 8.24).

Respiratory adaptations to endurance training

Respiratory adaptations to endurance training include an improved economy of ventilation, and a higher maximum voluntary ventilation (MVV, Figure 6.51), due presumably to improvements in respiratory muscle endurance and economy. An improved economy of ventilation means that respiratory muscles consume less oxygen at any given level of ventila-

tion; this improves the economy of exercise because it permits a greater fraction of the oxygen uptake to be consumed by working muscles.

However, most pulmonary function test parameters, such as lung volumes (Figure 6.48) and expiratory airflows (Figure 6.50), are essentially unchanged by endurance training.

Mitochondrial adaptations to endurance training

Mitochondrial adaptations to endurance training include increases in the number and size of mitochondria and alterations in mitochondrial enzyme composition. These adaptations improve the capacity of trained muscles to oxidize pyruvate, fatty acids, and ketones in the aerobic pathways of the Krebs cycle (Figure 9.26) and electron transport chain. In contrast, endurance training does not increase the activity of enzymes of the ATP-PCr system (creatine kinase, myokinase) or the glycolytic system (phosphofructokinase); this result is compatible with the view that endurance training does not improve muscle strength (Figure 9.3).

Endurance training also increases the resting levels of substrates for the oxidative system (intracellular glycogen and triglycerides) (Figure 9.26). Higher substrate concentrations

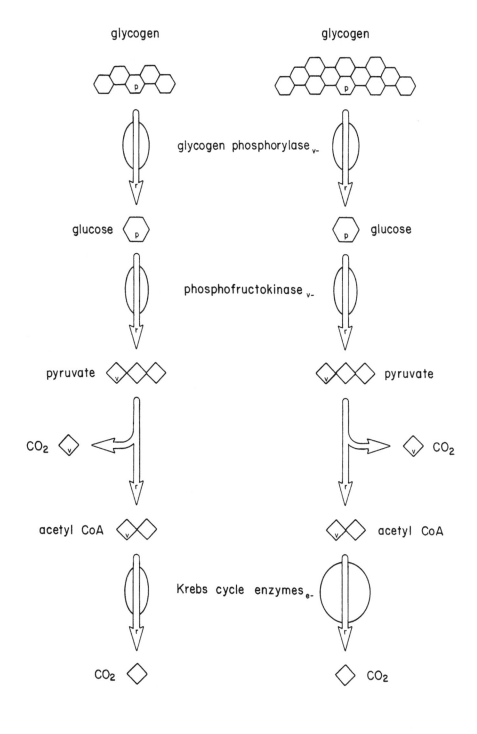

glycogen glycogen

glycogen phosphorylase v-

glucose glucose

phosphofructokinase v-

pyruvate pyruvate

CO_2 CO_2

acetyl CoA acetyl CoA

Krebs cycle enzymes e-

CO_2 CO_2

untrained endurance trained

Figure 9.26 Effect of endurance training on the oxidative system. For each condition, color and compare the molecules of glycogen, the arrows that indicate the pathway of glycogenolysis, the molecules of glucose, the arrows that indicate the pathway of glycolysis, the moleucles of pyruvate, the arrows that indicate the conversion of pyruvate to acetyl CoA, the moleces of acetyl CoA, the arrows that indicate the pathway of the Krebs cycle, and the molecules of CO_2. Observe that endurance training (right panel) increases muscle glycogen (indicated by larger molecule). Observe also that endurance training increases the activities of Krebs cycle enzymes (indicated by larger symbol for enzymes). These adaptations to endurance training enhance the capacity of the oxidative system to supply ATP for muscle contraction. Compare this figure with Figure 9.15.

coupled with increased activity of oxidative enzymes enables the oxidative system of trained muscles to produce more ATP. At any given level of submaximal exercise, therefore, trained muscles derive more of their energy from aerobic sources of ATP (oxidative system) and less of their energy from anaerobic sources of ATP (ATP-PCr and glycolytic systems) than do untrained muscles.

Reduced activity of the ATP-PCr system enables trained muscles to exhibit lower rates of phosphocreatine depletion (Figure 3.2). Reduced activity of the glycolytic system enables trained muscles to exhibit lower rates of glycogen depletion and lactic acid production than do untrained muscles.

Effect of endurance training on O₂ uptake

Endurance training increases the oxidative capacity of muscle, thereby enabling trained muscle to consume O₂ at a higher rate than untrained muscle. Endurance training also increases the *myoglobin* content of skeletal muscle, whose main function is to transport O₂ from the cell membrane to the mitochondria.

These improvements in mitochondrial function and myoglobin content explain why trained persons exhibit higher maximal rates of O₂ uptake during exercise than their untrained counterparts (Figure 9.22). They also explain why trained persons attain steady-state levels of oxygen consumption in a shorter period of time; this reduces the O₂ deficit incurred during the initial transient period of exercise (Figure 3.9).

Effect of endurance training on endocrine response to exercise

Endurance training decreases sympathetic activity and lowers the plasma levels of epinephrine and norepinephrine associated with any given level of submaximal exercise (Figure 9.27). Lower catecholamine levels reduce the stimulation of adrenergic receptors in the pancreas and thereby blunt the insulin and glucagon responses to exercise; these changes lead to a smaller decrease in blood levels of insulin and a smaller increase in blood levels of glucagon. As an outcome, trained persons have higher blood levels of insulin and lower blood levels of glucagon than do untrained persons at the same exercise intensity. These hormonal adaptations to endurance training cause less stimulation of glycogenolysis, which, in turn, leads to lower rates of glycogen depletion.

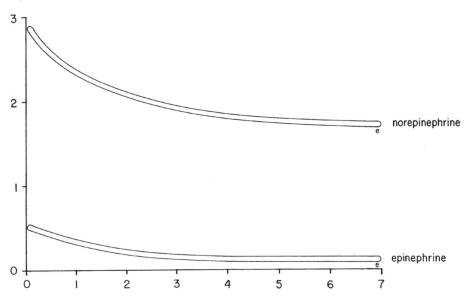

PLASMA CONCENTRATION (ng/mL)

TRAINING DURATION (weeks)

Figure 9.27   Effect of endurance training on blood levels of catecholamines. Color the lines that depict the plasma levels (in ng/mL) of norepinephrine and epinephrine plotted against training duration (in wk). These data show that endurance training lowers the blood levels of catecholamines at any given level of submaximal exercise. Lower blood levels of catecholamines result in less stimulation of glycogen breakdown in liver and muscle, less stimulation of glucagon release, and less inhibition of insulin release. Note that these hormonal adaptations to endurance training lead to lower rates of glycogen depletion which, in turn, permit exercise to continue for a longer period of time. Compare this figure with Figure 7.19. Modified from W. W. Winder et al. *J Appl Physiol* 45:370, 1978.

Effect of endurance training on fuel utilization

In light of the above considerations, metabolic adaptations to endurance training include a slower depletion of muscle and liver glycogen stores. Because glycogen stores are indispensable for prolonged strenuous exercise, glycogen depletion is associated with fatigue that forces either a cessation of exercise or a decrease in its intensity. For this reason, lower rates of glycogen depletion permit exercise to continue for a longer period of time.

This glycogen-sparing effect of training is due to a lower rate of carbohydrate utilization as a source of energy, which is offset by a higher rate of fatty acid utilization (Figure 9.28). Increased oxidation of fatty acids in the trained state, therefore, plays a major role in bringing about the slower depletion of glycogen stores during submaximal exercise. Increased fatty acid oxidation in trained muscles is due to higher resting levels of intracellular fat stores (muscle triglycerides) coupled with improved capacities for: (1) fatty acid uptake from the blood; (2) fatty acid transport from the cytoplasm into the mitochondria; and (3) fatty acid breakdown into 2-carbon units that can enter the Krebs cycle as acetyl CoA (β-oxidation).

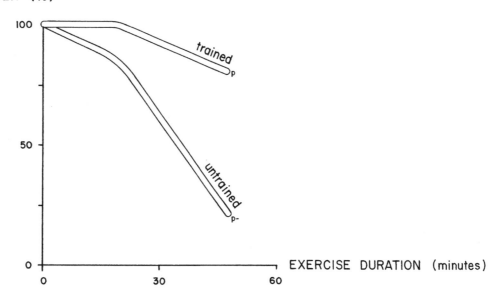

Figure 9.28   Effect of endurance training on fuel utilization. Color and compare the lines that plot liver glycogen (% pre-exercise value) against exercise duration (in min) in a group of endurance trained (upper line) and untrained (lower line) rats performing the same treadmill exercise protocol. Note that the liver glycogen levels of the trained rats are significantly higher than those of the untrained rats throughout the exercise period. These findings indicate that endurance training leads to a lower rate of carbohydrate utilization, which is offset by a higher rate of fatty acid utilization. Stated another way, increased oxidation of fatty acids in the trained state brings about a slower depletion of glycogen stores during submaximal exercise. Modified from K. M. Baldwin et al. *Pflug Arch* 354:206, 1975.

Effect of endurance training on blood lactate levels

Endurance training lowers the muscle and blood levels of lactate associated with a given level of submaximal exercise. Endurance training also increases the lactate threshold, defined as the workload at which lactate begins to accumulate in the blood. Because lactate buildup in muscle is associated with fatigue, a higher lactate threshold is associated with a capacity to sustain a higher intensity of continuous submaximal exercise (Figure 9.29).

Blood levels of lactate represent the balance between the rate at which lactate is added to the blood and the rate at which lactate is removed from the blood (Figure 3.13). The lower levels of blood lactate that result from training are due to a lower rate of lactate production coupled with a higher rate of lactate removal. Lower rates of lactate production could be due to: (1) greater aerobic production of ATP; (2) lower blood levels of catecholamines, which lead to lower rates of glycogen breakdown in liver and muscle; (3) reduced reliance on carbohydrate metabolism; and (4) changes in the isozymes of lactate dehydrogenase to forms that favor the

BLOOD LACTATE (mmol/L)

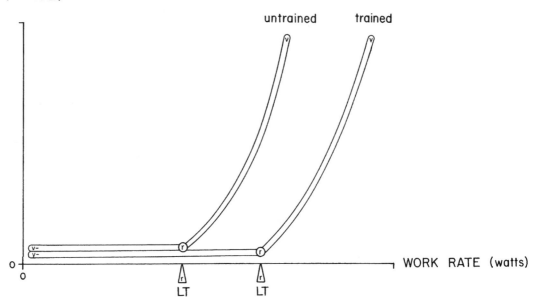

Figure 9.29 Effect of endurance training on blood lactate levels. Color the lines that depict blood levels of lactate (in mmol/L) plotted against work rate (in watts). Lines fitted to data obtained during a graded exercise test in the same person before (untrained) and after (trained) an endurance training program. Identify the lactate threshold (LT), defined as the exercise intensity beyond which blood levels of lactate rise above the resting level. Observe that endurance training increases the lactate threshold. Because the lactate threshold corresponds to the highest level of exercise intensity that can be sustained in the absence of a concomitant buildup of blood lactate, a higher lactate threshold is associated with a capacity to sustain a higher level of continuous submaximal exercise. Compare this figure with Figure 3.12.

conversion of lactate to pyruvate. Increased rates of lactate removal could be due to increased blood flow to the liver, which aids in lactate clearance, and to enhanced uptake of lactate by cardiac and skeletal muscle.

Longitudinal changes with endurance training

Increases in $\dot{V}O_2$max with endurance training are due to the combined effects of a number of factors, including: (1) a higher capillary-to-fiber ratio; (2) increased concentrations of Krebs cycle enzymes; (3) enhanced oxidative potential of fast-twitch fibers; and (4) increased cross-sectional area of slow-twitch fibers, indicating a preferential hypertrophy of the type I muscle fibers.

These factors exhibit different time courses. For example, Krebs cycle enzymes continue to increase over twenty-four months of training, while the cross-sectional area of slow-twitch fibers attains steady-state levels in approximately two months (Figure 9.30). In accordance with the reversibility principle, gains in aerobic capacity are quickly lost when training stops.

PERCENT INCREASE

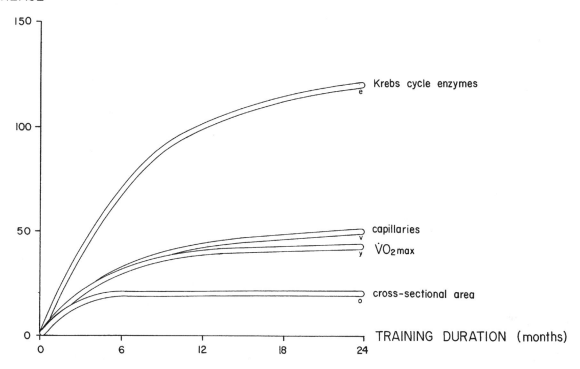

Figure 9.30 Longitudinal changes with endurance training. Color the lines that plot the percent increases in Krebs cycle enzymes, capillary density, V̇O₂max, and muscle cross-sectional area against training duration (in months). Compare the relative magnitudes and time courses of the different responses to endurance training. Observe that the increase in V̇O₂max with endurance training is due to the combined effects of a number of factors, including increased concentrations of Krebs cycle enzymes, a higher capillary density in trained muscles, and an increased cross-sectional area (hypertrophy) of type I muscle fibers. In accordance with the reversibility principle, these gains in aerobic capacity are quickly lost when training stops. Modified from B. Saltin et al. *Ann NY Acad Sci* 301:3, 1977.

chapter **ten**
nutrition

Nutrition is the scientific study of the metabolism of foods and the ways in which the diet, or habitual pattern of food intake, affects physiological function. Physical performance and health can be strongly influenced by an individual's nutritional practices.

Nutrients

The components of food may be grouped into six different categories, called *nutrients*, according to their chemistry and function. In order to be classified as a nutrient, a food component must be able to be digested, absorbed, transported through the blood, taken up into cells, and metabolized. Substances that fail to meet all of these criteria, such as dietary fiber and some food additives, are not considered to be nutrients.

The categories of nutrients are carbohydrates, fats, proteins, vitamins, minerals, and water (Figure 10.1). A substance also must be found to have a physiological function in order to be considered to be a nutrient. For example, even though the minerals gold and silver are found in human tissues, they are not classified as nutrients because they have no known biological function.

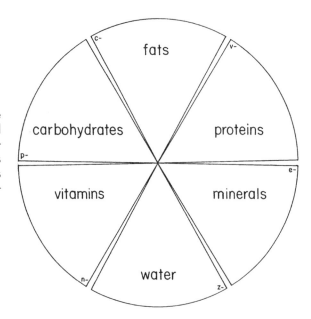

Figure 10.1 Categories of nutrients. Color the sections of the circle representing the six categories of nutrients; carbohydrates, fats, and proteins function as fuels, while vitamins, minerals and water serve non-fuel functions. Note that each class of nutrient, except for water, includes a number of different compounds; for example, the category of vitamins includes thirteen known substances or groups of related substances having common biological effects.

Nutrient requirements

For many of the nutrients, recommendations have been established that specify the amount to be consumed each day by healthy individuals. The Food and Nutrition Board of the National Research Council of the United States has, since 1941, published and periodically revised such standards. The *Recommended Dietary Allowance* (RDA) lists values for recommended daily intakes of energy (kcal), protein, and a number of vitamins and minerals. These standards are based on the results of scientific studies that are extrapolated to the general healthy population.

One way of determining the amount of a nutrient needed in the diet is to test different levels of intake, one at a time, over many weeks and to monitor the development of adverse symptoms, which are signs of inadequate intake (deficiency) of the nutrient. Deficiency of a particular nutrient is associated with a constellation of biochemical and physiological abnormalities, known as *deficiency signs* (Figure 10.2). For example, lack of vitamin C (ascorbic acid) produces fragile capillaries, poor formation of scar tissue, and decreased synthesis of certain neurotransmitters. The amount of time needed for a nutrient deficiency to cause abnormalities depends on the amount of the nutrient stored in the body and on the severity of the dietary deficiency. For example, signs of vitamin C deficiency could appear after a few weeks of no vitamin C intake, whereas signs of vitamin A deficiency might only develop after many months of no vitamin A intake.

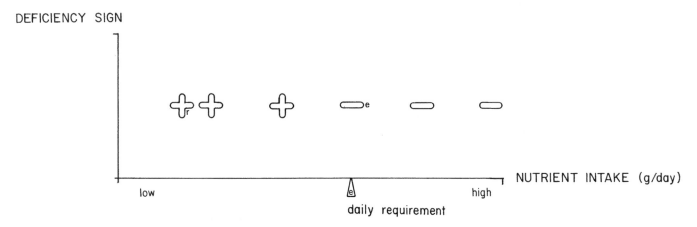

DEFICIENCY SIGN

NUTRIENT INTAKE (g/day)

low

high

daily requirement

Figure 10.2   Nutrient requirements. Color the plus and minus signs plotted against nutrient intake (in g/day), noting that "plus" indicates the presence of deficiency signs whereas "minus" indicates the absence of deficiency signs. Color the arrowhead labeled daily requirement, noting that it represents the minimal intake needed to prevent the development of deficiency signs. Each individual has his or her own daily requirement for each nutrient and these levels may differ widely among individuals.

The recommended daily intakes for protein, vitamins, and minerals incorporate a large margin of error, so that their RDAs overestimate the actual requirement of approximately 98% of the population and underestimate it for the remaining 2% of the population (Figure 10.3).

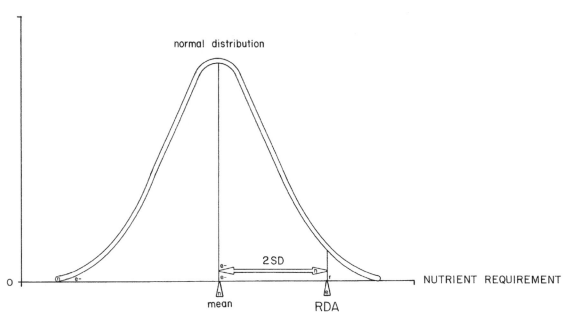

NUMBER OF PERSONS

normal distribution

2 SD

NUTRIENT REQUIREMENT

0

mean

RDA

Figure 10.3   Determination of the recommended dietary allowance (RDA). Color the normal distribution, which plots the number of persons in the population against their actual daily requirement for a particular nutrient. Observe that the curve reaches its peak (highest number of persons) at the mean requirement of the population (arrowhead labeled mean). Note that most people need the mean requirement, and that progressively fewer people need more or less than the mean requirement. Color the arrow labeled 2SD and the arrowhead labeled RDA, noting that the RDA is calculated by adding a generous margin of error (two standard deviations, 2SD) to the mean. Observe that the RDA overestimates the daily nutrient requirement in about 98% of the population (large area at left of RDA) and underestimates it in the remaining 2% of the population, (small area at right of RDA).

Dietary Reference Intake

The *Dietary Reference Intake* (DRI) is a group of published standards that is comprised of the RDA (described above), Estimated Average Requirements, Adequate Intakes (AI), and Tolerable Upper Intake Levels. The DRI represents an expansion and updating of recommendations for nutrient intake because it addresses requirements for all known nutrients, including those for which there is no RDA, as well as the upper limits of safe supplementation.

The *Estimated Average Requirement* establishes the intake of a nutrient needed to fulfill a particular function, not its complete set of functions as in the RDA. In contrast to the RDA, which satisfies the needs of about 98% of the population (Figure 10.3), the Estimated Average Requirement only lists the mean (average) requirement and so only satisfies the needs of about 50% of the population. Since for some nutrients there is insufficient information to establish an RDA or an Estimated Average Requirement, the value called *Adequate Intake* (AI) is used. This is the average amount of a given nutrient that is consumed by healthy people. *Tolerable Upper Intake Levels* indicate the intake above which toxicity is likely to occur; these values are used to assess the safety of nutritional supplements.

Factors affecting nutrient requirements

The actual amount of each nutrient that an individual requires is influenced by a number of factors, including genetics, body size, age, energy expenditure, and the composition of the diet. Genetic factors cause people to inherit different abilities to utilize or to recycle nutrients. The requirement for some nutrients, like protein, is proportional to body weight. Age is a consideration inasmuch as infants and children may need disproportionately more of a nutrient to meet the demands of tissue growth. Because energy expenditure can vary dramatically, energy requirements (in kcal) differ greatly among individuals. The composition of the diet is another relevant consideration, because the RDAs for nutrients involved in fuel usage—such as the vitamins thiamin, riboflavin, and niacin—depend on the number of calories that an individual consumes per day. Moreover, interactions between substances in the diet can influence the amount of a nutrient that should be consumed, because dietary components can enhance or inhibit the utilization of nutrients. For example, vitamin C promotes the absorption of iron whereas black tea hinders it, so that people with low vitamin C intakes and high tea consumption would have a higher iron requirement than people with the opposite pattern of intake.

In addition to the above considerations, a person's physical state can affect nutrient requirements. Requirements can be influenced by occupation, climate, and type of physical activity. The RDA for most nutrients is increased during pregnancy, and requirements may be altered by disease. In short, there is great variability among people in their actual nutrient requirements. The DRI addresses this variability by providing standards for different uses and, in the case of the RDA, by establishing a purposely high recommendation.

Nutritional support of exercise performance

Long-term nutritional practices can influence athletic performance because an individual's diet can affect health as well as body composition. For example, deficiency of iron produces anemia, which could limit performance by reducing the oxygen content of arterial blood. Short-term dietary practices can also influence athletic performance. For example, provision of fuels and fluid during exercise can improve endurance by replenishing blood glucose and by preventing dehydration.

Nutritional supplements

Nutritional supplements are utilized by many athletes in hope of enhancing performance. Some products consist of high concentrations of protein, vitamins, or minerals so that one serving would provide many times the RDA for those nutrients. Other products contain concentrated extracts of plants or substances chemically derived from them, which are thought to enhance physical function. Note that all are classified as supplements, or additions, to the diet. They are not substitutes for a healthful diet.

Characteristics of a healthful diet

Foods are complex substances. They contain not only the six categories of nutrients listed above but also many other materials that influence bodily function and risk of disease. Naturally occurring chemicals in plants *(phytochemicals)* affect absorption of vitamins and minerals; some phytochemicals are absorbed themselves and influence metabolism. *Dietary fiber,* the unabsorbed polysaccharide in plants, influences the growth of microorganisms in the large intestine that metabolize bile and other substances that affect development of cancer and cardiovascular disease. Highly processed foods, food extracts, and nutritional supplements are missing known and unknown compounds, found in unprocessed foods, that affect physiological function. For this reason, a healthful diet should consist of a large variety of relatively unprocessed foods.

A healthful diet should meet the RDA for all nutrients. Because the RDA is an overestimate of the needs of most people, intake of nutrients below the level of the RDA does not necessarily mean that deficiency signs will develop. Furthermore, since there is storage of nutrients in the body (which can range from a few days' to several years' supply, depending on the nutrient), a particular day's intake does not have to meet the RDA. However, since we do not know our personal requirements, it is prudent to use the RDA as a standard and to strive to meet its level for each nutrient.

Dietary assessment

The adequacy of one's diet can be assessed by recording, for several days, the amounts of all food and beverages consumed each day. This technique requires measurement of the weights or volumes of the items, or use of information on packages, to determine the number of portions of each food item that were actually consumed. The total daily intake of each nutrient or intake of energy (kcal) can then be calculated by multiplying the number of portions of each food item consumed per day by the nutrient or energy content of each portion; these latter values appear in published tables of food composition (Figure 10.4). This procedure permits the total daily intake of each nutrient to be obtained and compared to the RDA for the nutrient. Intakes that are chronically less than two-thirds of the RDA should be increased by dietary change.

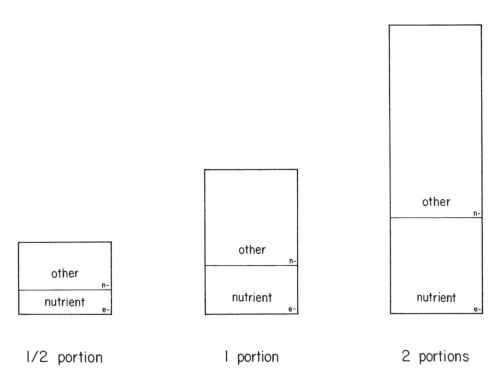

1/2 portion   1 portion   2 portions

Figure 10.4   Assessment of nutrient intake. The amount of a particular nutrient in a food can be estimated by using a table of food composition in which the amount of each nutrient contained in a specified amount (portion) of a food is listed. Color the single portion of the food, noting the amount of the nutrient contained in one portion (middle panel). Repeat this process for the ½-portion serving (left panel) and the 2-portion serving (right panel), noting that the amount of the nutrient has also been halved and doubled, respectively. These examples demonstrate that the total daily intake of a given nutrient can be calculated by multiplying the number of portions of each food item consumed per day by the nutrient content of each portion; these latter values appear in published tables of food composition. The nutritional adequacy of an individual's diet can be assessed by calculating the total amount of each nutrient in all of the foods consumed, and then comparing the values obtained with the RDA for each nutrient.

Energy requirements

The amount of energy (kcal) needed per day is one requirement that individuals can measure for themselves. Energy intake can be calculated through the dietary assessment technique described above. If energy intake is chronically inadequate, body weight loss will result; if energy intake is chronically excessive, body weight gain will result. The daily energy intake that supports a stable body weight (assuming good health and normal water balance) is the individual's energy requirement.

Increased physical activity (thermic effect of exercise, TEE, Figure 3.26) raises total energy expenditure and therefore raises the dietary energy requirement. If the individual simply increases the number of portions in an already healthful diet, then the intake of energy and of all nutrients will be increased proportionally. Athletes engaged in extreme activities (e.g., ultramarathons) may fail to eat adequate amounts of their normal diet to meet energy needs during the event and could require high-energy (high kcal/g) supplements.

In addition to the dietary assessment technique described above, the energy content of the diet (in kcal) also may be calculated by multiplying the amounts of carbohydrate, fat, and protein consumed per day (in g) by their corresponding physiological fuel values (in kcal/g, Figure 3.15). The optimal proportions of carbohydrate, fat, and protein in a diet depend on the nature and amount of physical activity that an individual performs as well as other considerations such as cardiovascular disease risk.

Carbohydrate intake

Carbohydrate is found in the diet in sugars, starches, and dietary fiber; the last category is not absorbed and so provides no energy value. Carbohydrate has several advantages compared with fat as a dietary energy source: (1) it is more rapidly absorbed; (2) it maintains blood levels of glucose,

thereby sparing glycogen and protein from breakdown; (3) it replenishes glycogen stores in muscle and liver; and (4) it is the only fuel that can be used by the glycolytic system (Figure 3.1).

High carbohydrate diets

A diet in which carbohydrate, in any form, contributes more than 50% of the total kcal is considered to be high in carbohydrate (Figure 10.5). If the individual's energy intake were 2000 kcal, carbohydrate intake would be at least 1000 kcal, which is provided by 250 grams of starch and/or sugar (carbohydrate yields 4 kcal/g). Athletes involved in endurance events may require much higher energy intakes; ultramarathon athletes, for example, may consume more than 4000 kcal per day. A 50% carbohydrate diet in these elite competitors would therefore consist of over 500 g of carbohydrate per day. Individuals who consume fewer kcal may utilize diets with higher carbohydrate compositions, sometimes as high as 80% of kcal, to achieve high carbohydrate intakes (Figure 10.6). As long as protein, fat, and other nutrient requirements are met, extremely high carbohydrate diets can be nutritionally adequate.

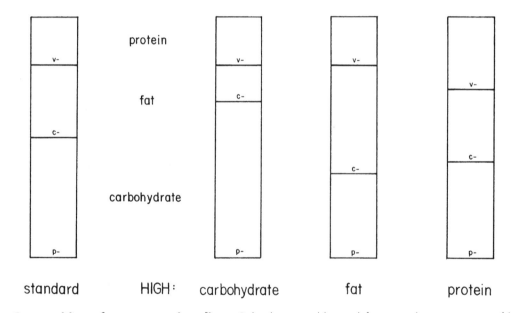

Figure 10.5 Composition of representative diets. Color the vertical bar at left, noting the percentages of kcal provided by protein (20%), fat (30%), and carbohydrate (50%) in a standard diet that is recommended for the general population to reduce risk of cardiovascular disease. Repeat this process for a high carbohydrate diet (65% kcal as carbohydrate, 15% kcal as fat, 20% kcal as protein), a high fat diet (35% kcal as carbohydrate, 45% kcal as fat, 20% kcal as protein), and a high protein diet (40% kcal as carbohydrate, 30% kcal as fat, 30% kcal as protein). Observe that in order to keep the total energy content (kcal) of the diet constant, an increase in the intake of any component must be offset by corresponding decreases in intakes of the other components. This consideration explains why high carbohydrate diets are usually low fat diets.

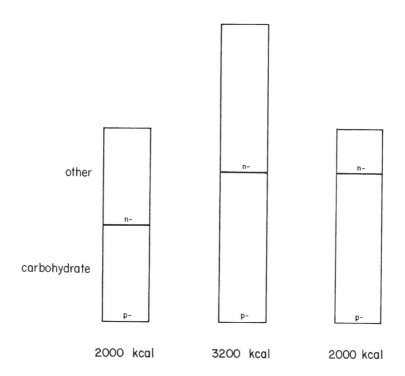

2000 kcal   3200 kcal   2000 kcal

Figure 10.6 High carbohydrate diets. Color the bar at left, noting that its height indicates the total energy content of this diet (2000 kcal) and that 50% of these kcal (1000 kcal) are provided by carbohydrate (lower portion) and the remaining 50% (1000 kcal) are provided by other nutrients (upper portion). Color the middle bar, noting that it depicts a higher energy diet (3200 kcal) in which 50% of the energy (1600 kcal) also comes from carbohydrate. Color the bar at right, noting that it depicts a diet with the same total energy content as in the left panel (2000 kcal) and the same number of carbohydrate kcal (1600 kcal) as in the middle panel and that this results in a diet in which 80% of the energy comes from carbohydrate. These examples illustrate that higher carbohydrate intakes can be achieved either by increasing the total intake of a diet with a given composition (middle bar) or by increasing carbohydrate intake at the expense of fat and/or protein intake so that total kcal intake can remain unchanged (right bar).

Another way of expressing carbohydrate requirement is on a body weight basis. Between 6 and 10 g of carbohydrate per kg of body weight are recommended; the higher levels are recommended for competitive endurance athletes. This method bypasses the need to adjust the % kcal recommendations for those individuals who have lowered their energy intake to lose weight.

Form of dietary carbohydrate

From a nutritional perspective, the best sources of dietary carbohydrate are minimally processed grains, vegetables, and fruits. These foods have high carbohydrate contents (kcal from carbohydrate expressed as a percent of total kcal) and are rich sources of vitamins, minerals, dietary fiber, and phytochemicals. The lack of these additional food components may make commercial "sports" candy bars and other supplements inferior substitutes for unprocessed foods.

Effect of dietary carbohydrate on glycogen storage

Dietary carbohydrate is necessary for the maintenance of muscle glycogen stores, which are indispensable for prolonged strenuous exercise. Ingested carbohydrate is a source of blood glucose, from which glycogen is synthesized. Ingestion of carbohydrate also increases insulin release, which stimulates the pathway of glycogen synthesis. For these reasons, high carbohydrate diets promote glycogen synthesis (Figure 10.7). Conversely, adherence to the very low carbohydrate diets that are advocated popularly for rapid weight loss (< 50 g carbohydrate/day) leads to the depletion of glycogen stores in liver and muscle. Low levels of muscle glycogen diminish an individual's capacity to perform physical activities that rely heavily on glycogen stores, such as high-intensity exercises or long-duration exercises.

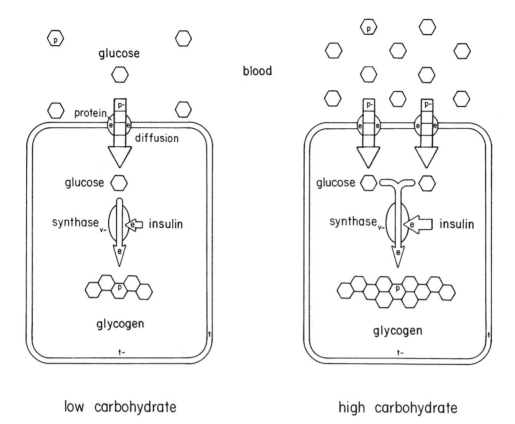

low carbohydrate   high carbohydrate

Figure 10.7   Effect of carbohydrate intake on glycogen synthesis. Color the molecules of glucose in the blood and their facilitated diffusion into the muscle cell at left, which depicts conditions with a low carbohydrate diet. Color the reaction in which glycogen is synthesized from glucose through the action of the enzyme glycogen synthase. Color the molecules of glucose in the blood and their facilitated diffusion into the muscle cell at right, which depicts conditions with a high carbohydrate diet. Color the reaction in which glycogen is synthesized from glucose through the action of glycogen synthase. Compare the two panels, observing that the high carbohydrate diet is associated with higher blood levels of glucose (higher density of hexagons), improved uptake of glucose (more transport proteins in membrane), increased stimulation of glycogen synthase by insulin (larger horizontal arrow indicating higher blood levels of insulin), and greater synthesis of glycogen (larger molecule). Compare this figure with Figure 7.23.

Glycogen loading

The direct relationship between carbohydrate intake and glycogen storage provides the rationale for the technique of *glycogen loading* (also called carbohydrate loading or supercompensation), which is intended to prolong high-level performance. The underlying principle of carbohydrate loading, regardless of the particular regimen that is followed, is to deplete glycogen stores in the muscles that are most utilized in the activity and then to refill (replete) them with a greater amount of glycogen (Figure 10.8). About a week before the event, the athlete consumes a low carbohydrate diet (e.g., 2 g

of carbohydrate per kg body weight, 2 g/kg) and performs high-intensity exercise to exhaustion. A few days before the event, the athlete switches to a high carbohydrate diet (e.g., 10 g/kg) and dramatically reduces training intensity, in some cases to no training on the day before the event.

Training is a necessary feature of the carbohydrate loading technique; only those muscles that are trained during the regimen exhibit enhancement of glycogen storage. A high carbohydrate diet, by itself, does not cause glycogen loading in a sedentary individual.

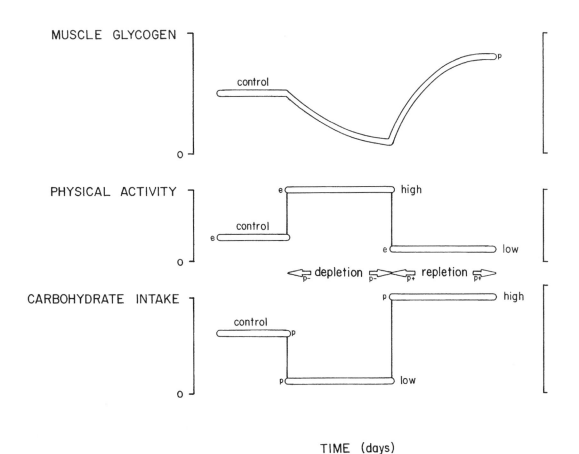

Figure 10.8 Glycogen loading technique. Color the lines that plot muscle glycogen content (top panel), physical activity (middle panel), and carbohydrate intake (bottom panel) against time (in days). Note that the glycogen loading technique involves a period of glycogen depletion followed by a period of glycogen repletion. Observe that glycogen depletion (downward curve, top panel) occurs in response to high levels of physical activity (middle panel) coupled with low levels of carbohydrate intake (bottom panel). Observe also that glycogen repletion (upward curve, top panel) occurs in response to low levels of physical activity (middle panel) coupled with high levels of carbohydrate intake (bottom panel). Note that the final level of muscle glycogen (right end of top line) exceeds the initial (control) level of muscle glycogen (left end of line), indicating that this procedure increases the absolute amount of glycogen stored in muscle. Glycogen loading occurs only in muscles that are exercised during the depletion period.

Carbohydrate intake before and during exercise

Fasting (including an overnight fast) depletes glycogen stores and may therefore interfere with optimal performance. For this reason, a high carbohydrate meal (like breakfast) should be eaten a few hours before an athletic event to replete glycogen stores.

Consumption of a high carbohydrate snack within 30 minutes of the onset of physical activity may diminish initial performance because of gastrointestinal distress or because of transient *hypoglycemia* (lower than normal concentration of blood glucose) that results from glucose-stimulated insulin release (Figure 10.9). Hypoglycemia does not occur when the same amount of carbohydrate is consumed after the onset of exercise, because the catecholamines that are released during exercise suppress the release of insulin and therefore its effect on blood glucose (Figure 7.19).

During exercise, muscle metabolizes glucose obtained from the breakdown of its glycogen stores and glucose that it takes up from the blood. Glucose is supplied to the blood by the liver through the breakdown of liver glycogen (glycogenolysis) and through the synthesis of glucose from noncarbohydrate sources (gluconeogenesis) as well as by the absorption of ingested carbohydrate from the gastrointestinal system. Thus, carbohydrate intake during exercise can mitigate the decline in blood glucose during prolonged activities and bring about a slower depletion of glycogen stores in liver and muscle. For these reasons, carbohydrate ingestion during exercise can prolong its duration.

BLOOD GLUCOSE

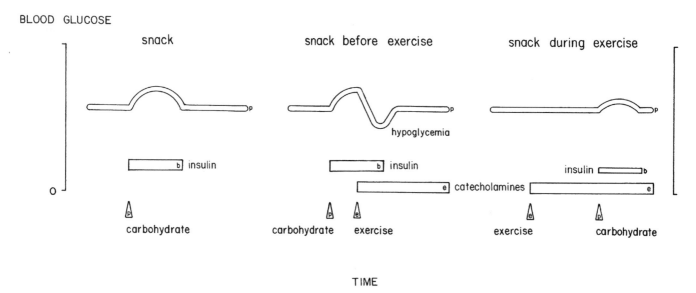

Figure 10.9   Effect of carbohydrate ingestion on blood glucose during exercise. Color the panels from left to right, noting that the top lines indicate blood glucose levels plotted against time. Observe in the left panel that the consumption of a high carbohydrate snack (arrowhead labeled carbohydrate) causes a subsequent rise in blood glucose levels above the horizontal baseline. Color the horizontal band (labeled insulin) representing the magnitude (height of band) and duration (width of band) of insulin release. Observe in the middle panel that the consumption of the same carbohydrate snack (arrowhead labeled carbohydrate) 30 minutes prior to the onset of exercise (arrowhead labeled exercise) causes an initial rise in blood glucose followed by a fall in blood glucose to below the baseline level (transient hypoglycemia). Color the horizontal bands that indicate the release of insulin and catecholamines, noting that insulin release precedes catecholamine release because the snack was consumed before exercise began. Blood glucose levels are lowered both by the action of insulin and by increased uptake of glucose by exercising muscle. Observe in the right panel that the consumption of the same carbohydrate snack (arrowhead labeled carbohydrate) after the onset of exercise (arrowhead labeled exercise) does not cause transient hypoglycemia. Color the horizontal bands that indicate the release of insulin and catecholamines, noting that catecholamine release precedes insulin release because the snack was consumed after exercise began. Observe also that the magnitude of insulin release is smaller (narrower band) because catecholamines suppress insulin release. These considerations explain why the consumption of a high carbohydrate snack within 30 minutes before the onset of exercise might prevent optimal performance.

The rate of absorption of foods consumed during exercise is a consideration in their selection. The *Glycemic Index* of a food is a measure of its ability to make blood levels of glucose rise; foods with a high Glycemic Index cause blood glucose concentration to rise rapidly and attain the level produced by the same amount of carbohydrate consumed as pure glucose. In general, foods with higher protein, fat, and dietary fiber contents are associated with lower rates of carbohydrate absorption and therefore have a lower Glycemic Index. In order to maintain blood glucose levels during continuous physical activity, foods with a high Glycemic Index should be consumed within the first hour of exercise, before blood levels of glucose begin to fall.

Postexercise carbohydrate intake

Carbohydrate intake is required to replete liver and muscle glycogen stores. The period immediately following the cessation of exercise is optimal for glycogen synthesis (Figure 10.10) because: (1) blood flow and therefore glucose delivery to muscle is still high; (2) exercise-stimulated uptake of glucose is still high; and (3) the enzyme glycogen synthase is more sensitive to insulin in the postexercise period than at other times. For these reasons, the consumption of a given amount of glucose leads to the formation of more muscle glycogen in the postexercise state than in the resting state

(Figure 10.11). Therefore, glycogen repletion is best served by the consumption of carbohydrate immediately after exercise.

Any form of carbohydrate is effective in promoting postexercise glycogen repletion; it is the amount of carbohydrate that is important. Carbohydrate in foods with lower fat, protein, and fiber contents are absorbed more rapidly, so such high Glycemic Index foods may be more efficient in increasing muscle glycogen content during the early postexercise period.

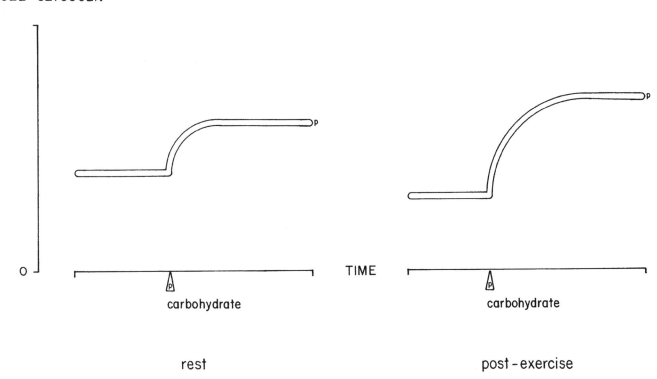

MUSCLE GLYCOGEN

TIME

rest

post-exercise

Figure 10.10 Postexercise glycogen synthesis. Color the lines that show muscle glycogen plotted against time in the resting state (left panel) and the postexercise state (right panel). Note the times at which a high carbohydrate meal is ingested (arrowheads labeled carbohydrate). Observe that the pre-meal (baseline) level of muscle glycogen is higher in the resting state than in the postexercise state. Observe also that the post-meal level of muscle glycogen is higher in the postexercise state than in the resting state. These findings demonstrate that glycogen repletion is best served by the consumption of carbohydrate immediately following exercise when blood flow to muscle is still high and the enzyme glycogen synthase is more sensitive to insulin.

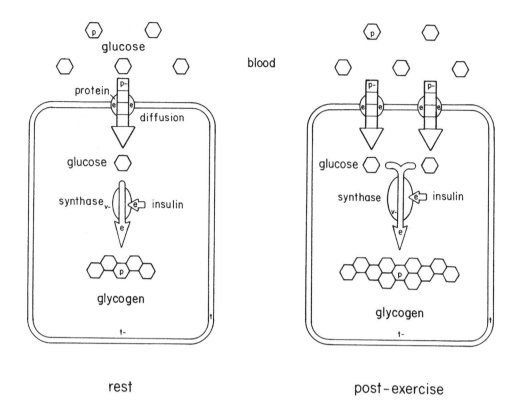

rest

post-exercise

Figure 10.11   Mechanism of postexercise glycogen synthesis. Color the molecules of glucose in the blood and their facilitated diffusion into the muscle cell at left, which depicts conditions in the resting state. Color the reaction in which glycogen is synthesized from glucose through the action of the enzyme glycogen synthase. Color the molecules of glucose in the blood and their facilitated diffusion into the muscle cell at right, which depicts conditions in the postexercise state. Color the reaction in which glycogen is synthesized from glucose through the action of glycogen synthase. Compare the panels, observing that the postexercise state is associated with equivalent levels of blood glucose (equal density of hexagons), improved uptake of glucose (more transport proteins in membrane), equivalent levels of insulin (same size arrows), increased sensitivity of enzyme to insulin (bigger icon for enzyme), and greater synthesis of glycogen (larger molecule). The greater stimulation of glucose uptake and glycogen synthesis by insulin that occurs during the immediate postexercise period is evidence of the greater insulin sensitivity in muscle that is produced by exercise. Because of this effect, exercise is a useful therapy for controlling blood glucose levels in obesity and type 2 diabetes mellitus. Compare this figure with Figures 7.23, 10.7, and 10.10.

Fat intake

Fat is a necessary component of the diet. Its three main functions are to provide a concentrated source of energy, to enable fat-soluble vitamins to be absorbed, and to supply the precursors (called essential fatty acids) for synthesis of regulatory compounds called eicosanoids.

Storage of fat in adipose tissue does not require consumption of fat from the diet. Dietary carbohydrate can be converted to fat, as occurs during weight gain on high carbohydrate diets. Because fat is a more concentrated source of kcal than carbohydrate (Figure 3.15), high fat diets tend to be high-energy (kcal) diets that will cause weight gain unless energy expenditure is also high.

Dietary fat is needed for the fat-soluble vitamins, A, D, E, and K to be dissolved, emulsified, and absorbed in the intestine and for them to be transported to tissues in lipoprotein particles (Figure 2.34). It is estimated that between 15 and 40 g of fat (equivalent to 135 to 360 kcal) per day must be consumed for adequate absorption and transport of fat-soluble vitamins.

Polyunsaturated fatty acids

Polyunsaturated fatty acids are needed in the diet because they serve as precursors for the synthesis of locally acting hormones called eicosanoids. Polyunsaturated fatty acids have two or more carbon-to-carbon double bonds (Figure 2.28); the locations of the double bonds vary. Polyunsaturated fatty acids in which the first carbon-to-carbon double bond is at the third carbon from the CH_3 (methyl, or omega) end are called *omega-3 polyunsaturated fatty acids* (Figure 10.12); these are found mainly in coldwater fish such as salmon, tuna, and mackerel or in their extracted oils. *Omega-6 polyunsaturated fatty acids* have their first double bond at the sixth carbon from the methyl end; they are found in plant oils such as corn, safflower, and sunflower oils.

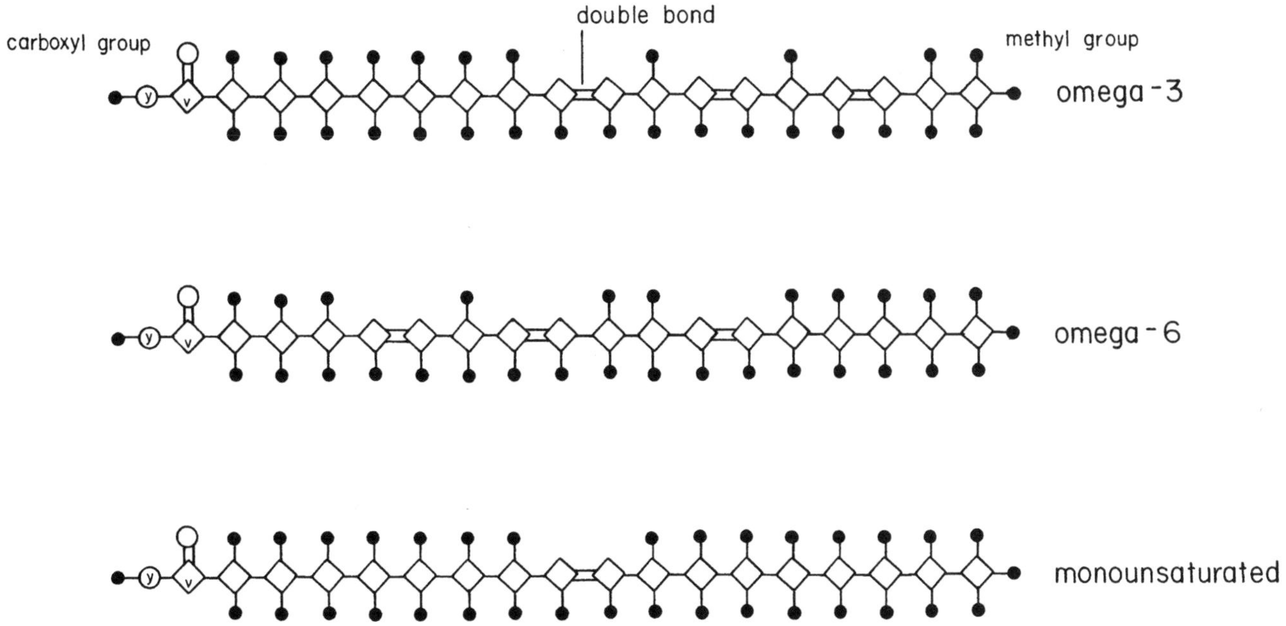

Figure 10.12 Structures of unsaturated fatty acids. Color the carbon (diamonds) and oxygen (open circles) atoms and identify the hydrogen atoms (filled circles) in the top structure (α-linolenic acid); identify its carboxyl (COOH) end and its methyl (CH₃) (or omega) end. Count its carbon atoms and its carbon-to-carbon double bonds, noting their positions relative to the omega end of the molecule. Because the carbon-to-carbon double bond nearest the omega end is at the third carbon, it is called an omega-3 fatty acid. Repeat this process for the middle structure (γ-linolenic acid), which is called an omega-6 fatty acid because its carbon-to-carbon double bond nearest the omega end is at the sixth carbon. These compounds are classified as polyunsaturated fatty acids because they have at least two carbon-to-carbon double bonds. Next, color the bottom structure (oleic acid), counting its carbon atoms and observing the placement of its carbon-to-carbon double bond. Because it has one carbon-to-carbon double bond, it is a monounsaturated fatty acid. Omega-3 and omega-6 polyunsaturated fatty acids are classified as essential fatty acids because the body cannot form double bonds within nine carbons from the methyl end of a fatty acid. Monounsaturated fatty acids are not essential fatty acids because they can be synthesized in the body. Compare this figure with Figure 2.28.

Essential fatty acids

The omega-3 and omega-6 polyunsaturated fatty acids cannot be synthesized in the human body and therefore must be obtained from the diet. For this reason, they are called *essential fatty acids.* Daily intake of essential fatty acids should provide about 2% of the total energy intake. For a person consuming 2000 kcal/day, total essential fatty acid intake should be about 4.5 g/day (providing 40 kcal); 25% of this amount (about 1 g) should be comprised of omega-3 polyunsaturated fatty acids. Although the requirement for athletes, based on energy intake, is the same as for the general population, some athletes use supplements of omega-3 polyunsaturated fatty acids for their anti-clotting and purported vasodilatory effects.

Both omega-3 and omega-6 polyunsaturated fatty acids are converted by cells to a variety of 20-carbon compounds called *eicosanoids* (eicosa means 20), which include prostaglandins, prostacyclins, thromboxanes, and leukotrienes. The eicosanoids regulate a number of processes that occur within cells and outside of cells. For example, blood clotting is stimulated by some of these compounds but inhibited by others, so that the relative amounts of the different types of these compounds determine the net effect. Various eicosanoids regulate the contraction of vascular and bronchial smooth muscle, the function of the immune system, and the secretion of hormones.

High fat diets

Although a high carbohydrate diet increases the usage of carbohydrate as a fuel, a high fat diet (> 40% of kcal as fat) does not increase the usage of fat as a fuel. Thus, RQ values, a measure of fuel utilization (Figure 3.20), are raised by high carbohydrate diets but are not lowered by high fat diets (when the dietary content of the other fuels is held constant).

Since normal blood levels of glucose must be maintained for proper function of the nervous system, diets that are high in fat but low in carbohydrate can lead to increased protein breakdown to provide the substrates for glucose synthesis by gluconeogenesis (Figure 2.26). Because high fat diets do not promote glycogen storage (Figure 10.13), they are not optimal for activities that are limited by glycogen depletion, such as high-intensity or long-duration exercises. Since the amount of fat in the diet does not appear to influence the amount of fat mobilized from adipose tissue during exercise, high fat diets do not appear to improve performance in endurance exercise, although benefits have sometimes been reported for prolonged low-intensity exercise.

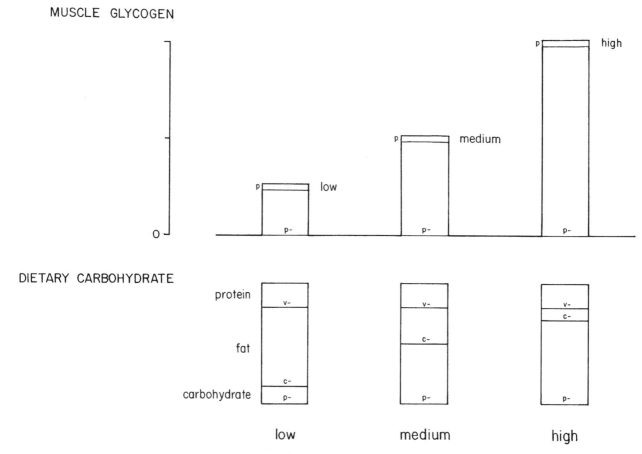

Figure 10.13 Effect of diet composition on glycogen storage. Color the bars that represent the compositions of a low (15% kcal as carbohydrate), medium (50% kcal as carbohydrate), and high (70% kcal as carbohydrate) carbohydrate diet (bottom panel). Observe that the total energy (height of bars) and protein contents of the diets are the same. Color the graph above each bar, which depicts the muscle glycogen level associated with the diet beneath it. Observe that low carbohydrate (high fat) diets lead to low levels of muscle glycogen (left panel) and, at the opposite extreme, high carbohydrate diets lead to high levels of muscle glycogen (right panel). Because glycogen depletion occurs during weight loss, this relationship between carbohydrate intake and muscle glycogen content can be observed only when there is adequate energy intake.

Dietary sources of fat

Fat is a component of most foods; the highest fat concentration is found in oils (~100% fat). The fat in foods may be visible, as in the adipose tissue included in many cuts of meat, or perceived through its texture or flavor, as when frying provides a crispy texture. However, the fat contents of many foods are often unappreciated by consumers; foods categorized as sweet (cookies, ice cream) may be high in fat, and meals purchased in fast-food restaurants are typically high in fat.

Intake of saturated fat is associated with increased risk of cardiovascular disease; it is recommended that less than 10% of a person's energy intake come from saturated fat each day. Although regular exercise decreases one's risk of cardiovascular disease, it may not compensate for the disease-promoting effect of a high saturated fat diet. Diets rich in *monounsaturated fats* (fatty acids having one carbon-to-carbon double bond) (Figure 10.12) and polyunsaturated fats lower one's risk of cardiovascular disease. However, intake of even unsaturated fat should not exceed 30% of kcal, since high intakes of polyunsaturated fat are associated with increased prevalence of some forms of cancer.

Protein intake

Dietary protein provides amino acids for fuel and for building body protein. The amino acids that are made in adequate quantities in the body are called *nonessential amino acids,* and those that must be provided by the diet are called *essential amino acids.* Thus, adequate intake of protein not only involves the total amount of protein but also the amounts of the specific essential amino acids (Figure 10.14).

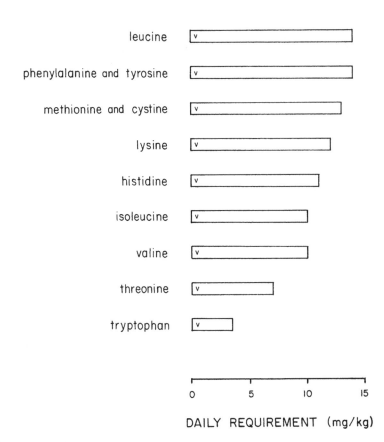

leucine

phenylalanine and tyrosine

methionine and cystine

lysine

histidine

isoleucine

valine

threonine

tryptophan

0　　5　　10　　15

DAILY REQUIREMENT (mg/kg)

Figure 10.14　Essential amino acid requirements. Color the horizontal bar, next to the name of each essential amino acid, that represents the amount (mg/ kg of body weight) of the particular amino acid that is required in the diet each day. Observe that the amounts vary among amino acids. Note that some amino acids are grouped together, since intake of one decreases the need for the other—that is, tyrosine can be synthesized from phenylalanine, and cystine can be synthesized from methionine.

Essential amino acids

In adults, the essential amino acids are leucine, isoleucine, valine, phenylalanine, tryptophan, methionine, histidine, lysine, and threonine. They are required in the diet in certain proportions; dietary proteins that contain all of the essential amino acids in these approximate proportions are called *complete,* or *high-quality,* proteins. Dietary proteins that are low in an essential amino acid relative to its required proportion (which would be called the *limiting amino acid* for that protein source) are called *incomplete,* or *low-quality,* proteins (Figure 10.15).

Dairy products, eggs, meat, fish, and poultry are sources of complete protein, whereas most plant-derived foods are sources of incomplete protein. However, by eating two plant sources chosen so that the limiting amino acid in one source is provided by the other source, a meal can be composed that has the correct proportions of all of the essential amino acids. This practice, utilized by vegetarians, is called *complementation of protein.*

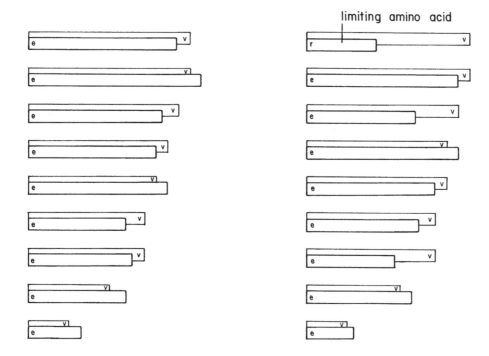

complete protein · · · · · · · · · · · · · · incomplete protein

Figure 10.15   Complete and incomplete proteins. Color the bars that represents the amount of each essential amino acid contained in a complete protein source (left panel) and in an incomplete protein source (right panel), noting that for each amino acid the bar is superimposed on the corresponding amino acid requirement depicted in Figure 10.14. Observe that in the complete protein the relative amounts of the essential amino acids are similar to their requirements. Observe also that the amounts of some amino acids are far below the requirement in the incomplete protein, while the amounts of others meet or exceed the requirement. The essential amino acid whose amount falls most below its requirement is known as the limiting amino acid for that protein source (top bar, right panel). In order to satisfy the daily protein requirement using this incomplete protein, the individual would have to consume enough of it to provide the daily requirement of the limiting amino acid and, in the process, would therefore consume amounts of the other amino acids that greatly exceed their requirements. The implication is that a greater amount of incomplete protein than complete protein is needed to fulfill protein requirements.

Protein requirements

The amount of protein required each day depends upon the quality of protein consumed. High-quality protein is used more efficiently, since it supplies the correct proportions of the essential amino acids needed for protein synthesis. In other words, it is necessary to consume a greater amount of low-quality protein than high-quality protein to meet the requirements for essential amino acids (Figure 10.16).

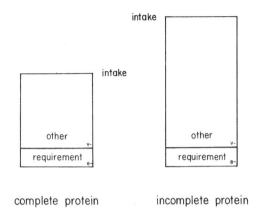

complete protein   incomplete protein

Figure 10.16 Protein requirements. Color the rectangle at left that depicts an amount of complete protein (height of rectangle) in a particular food, noting that it contains the amount of essential amino acids required for the day (requirement). Next color the rectangle at right that illustrates that a larger amount of incomplete protein (higher rectangle) is needed to provide the same amount of essential amino acids (requirement). Observe that more nonrequired (other) amino acids must be consumed when incomplete protein is used than when complete protein is used; this occurs because more of the incomplete protein must be consumed to meet the requirement for its limiting amino acid (Figure 10.15). The excess of other amino acids that are consumed in incomplete protein can be used as a fuel; the amino groups removed from these amino acids in the process are excreted as urea.

Protein requirements can be assessed by measuring a person's *nitrogen balance* under specified conditions. The method compares nitrogen intake in the diet with nitrogen excreted in urine and other nitrogen-containing substances (Figure 10.17). Nitrogen intake can be calculated from dietary protein intake by assuming that 1 g nitrogen corresponds to 6.25 g protein. Nitrogen output can be quantified by measuring the nitrogen in urea (plus other urinary nitrogen), feces, hair and nail growth, as well as in sweat, shedded skin, and lost blood.

Positive nitrogen balance is a condition in which nitrogen intake exceeds nitrogen output, indicating that there is a net addition of protein to the body. This occurs during childhood growth, body building, weight gain, and pregnancy. Negative nitrogen balance occurs when there is a net loss of protein from the body, as occurs when weight is lost or when protein intake is inadequate. Nitrogen balance (zero balance) is the usual state for healthy adults who are neither gaining nor losing weight.

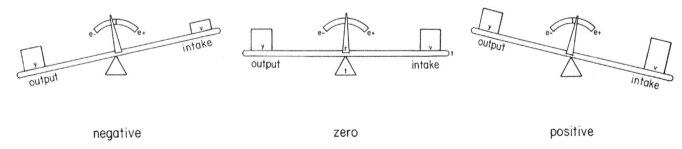

negative   zero   positive

Figure 10.17 Nitrogen balance. Color the balance, the pointer, and the nitrogen scale. For each condition, color and compare the rectangles that depict the rate (g/day) at which nitrogen is removed from the body (output, left side of balance) and the rate at which nitrogen is added to the body (intake, right side of balance). Observe that nitrogen balance is negative when output exceeds intake (left panel), zero when output equals intake (middle panel), and positive when intake exceeds output (right panel). Zero nitrogen balance occurs in adults who are not gaining or losing weight and who have an adequate protein intake. Negative nitrogen balance occurs when amino acids are lacking in the diet either because the total amount of protein is too low or because intake of limiting amino acids is inadequate; negative balance also usually occurs during weight loss. Positive nitrogen balance occurs during growth, weight gain, or other addition of lean body mass, (e.g., body building) when protein intake is adequate. Note that increased protein intake alone does not cause positive nitrogen balance, since increased intake is matched by increased nitrogen output in urea unless other factors (e.g., hormonal signals) promote protein retention.

Assessment of protein requirements

An individual's protein requirement can be assessed by determining the lowest intake of high-quality protein needed to offset the level of nitrogen output (Figure 10.18). If too little protein is consumed, nitrogen output will exceed nitrogen intake and negative nitrogen balance will result. This technique requires that the subject consume a particular level of protein for several weeks because more efficient recycling of amino acids occurs as one adapts to a low protein diet.

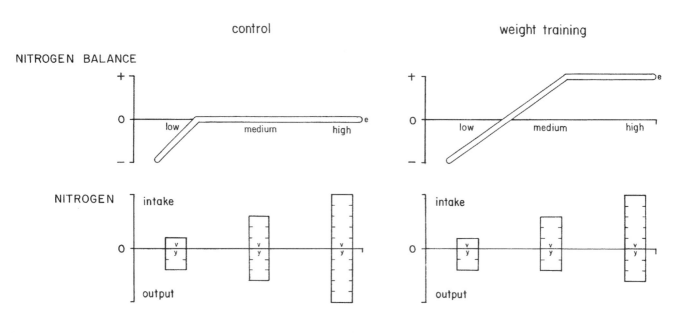

Figure 10.18 **Effect of protein intake on nitrogen balance.** Color the line in the upper left panel that represents nitrogen balance at different levels of protein intake in the control (non-weight training) condition. Observe that nitrogen balance is negative at low (deficient) levels of protein intake, zero at medium levels of protein intake, and zero at high levels of protein intake. The graph below plots the levels of nitrogen intake and output that correspond to each of these conditions. Note that nitrogen intake is depicted as a bar graph above the x-axis and nitrogen output is depicted as a bar graph below the x-axis. Observe that negative nitrogen balance at low protein intake (top panel) occurs because nitrogen output (2 units) exceeds nitrogen intake (1 unit). Observe also that zero nitrogen balance occurs at the medium and high levels of protein intake because these levels of nitrogen intake (3 units for medium and 5 units for high) are matched by equal levels of nitrogen output (also 3 and 5 units, respectively). Color the line in the upper right panel that represents nitrogen balance at different levels of protein intake in a person engaged in a weight training program involving resistance exercises. Observe that nitrogen balance is negative at low levels of protein intake, positive at medium levels of protein intake, and more positive at high levels of protein intake. Color the graph beneath, comparing the levels of nitrogen intake and nitrogen output that correspond to each of these conditions. Observe that negative nitrogen balance occurs at low levels of protein intake because nitrogen output (2 units) exceeds nitrogen intake (1 unit). Also observe that positive nitrogen balance occurs at the medium and high levels of protein intake because intake exceeds output in each of these conditions (3 vs. 2 units for medium intake and 5 vs. 3 units at high intake). Identify the level of protein intake for which positive nitrogen balance reaches a plateau, noting that this level of protein intake represents the upper limit for building body protein. Compare this figure with Figure 10.17.

Protein requirements of healthy adults have been estimated using diets containing high-quality protein and ensuring that the subjects were neither gaining nor losing weight. The average requirement was found to be 0.47 g of protein per kg of body weight. To this value, a margin of error was added to account for variation among individuals and for variation in the quality of dietary protein, so that the resulting RDA for protein is 0.8 g/kg. Using this formula, the RDA for a 50 kg woman would be be 40 g protein. If her daily energy intake were 1800 kcal, her protein requirement would represent 160 kcal, or about 9% of her energy intake. This example illustrates that a diet that is 15% to 20% protein, which is often recommended, generally exceeds the RDA for protein content (Figure 10.5).

The RDA sets values for protein intake that prevent negative nitrogen balance in the general population. It does not set the optimal level for an adult body builder who should be in positive nitrogen balance when building muscle. The optimal level of protein intake can be measured by utilizing higher intakes of protein to determine the amount that supports the highest level of positive nitrogen balance. Since addition of protein to the body is supported by higher intakes but is not caused by them, the degree of positive nitrogen balance will eventually reach a limit and increase no further. Once the upper limit of protein intake is reached, additional intake of dietary nitrogen will be excreted in urea (Figure 10.18).

Protein requirements for endurance exercise

The RDA for protein is sufficient for individuals who participate in moderate-intensity exercise. As noted above, if a person using more energy consumes more of his usual, healthful diet to provide the kcal, then intake of all nutrients will be increased proportionally. Some studies have shown that endurance athletes require somewhat more than the RDA for protein (1.0 to 1.4 g/kg) in order to maintain nitrogen balance because their nitrogen output is higher than that of average individuals of the same body weight. The reason for this increased nitrogen output may be the additional use of amino acids as fuel by muscle during endurance exercise; the nitrogen-containing (amino) groups of the amino acids that are used as fuel are excreted as urea, causing an increase in nitrogen output.

Most healthy adults in the United States consume more than the RDA for protein, so that the higher recommendation for endurance training is likely to be provided by a normal diet. Using the example above, if the 50 kg woman were an en-durance athlete, she would need 50 to 70 g of protein, or 11% to 16% of kcal in the 1800 kcal diet as protein.

Protein requirements for strength training

Strength training leads to a net addition of protein to the body and therefore to positive nitrogen balance. Studies support a higher protein requirement for body builders than the RDA, between 1.8 and 2.6 g/kg, with the upper end of the range recommended for those participating in very high-intensity training. This level of intake may be provided by a normal diet without commercial supplements, for example, by utilizing foods with a high protein density like skim milk (8 g of protein per 80 kcal, or 40% of kcal as protein). Using these higher values for protein requirement, a 90 kg man with an energy intake of 3500 kcal would need between 162 and 234 g of protein, or 23% to 27% of kcal intake; this would be considered to be a high protein diet (Figure 10.5).

Upper limit for protein intake

Once protein intake is adequate to support the highest rate of protein accumulation that is promoted by training or by physiological signals (as in childhood growth), the excess protein that is ingested will be utilized as fuel. When amino acids are oxidized, their amino groups are removed, incorporated into urea by the liver, and excreted by the kidney in urine. The point at which the rate of urea excretion increases disproportionately to protein intake marks the upper limit beyond which additional protein intake is superfluous (Figure 10.19).

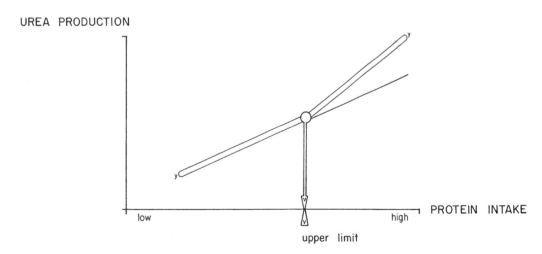

Figure 10.19 Upper limit of protein requirement. Color the line that plots urea production (a measure of nitrogen removal) against protein intake. Observe that a given increment in protein intake causes a proportional increment in urea production (straight line) until the upper limit of protein requirement is reached (arrowhead). Observe also that a given increment in protein intake in excess of the upper limit causes a greater increment in urea production (straight line with steeper slope). These results show that the excess protein is broken down for fuel and the amino groups are used to form urea. Thus, measurement of urea production at different levels of protein intake beyond the RDA can be used to determine the maximal level of dietary protein intake that will still contribute to training-induced addition of body protein. Compare this figure with Figure 10.18.

For individuals with impaired liver or kidney function, the processing of excess protein poses a physiological stress that could worsen their disease. In addition, high protein intakes (more than twice the RDA) have been associated with increased urinary loss of calcium from the body, perhaps increasing the risk of *osteoporosis* (loss of bone mass).

Vitamins

Vitamins are organic compounds, necessary in the diet in trace amounts, that have specific regulatory (as opposed to fuel) functions. Vitamins are classified by their solubility: Vitamins A, D, E, and K are fat-soluble, and the B vitamins and vitamin C are water-soluble. The B vitamins, grouped together because they were not initially distinguished from one another, consist of thiamin, riboflavin, niacin, vitamin B_6, folate, vitamin B_{12}, biotin, and pantothenic acid. Vitamin C, or ascorbic acid, differs from the B vitamins in that it does not contain nitrogen.

Vitamins have a wide variety of functions. They may supply the portion of coenzymes (such as hydrogen carriers, Figure 2.16) that cannot be synthesized by the body; this is a function of all of the B vitamins. Vitamins may also act as antioxidants, regulate gene expression in specific tissues, or regulate physiologic function in other ways. The variety of effects displayed by a given vitamin is due, in part, to the fact that it may exist in different chemical forms that have different functions.

An example of this variety of form and function is seen with vitamin A. The plant-derived precursor to vitamin A, β-carotene, acts as an antioxidant in lipid environments (e.g., lipoprotein particles). Retinal, a form of active vitamin A, comprises part of the pigments in photoreceptors in the retina (like rhodopsin) that are needed for sight. Vitamin A in the form retinoic acid is a regulator of gene expression. Because of the range of functions provided by a given vitamin, high intakes through supplementation could result in many, perhaps unexpected, effects.

Vitamin requirements

Recommendations for the amount of each vitamin to be consumed daily (RDA and AI) generally apply to physically active people. Consumption of more of a nutritious diet in order to meet higher energy needs should lead to increased vitamin intake. Since the RDA for many vitamins is not a fixed number but, in fact, varies with energy intake or protein intake, vitamin requirements may be met by using different amounts of a diet with a given nutrient density (mg/kcal). For example, the RDA for thiamin is 0.5 mg/1000 kcal; a basic diet plan providing that density of thiamin would be suitable for individuals with any level of energy intake.

Most studies evaluating the vitamin requirements of athletes support the adequacy of the RDA. Supplementation beyond the RDA does not reliably enhance performance unless the individual was deficient in the vitamin and is correcting the deficiency. The decision to use vitamin supplements should be based on the results of an evaluation of the individual's diet that provide information on the adequacy of intake of each vitamin. The use of supplements may be warranted when additional dietary sources are insufficient (due to health restrictions, expense, or esthetic considerations). For example, iron supplements (e.g., as ferrous sulfate) may be needed by young women who are vegetarians, since their iron requirement is high but their intake of good dietary sources of iron (liver, red meats) is low.

Antioxidants

Vitamin C, vitamin E, and β-carotene, as well as the mineral selenium, are antioxidant nutrients. Oxidation is a reaction that involves the removal of electrons from a compound (Figure 2.15); *antioxidants* protect other compounds from oxidation by donating their own electrons to the oxidizing compound (Figure 10.20). High rates of metabolic activity are associated with increased production of oxidizing compounds called *free radicals*. These compounds contain one or more unpaired electrons and are extremely reactive in their attempt to procure electrons from other molecules.

Antioxidants, including the nutrients listed above, can reduce the oxidative damage to lipids, proteins, and DNA caused by free radicals. For example, vitamin E protects polyunsaturated fatty acids in cell membranes and lipoprotein particles (like LDL) from oxidation; these effects help to maintain the integrity of cell membranes and to prevent the progression of atherosclerosis, respectively.

Because of the high rates of metabolic activity in exercise, it has been proposed that athletes need greater amounts of antioxidant nutrients in order to protect them from putative deleterious effects of the free radicals that are generated. This idea has some experimental support in that very high (20 · RDA) intakes of vitamin E may lessen muscle damage from exhaustive training. However, as is the case for many therapies, the link between antioxidant supplementation and improved function is still theoretical. It must be considered, for example, whether generation of free radicals could also be associated with beneficial responses, such as increased immune function.

Excessive vitamin intake

Excessive intake of nutritional supplements can produce toxicity syndromes, while high dietary intakes of nutrients almost never do, since very large amounts of food would have to be consumed in order to raise vitamin intake to toxic levels. Chronic consumption of vitamins A and D at levels of only 5

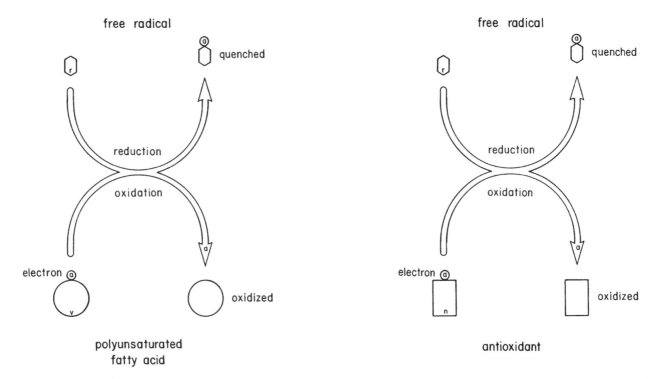

Figure 10.20 Function of antioxidants. Color the reaction in the left panel, noting that a free radical removed an electron from a polyunsaturated fatty acid. In this process, note that the free radical is reduced (quenched), while the polyunsaturated fatty acid is oxidized. Color the reaction in the right panel, noting that a free radical removed an electron from an antioxidant instead, thereby sparing the polyunsaturated fatty acid from oxidation. Observe that antioxidants are compounds that prevent oxidation (loss of electrons) of other compounds by donating their own electrons to oxidizing compounds, such as free radicals. Antioxidants, therefore, protect other compounds (such as polyunsaturated fatty acids) from oxidation and thereby preserve their structure and function.

to 10 times the RDA can produce dangerous toxicity syndromes. Note that β-carotene, a form of vitamin A found in plants, can be consumed safely in large quantities in the diet (but perhaps not so in supplement form). Regular consumption of large doses of other vitamins, including some water-soluble vitamins, can produce deleterious effects; the multiples of the RDA that produce toxicity vary widely among nutrients. For these reasons, unless an individual has been diagnosed with a vitamin deficiency and must consume a high dose of the vitamin for a specified period, habitual intakes of nutrients that are more than twice the RDA are not recommended.

Much of what vitamins do is yet undiscovered; this becomes more apparent as more of their actions are understood. Diseases that may take decades to develop, like cardiovascular disease and cancer, may be influenced by the level of intake of these potent nutrients over periods of years. Consumption of amounts that are far greater than what could be obtained from the diet alone (as in nutritional pharmacology) is a new phenomenon; its long-term effects are unknown. Consumers of vitamin supplements should be knowledgeable about the benefits and risks of using doses that greatly exceed the RDA.

The interactions among the concentrated components in nutritional supplements should also be considered. Little information is available about the bioavailability (usability) of nutrients in multivitamin and mineral preparations. For example, inclusion of minerals, like iron, in supplements may oxidize some vitamins and diminish their biological activity.

Mineral requirements

The mineral requirements of athletes do not appear to be greater than those of the general population. However, since young athletes are in a stage of growth and development, they are at risk for nutritional deficiencies. Not only may their requirements be greater than those of adults, their dietary habits may be more extreme. Intakes of the minerals iron and calcium tend to be deficient in individuals, including athletes, who restrict their food intake to maintain low body weights.

Female athletes of child-bearing age are at risk for iron deficiency both because of their high iron requirement (15 mg/day for females vs. 10 mg/day for males) and because of their low dietary iron intake (compared with males). Iron deficiency can eventually cause anemia, which can lead to a decrease in exercise capacity and an increase in the cardiac output associated with any given level of continuous exercise. Iron supplementation can correct these deficiency signs.

Female athletes who maintain a lower than normal level of body fatness may develop *amenorrhea* (absence of menstrual periods). In this condition, circulating levels of estrogens are low. Low estrogen levels in females lead to loss of bone mass (osteoporosis), which increases risk of bone fracture. The triad of food restriction, amenorrhea, and osteoporosis is relatively common among young female athletes. Treatment may include estrogen therapy and supplementation with calcium, phosphorus, magnesium, and vitamin D, as well as promotion of weight gain.

Exercise, along with consumption of the RDA for calcium, phosphorus, and vitamin D, promotes accretion of bone mass in young individuals and so can be protective against later development of osteoporosis. Dairy products (including low-fat varieties) are rich sources of calcium and phosphorus; calcium-fortified food products, such as orange juice, are also protective.

Mineral supplementation

As is the case for vitamin supplementation, an individual's mineral intake should first be evaluated by examining the mineral content of the diet and comparing it to the RDA or AI. Absorption of minerals is strongly influenced by other dietary components consumed at the same time. Mineral absorption is generally decreased, for example, by dietary fiber and phytic acid, which are found in whole grains.

Supplements are concentrated sources of minerals; their absorption is also affected by other substances in the diet or in the supplement itself. When a supplement is required, conditions that optimize its absorption should be utilized; for example, consumption of vitamin C along with iron can increase iron absorption fourfold.

Excessive mineral intake

The use of mineral supplements has not been shown to improve performance in individuals unless the increased intake was correcting a mineral deficiency (Figure 10.21). This generalization holds true for the popular supplement, chromium picolinate, which is purported to increase lean body mass during weight training.

As is the case for vitamins, toxic intakes of minerals are rarely provided by the diet. Most toxicity, both acute and chronic, results from the intake of supplements or from environmental hazards. Mineral toxicities have been shown to be responsible for serious pathologies. For example, excessive iron storage in the condition hemochromatosis, which is due to the combined effects of high iron intakes and a genetic predisposition to increased efficiency of iron absorption, can lead to cardiac and hepatic failure, diabetes mellitus, and blindness. Given the risk of toxicity, mineral intake beyond the RDA should be undertaken only to correct deficiency states.

MINERAL STATUS

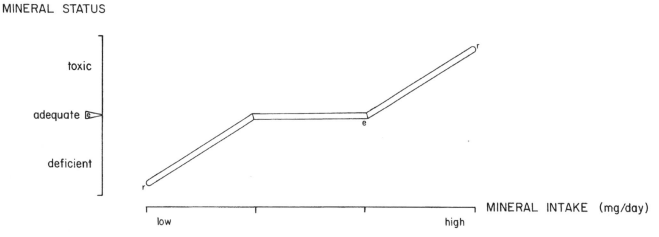

Figure 10.21 **Mineral status.** Color the line that shows the relationship between mineral intake and mineral status. Observe that at low intakes (compared to the requirement) the individual's status is deficient and he or she may show deficiency signs (Figure 10.2) for the mineral in question (e.g., anemia). Observe also that at high intakes (compared to the requirement) the individual may show signs of toxicity for the mineral in question (e.g., hemochromatosis or iron overload). Note that at intakes near the requirement for the mineral, the individual's status is adequate and characterized by lack of deficiency signs. Mineral intake in excess of the requirement does not improve status but increases risk of toxicity since regulation of body mineral absorption and excretion may not provide adequate protection.

Fluid requirements

Healthy individuals generally require an intake of at least 2 liters of water per day in order to replace the water lost in urine, sweat, feces, and expired air (Figure 10.22). Exercise increases heat production and therefore promotes water loss through the production of sweat. Excessive sweat loss can lead to dehydration and higher sodium concentrations in extracellular fluid (Figure 8.23). These conditions stimulate the *osmoreceptor–thirst mechanism* to increase the consumption of fluids and thereby compensate for the water lost in sweat. However, because osmoreceptors are stimulated by dehydration, the thirst mechanism is activated too late to prevent dehydration. For this reason, fluid intake during exercise should anticipate and correct fluid loss before dehydration occurs and the sensation of thirst arises.

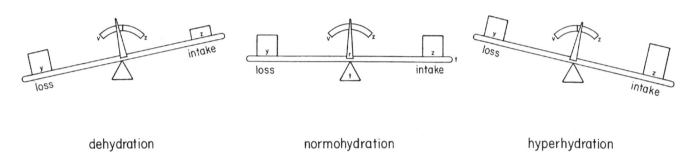

dehydration   normohydration   hyperhydration

Figure 10.22 **Water balance.** Color the balance, the pointer, and the hydration scale. For each panel, color and compare the rectangles that indicate water loss (left side of balance) and water intake (right side or balance). Observe that dehydration occurs when water loss exceeds water intake (left panel), normohydration occurs when water loss equals water intake (middle panel), and hyperhydration occurs when water intake exceeds water loss (right panel). Water intake consists of water in beverages and food and metabolic water (produced in the electron transport chain). Water loss refers to water lost in urine, sweat, feces, and expired air. Healthy individuals with free access to fluids usually maintain a state of normohydration (middle panel).

Various protocols for fluid replacement have been developed. Fluid intake should be increased before, during and after exercise. Fluid intakes of about 500 mL are recommended about 30 minutes before exercise, followed by 250 mL every 15 minutes during exercise, and liberal fluid consumption during the recovery period. Caffeine-free beverages are recommended because caffeine increases urinary water loss.

Composition of fluid replacement

The choice of beverage for fluid replacement should take into account the effects of carbohydrate and salts on fluid absorption, electrolyte composition of body fluids, and blood glucose level. In general, the more concentrated the solution, the more slowly it will leave the stomach, and the more slowly water will be absorbed. For this reason, carbohydrate concentrations greater than 10% (as found in soda or orange juice) that retard gastric emptying and delay absorption are not recommended for use before or during exercise. Glucose, fructose, sucrose, and glucose polymers (short chains averaging six glucose units) are all forms of carbohydrate that are equivalent in their effects on gastric emptying, despite their different osmotic effects (Figure 10.23). There are also no appreciable differences among these carbohydrate sources in their ability to maintain normal blood glucose levels, to spare muscle glycogen, or to extend the duration of exercise.

Beverages can provide salts to replace the electrolytes (Na$^+$, K$^+$, and Cl$^-$) lost in sweat. The sodium (Na$^+$) content of most diets far exceeds nutritional requirements, so that no additional salt intake is necessary during short periods of exercise. However, salt replacement is important in events lasting several hours. After a first drink of plain water, later beverages should contain about 2.5 g of NaCl (provided by a half teaspoon of table salt) per liter; this concentration more than compensates for sodium loss in sweat.

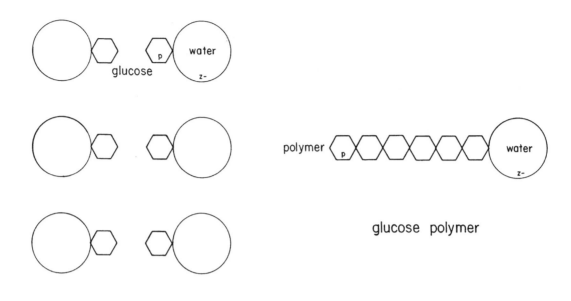

Figure 10.23 Osmotic effects of glucose and glucose polymers. Color the six molecules of glucose and the six water droplets that hydrate them (left panel). Color the polymer of six glucose molecules linked together (also known as an oligosaccharide) and the one water droplet that hydrates it (right panel). Observe that individual molecules of glucose are associated with more water than is the same number of glucose molecules contained in a polymer. In other words, the osmotic effect of individual glucose molecules is greater than the osmotic effect of the same number of glucose molecules within polymers. Because fluids with high osmotic effects are absorbed more slowly than fluids with low osmotic effects, some athletes consume beverages that contain glucose polymers to promote faster absorption of water and to reduce gastrointestinal discomfort during an event.

Nutritional supplements as ergogenic aids

An *ergogenic aid* is a substance used to enhance maximal exercise performance. For example, an effective ergogenic aid could increase power output during weight lifting or increase the maximal distance that a person could run at a given speed. Ergogenic aids could be hormones, blood transfusions, or even specialized footgear. Increased intakes of nutrients, as foods or as concentrated supplements, may be utilized as ergogenic aids. Other substances that can be derived from foods, which have not be identified as essential in the normal diet, may also be classified as ergogenic aids.

Under the Dietary Supplement Health and Education Act of 1994, products derived from foods may be sold as nutritional supplements without having to comply with regulations that apply to food and drugs. Supplement manufacturers are permitted to make health claims about products without provision of proof; the Food and Drug Administration (FDA) has the burden of proving the claim wrong. Unlike the case for regulation of food and drugs, the supplement manufacturer does not have to show proof of product safety in advance of

marketing it; the FDA must prove that the product is unsafe before it can be recalled. Therefore, these supplements are regulated much less stringently than are drugs or foods. For these reasons it is important for consumers of nutritional ergogenic aids to be knowledgeable about products before using them.

Evaluation of nutritional ergogenic aids

In order to choose a product that is safe and effective, it is necessary to know the identity and potency of the active component and the dosage of the product that will provide the desired amount of the component. The scientific literature on the topic should be evaluated; promotional information in magazines or on the internet may leave out information on effective dosage, side effects, or the necessary conditions for the product's effectiveness. Scientific articles must be consulted in order to establish the effect for which the product has been shown to work. For example, the substance may have been only shown to be effective in laboratory animals, but information in humans may be unconvincing. Finally, users of poorly studied products must realize that there is a risk of negative consequences; substances can have multiple effects, some of which may not yet have been identified. Descriptions of several promising ergogenic aids follow.

Creatine monohydrate

Creatine is a nitrogen-containing compound formed from portions of the amino acids glycine, arginine, and methionine. It is synthesized in liver and kidney and it is found in the diet in meat. Creatine is concentrated in skeletal muscle where it functions as part of the ATP-PCr (phosphagen) system. Supply of more creatine to muscle is believed to increase formation of phosphocreatine and thereby enable the ATP-PCr system to supply more energy to muscle during high-intensity exercise (Figure 10.24).

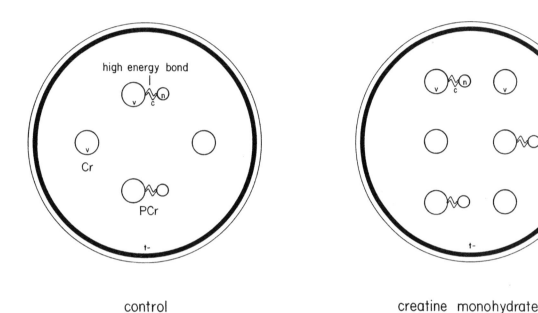

control   creatine monohydrate

Figure 10.24   Effect of creatine monohydrate supplementation. Color the molecules of phosphocreatine (PCr) and free creatine (Cr) in a muscle cell before (left panel) and after (right panel) creatine monohydrate supplementation. Observe that creatine supplementation increases the concentrations of PCr and Cr, and thereby increases the rate at which the ATP-PCr system can supply ATP for high-intensity, short-duration activities. Compare this figure with Figures 3.2, and 9.14.

Appropriate regimens of creatine monohydrate supplementation (i.e., 20 g/day, divided into 4 doses) have been shown to increase muscle creatine content up to a limit; the greatest effects are seen in individuals, such as strict vegetarians, who have low muscle creatine content beforehand. Other studies have reported improved performance in high-intensity, short-duration activities, such as power lifting or sprinting. Creatine supplementation does not improve endurance, but it may promote an increase in lean body mass. Part of this latter effect is due to increased water retention, and part is due to increased accumulation of muscle protein.

Supplementation with creatine has not been found to produce acute toxic effects, but the effects of long-term use in different populations are not known. Since it does increase urinary excretion of creatinine, a nonreusable compound formed from creatine, individuals with impaired kidney function should avoid high intakes of creatine because it increases the kidney's solute load.

β-hydroxy β-methylbutyrate

β-hydroxy β-methylbutyrate (HMB) is a compound synthesized in the body from the branched-chain amino acid leucine. Originally studied by the meat industry for its ability to increase muscle mass in livestock, HMB has been shown to enhance accretion of lean body mass in people engaged in resistance training. At daily intakes of about ten times that synthesized in the body, HMB supplementation has been shown to increase lean body mass and, in some studies, to increase strength. Its mechanism of action is theorized to be inhibition of protein degradation. Long-term effects in humans are not known.

Conjugated linoleic acid

Conjugated linoleic acid (CLA) is a fatty acid that is used as a dietary supplement in order to increase lean body mass while decreasing adipose tissue mass. CLA is an isomer of the essential fatty acid linoleic acid, but the two substances differ in the placement of their carbon-to-carbon double bonds (Figure 10.25). In CLA the carbon-to-carbon double bonds are two carbons apart; this arrangement produces conjugated double bonds.

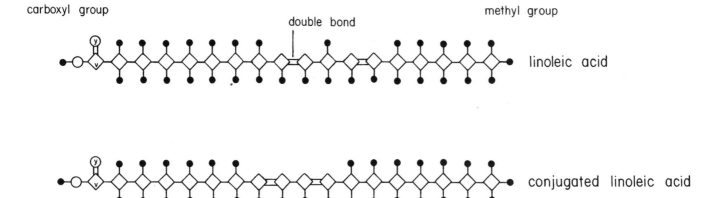

Figure 10.25 **Structure of conjugated linoleic acid.** Color the carbon (diamonds) and oxygen (open circles) atoms and identify the hydrogen atoms (filled circles) in the top structure (linoleic acid). Identify the carboxyl group (COOH), the methyl group (CH$_3$), and count the carbons, observing the locations of the carbon-to-carbon double bonds. Repeat this process for the bottom structure (conjugated linoleic acid); note that double bonds that are two carbons apart are known as conjugated double bonds. Compare the number and locations of their carbon-to-carbon double bonds and compare these fatty acids with those shown in Figures 2.28 and 10.12. Although these two compounds are very similar in structure, they are treated differently in the body and produce different effects. Supplementation with conjugated linoleic acid may influence the amount of fat stored in adipose tissue and may affect other aspects of cellular development.

CLA has been studied mainly for its effects on the metabolism of lipoprotein particles, and its protection against certain cancers, atherosclerosis, and diabetes. In the course of this work, it was observed that CLA caused a decrease in adipose tissue mass and an increase in lean body mass in laboratory rodents. However, there is little evidence that CLA affects body composition or strength in humans.

CLA is an example of a substance that may influence athletic performance but could have other far-ranging effects. CLA is known to bind to and activate regulators of gene expression and to influence cell differentiation. Diets high in CLA (1% of kcal) stimulate synthesis of hepatic proteins involved in fat metabolism. Use of CLA for body building could therefore result in widespread metabolic effects.

Most of the considerable scientific literature on CLA concerns work done in laboratory animals, not humans. Given that a large variability in the effects of CLA is seen among rodent species and strains, extrapolation of these results to humans must be done with caution.

Ginseng

Ginseng is the name used for a number of herbal preparations from several plants. These preparations differ widely in their content of active components, known as *ginsenosides;* some products have been shown to contain no ginsenosides. Standardized preparations of the ginseng root are available, however, thereby permitting consumption of known doses.

One variety of ginseng, called Chinese or Korean ginseng (Panax ginseng) has been used for many centuries in Asia where it has been attributed with many health-promoting effects. Among the purported effects related to exercise are improved aerobic capacity, decreased heart rate, preservation of glycogen stores through increased fat usage, and lower blood lactate levels. However, more controlled studies on ginseng must be conducted before these effects can be accepted. Other forms of ginseng (e.g., Siberian ginseng) have also been reported to improve athletic performance.

No mechanism has been elucidated for the actions of ginseng. Although the herbal preparation is widely regarded as safe due to its centuries of usage, it does have estrogenic properties which could produce undesired side effects.

Coenzyme Q

Coenzyme Q (or coenzyme Q_{10} or ubiquinone) is used as a nutritional supplement for the purpose of increasing aerobic production of ATP and maximum oxygen consumption ($\dot{V}O_2max$). Coenzyme Q is an electron carrier found in the mitochondria. It carries electrons from certain mitochondrial dehydrogenases to cytochrome b, which is part of the electron transport chain (Figure 2.21). Coenzyme Q also functions as an antioxidant within the mitochondria (Figure 10.20). Its level in the cell can be increased by supplementation.

Coenzyme Q usage has been studied in subjects with cardiovascular disease and congestive heart disease where it has fostered improvement in cardiac function. Most studies have shown that long-term (several months) supplementation (~100 mg/day) enables endurance athletes to exhibit increased time to exhaustion, higher $\dot{V}O_2max$ values, and increased fat utilization. Thus, coenzyme Q supplementation appears to enhance aerobic metabolism during exercise. The literature on the use of coenzyme Q in human subjects is considerable and supports its low toxicity.

chapter **eleven**
body composition and weight control

Adherence to a program of regular physical activity can lead to a reduction in body weight and a change in the relative proportions of muscle mass and fat mass. These changes can be beneficial for health, performance, and appearance.

Obesity

Obesity is defined as an excess of body fatness. The percent of body mass due to fat that is determined to be excessive is based upon the relationship observed between body fatness and mortality or risk of a given disease (Figure 11.1). Risks

of cardiovascular disease, hypertension, type 2 diabetes mellitus, osteoarthritis, gall bladder disease, and many types of cancer are increased by obesity. The risk becomes greater with increasing degree of obesity.

Obesity is not the same as excessive body weight. Body weight may be elevated not only due to excess body fat but also due to increased muscle mass or body water content; knowledge of an individual's body composition is therefore necessary to assess obesity. It is the amount and location of body fat, not an individual's weight, that confers risk of disease.

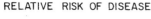

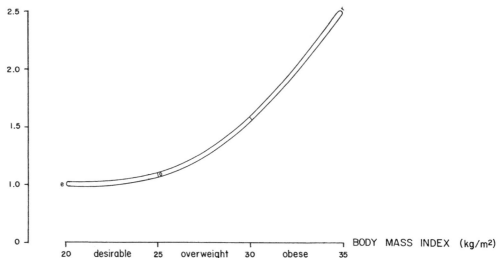

Figure 11.1 Effect of obesity on disease risk. Color the line that plots relative risk of disease against Body Mass Index, calculated as (body mass in kg) /(height in meters)^2. Note that BMI values in the 20 to 25 range are considered desirable, 25 to 30 are classified as overweight, and 30 to 35 are classified as obese. The relative risk of disease compares an individual's (or subgroup's) probability of having a condition with that of the general population. For example, a person with a 50% greater risk would have a relative risk of 1.5. Observe that the relative risk of disease increases markedly in obesity.

Adipose tissue

Body fat is stored in cells, called *adipocytes*, each of which contains a droplet of triglyceride that may occupy most of the volume of the cell (Figure 11.2). Adipose tissue is comprised of adipocytes; it is found in discrete depots or fat pads in many different regions of the body. For example, adipose tis-

sue that is found beneath the skin but above the muscle layer is called the subcutaneous depot, the mesenteric depot is attached to the intestines, and the pericardial depot surrounds the heart (Figure 11.3). The term *visceral fat* may refer collectively to all adipose tissue except subcutaneous fat, or specifically refer to the mesenteric plus omental (below the stomach) fat depots.

Figure 11.2   Structure of an adipocyte. Color the cell membrane, the nucleus and its membrane, the cytoplasm, and the triglyceride droplet inside the cell. Observe that the triglyceride droplet occupies most of the cell's volume and that the cytoplasm is pushed to the side. This adipocyte or fat cell belongs to a depot of white adipose tissue; adipocytes in brown adipose tissue, such as those found around the aorta or in subscapular regions, have a number of separate triglyceride droplets and many mitochondria, whose cytochromes give it a brown appearance.

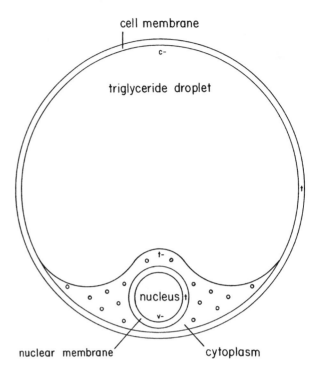

Figure 11.3   Fat depots. Color the outline of the body. Identify and color the subcutaneous fat pad (depot) beneath the skin, the pericardial fat depot surrounding the heart, and the mesenteric fat depot found along the length of the intestines. Note that fat depots vary greatly among individuals. In the case of the subcutaneous depot, its thickness varies among sites in a given individual so that, for example, it may be thick in the region around the hips and thighs but very thin in the hands and feet. Observe also that fat depots are discrete (as opposed to diffuse) regions of adipose tissue that are comprised of adipocytes (Figure 11.2).

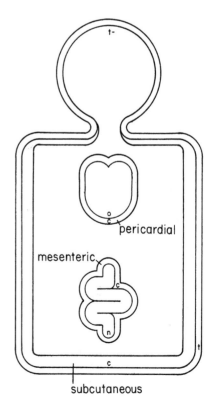

Fat pads can become larger through an increase in the total number of adipocytes (*hyperplasia*) or an increase in the size of individual adipocytes (*hypertrophy*); the enlargement of an adipocyte is due to accumulation of more stored triglyceride within the cell (Figure 11.4). Throughout life the total amount of adipose tissue, as well as the relative sizes of different fat pads, fluctuates. During infancy, childhood, and adolescence, individuals normally experience large increases in fat mass. Hormonal signals and prolonged periods of excess energy intake (overeating) can promote hyperplasia and hypertrophy of adipocytes.

Conversely, adipose tissue mass can also decrease during periods of a person's life. Individual adipocytes become smaller as their droplet of triglyceride is depleted (Figure 11.4). It does not appear, however, that fat mass is reduced by decreasing the number of adipocytes (except perhaps in advanced old age). In other words, loss of body fat appears to be accomplished by reduction in the size of individual adipocytes, rather than by reduction in their number.

Since hyperplasia in adipose tissue results in a permanent increase in the number of fat cells, individuals in whom excessive hyperplasia has occurred must shrink their fat cells to a subnormal size in order to lose excess body fat (Figure 11.4). Because a small adipocyte size is difficult to achieve and to maintain, adipose tissue hyperplasia is associated with a lifelong predisposition to obesity.

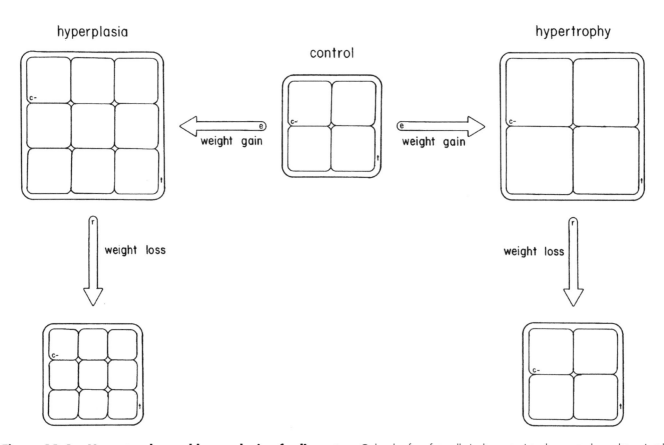

Figure 11.4   Hypertrophy and hyperplasia of adipocytes. Color the four fat cells (adipocytes) in the control condition (middle panel). Color the left arrow (labeled weight gain) and the larger fat depot labeled hyperplasia, observing that the increase in fat mass is due entirely to a greater number of fat cells. Color the downward arrow labeled weight loss and the smaller fat depot, noting that the return of the fat depot to its original size requires that fat cells become smaller than they were in the control state. Color the right arrow (labeled weight gain) and the larger fat depot labeled hypertrophy, observing that the increase in fat mass is due entirely to larger fat cells. Color the downward arrow labeled weight loss and the smaller fat depot, noting that the return of the fat depot to its original size requires that fat cells return to the same size that they were in the control state. Although fat mass returned to the control amount in both situations, weight loss following hyperplasia results in a greater number of smaller fat cells. Because such dramatic reductions in adipocyte size are difficult to achieve and maintain, adipose tissue hyperplasia is associated with a lifelong predisposition to obesity.

body composition

Regional distribution of body fat

Both the amount of excess body fat and the location of this excess are important in determining an individual's risk of disease and death. Two overall patterns of fat distribution are utilized in categorizing obesity: the *android pattern* and the *gynoid pattern* (Figure 11.5). In the android pattern, which is characteristic of men, body fat accumulates around the abdominal area, mainly in visceral fat pads, such as the omental (below the stomach) and mesenteric pads, although subcutaneous pads in the abdominal region may be enlarged as well. In the gynoid pattern, which is characteristic of women, there is enlargement of subcutaneous pads in the gluteal-femoral region (hip and thigh).

Excess accumulation of adipose tissue in the android pattern is associated with a greater risk of cardiovascular disease, hypertension, and type 2 diabetes than is the same amount of adipose tissue distributed in the gynoid pattern. One reason for this difference is that visceral fat exhibits a higher rate of lipolysis and therefore releases more fatty acids into the blood than does subcutaneous fat. The higher blood levels of free fatty acids in the android pattern produce adverse metabolic effects, including excessive output of VLDL particles (Fig 2.34) and glucose by the liver as well as resistance of tissues to the effects of insulin (insulin resistance).

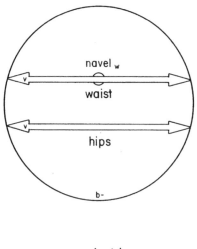
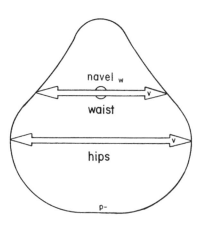

android   gynoid

Figure 11.5   Patterns of fat deposition. Color the left panel, which depicts the android (male) pattern of fat distribution, noting that the waist circumference is measured at the level of the navel (umbilicus) and the hip circumference at the broadest location below the waist. Color the right panel, which depicts the gynoid (female) pattern of fat distribution, noting that the waist circumference is also measured at the navel. Compare the relative magnitudes of the waist and hip circumferences (horizontal arrows), observing that in this case the waist-to-hip ratio (WHR) would be 1.0 (waist = hips) for the android pattern and 0.85 for the gynoid pattern (waist < hips). The WHR is used to categorize the pattern of body fat distribution among obese individuals.

Waist-to-hip ratio

The *waist-to-hip ratio* (WHR) is a useful parameter for assessing the pattern of fat distribution. Values for WHR are calculated by dividing the circumference over the navel (waist measurement) by the widest circumference below the waist (hip measurement) and expressing the ratio as a dimensionless number (Figure 11.5). Thus, the pattern of fat distribution is more android when the value of WHR is higher. Since even in lean individuals men have a higher WHR than do women, the value of WHR associated with increased disease risk is higher for men than for women: WHR > 1.0 in men and WHR > 0.85 in women are used as indicators of a pattern of body fat distribution associated with increased disease risk.

Because it is the size of the visceral fat depots that is associated with metabolic abnormalities, fat distribution reflects disease risk only in individuals who are obese; WHR>0.85 in a lean woman, a dancer for example, may be due to very low gluteal-femoral fat accumulation. Waist circumference alone, instead of WHR, also has been utilized in screening populations for risk of obesity-related disease; waist circumferences > 37 inches for men and > 32 inches for women are associated with increased morbidity (risk of disease).

Measurement of body fat

Indirect methods are used to estimate body fatness because it is not possible to directly measure body fat in a living person. Two models that are utilized in quantifying the fat composition of the body are the anatomical model and the chemical model (Figure 11.6). In the anatomical model, the body is partitioned into adipose tissue and nonadipose tissue; this latter component is known as *lean body mass*, which includes muscle, bone, blood, viscera, and neural tissue. Thus,

body mass = adipose tissue mass + lean body mass

In the chemical model, the body is partitioned into fat (lipid) and nonfat components, the latter is known as *fat-free mass*.

The fat component includes the triglyceride stored in adipose tissue as well as lipids in all cell membranes but not the aqueous portions of any cell (including adipocytes); the nonfat component includes the rest of the adipocyte and other cells, extracellular fluid, and bone. Thus,

body mass = fat mass + fat-free mass

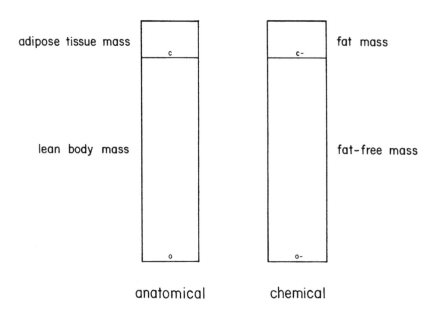

Figure 11.6   Models of body composition. Color the bars that represent the anatomical model (left panel) and the chemical model (right panel) of body composition. Observe that the anatomical model divides the body into adipose tissue mass and lean body mass. Observe also that the chemical model divides the body into fat mass and fat-free mass. Compare the relative proportions of these components of body composition.

Densitometry

Densitometry is a method of estimating body composition by determining the average density of the body, defined as the ratio of body mass to body volume (mass/volume). The method is based on the premise that adipose tissue mass has an average density of 0.9 g/mL and that lean body mass has an average density of 1.1 g/mL. It follows that the average density of the body reflects the relative contributions of adipose tissue and lean tissue to the total body mass (Figure 11.7). By determining body density and substituting the value in a formula, percent body fat can be calculated.

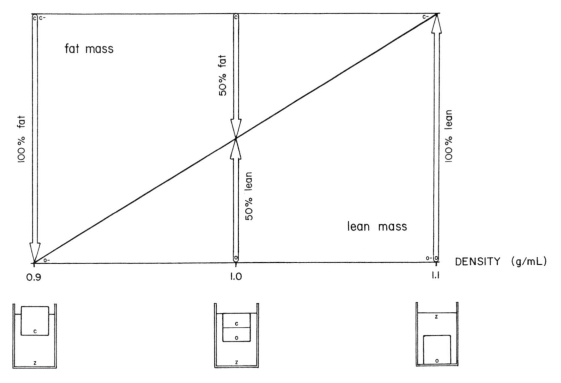

Figure 11.7   Effect of body composition on body density. Color the rectangle, noting that the area above the diagonal line represents fat mass (assumed density = 0.9 g/mL) and the area below the diagonal line represents lean (fat-free) mass (assumed density = 1.1 g/mL). This analysis enables a vertical line, corresponding to any given body density (such as the vertical arrows shown), to partition body mass into one component due to fat mass and one component due to lean mass. Note that the relative percentages of fat mass and lean mass can be visualized from the way in which the diagonal line divides the vertical line; the segment above the diagonal indicates fat mass and the segment below the diagonal indicates lean mass. Color the vertical arrows that correspond to a body density of 0.9 (100% fat, left side of figure), 1.0 (50% fat, 50% lean, middle of figure), and 1.1 (100% lean, right side of figure). Color the bottom panel, comparing the buoyancy associated with each of these assumed body densities. These theoretical considerations explain why measurements of body density can be used to determine body composition.

Body mass is measured directly on a scale and body volume is measured indirectly by the technique of hydrostatic (underwater) weighing (Figure 11.8). Objects weigh less in water because they experience a buoyant force that, according to Archimedes' principle, is equal to the weight of the water that is displaced by the object. For this reason, the difference between the weights of a body in air and in water is equal to the weight of the water that is displaced by the body (Figure 11.8).

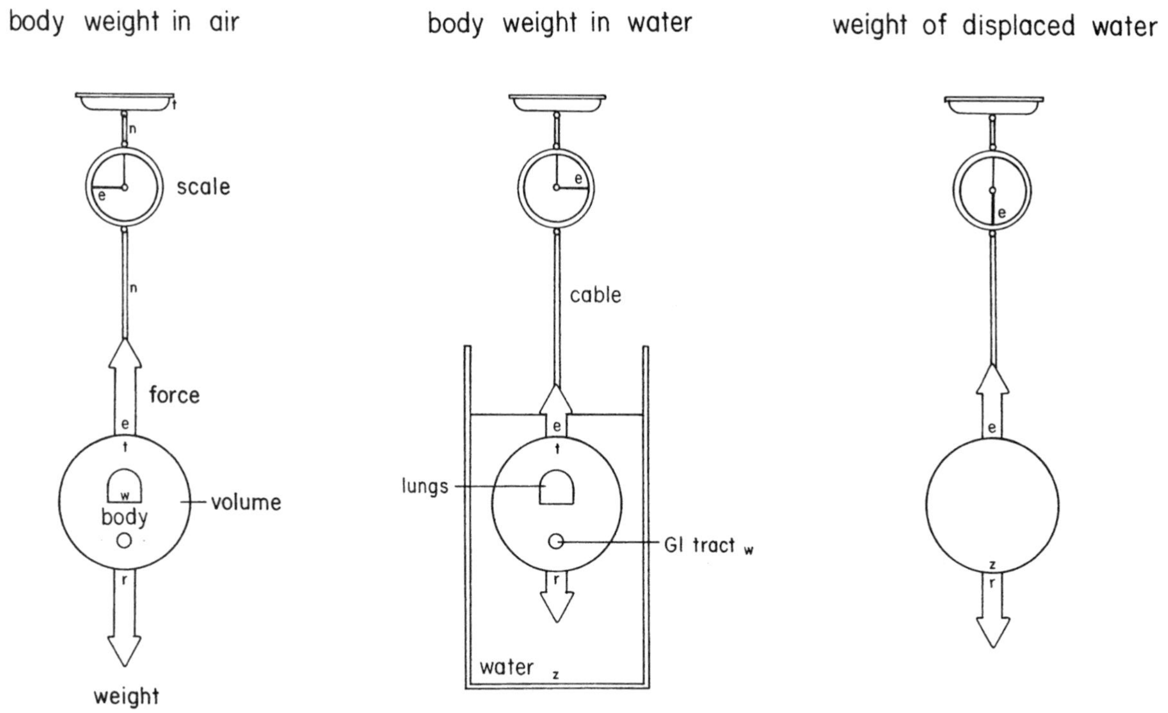

body weight in air   body weight in water   weight of displaced water

Figure 11.8 Principles of densitometry. Color the panels from left to right. For each panel, color the body, the upward force arrow, the downward weight arrow, and the scale. Compare the scale readings in each condition, noting that the weight of the body in air (left panel) is equal to the weight of the body in water (middle panel) plus the weight of the water displaced by the body, sometimes referred to as the buoyant force (right panel). Thus, the difference between the body weights in air and in water determines the volume of water that is displaced by the body. This example, which illustrates Archimedes' principle, forms the basis for the method of hydrostatic weighing to measure body volume. Note that measurements of body volume by this technique must be corrected to account for the volume of air contained in the lungs and GI tract.

Because water has a density of 1 g/mL, each gram of buoyant force indicates that a volume of 1 mL of water has been displaced. It follows that the difference between the weight of the body in air and water can be used to determine the volume of water that is displaced by the body during underwater weighing. Body volume is calculated by subtracting the volume of air in the lungs (residual volume, obtained by helium dilution, Figure 6.49) and the volume of air in the gastroin-

testinal tract (usually assumed to be 100 mL) from the volume of water displaced. The average body density, calculated by dividing the body mass by the body volume, is a measure of body composition. A low value of body density indicates a high percentage of body fat and a high value of body density indicates a low percentage of body fat (Figure 11.9).

body composition

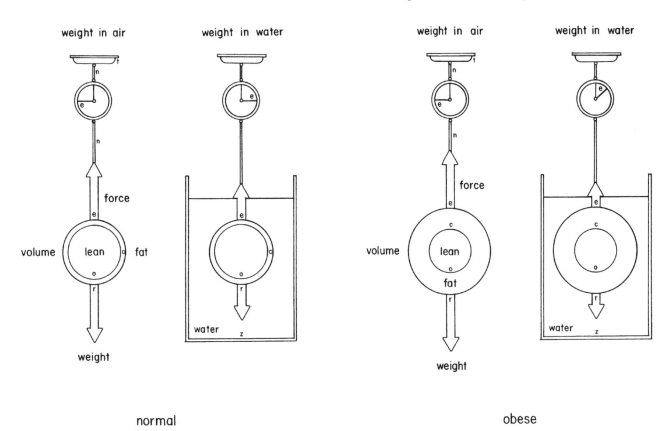

weight in air   weight in water   weight in air   weight in water

force

volume   lean   fat

weight

normal

force

volume   lean

fat

weight

obese

Figure 11.9   Effect of body composition on densitometry measurements. Color the panels from left to right. For each condition, color the body, the upward force arrow, the downward weight arrow, and the scale. Compare the scale readings in air (left side of each panel), noting that the normal (lean) (left panel) and obese (right panel) person have the same body weight in air. Compare the relative amounts of fat mass and lean (fat-free) mass, noting that the obese person has more body fat and therefore a larger body volume, a consequence of the fact that fat has a lower density than lean tissue. Compare the scale readings in water (right side of each panel), noting that the normal lean person weighs more in water (left panel) than does the obese person (right panel). Observe that the reason for this difference is that the obese person displaces more water during underwater weighing and therefore experiences a greater buoyant force. These examples explain why differences in body composition manifest themselves as corresponding differences in average body density. Compare this figure with Figure 11.7.

Skinfold thickness

Measurement of *skinfold thickness* is a convenient, inexpensive method used to estimate body fatness; the validity of this and other indirect techniques has been assessed by comparing their results with those obtained by densitometry in the same individual. In this technique the thickness of a fold of skin, plus the accompanying doubled-over subcutaneous fat, is measured using calipers equipped with specific tension settings. Skinfold thickness is usually measured at defined locations at the triceps, subscapular (below the level of the shoulder blades), and suprailiac (just above the iliac crest) regions, as well as at other sites (Figure 11.10).

The measured values of skinfold thickness may be substituted into equations (developed for each set of skinfold loca-

tions) that are used to estimate percent body fat. The skinfold values may also be compared with published values that are tabulated according to age and gender. Skinfold thickness values for each site are grouped into percentiles within each age and gender category, so that those thicknesses above the 85th percentile, for example, may be classified as indicative of obesity.

Skinfold thickness is a less reliable measure of body fatness than is densitometry. Because the regional distribution of body fat varies so widely among populations, increased thickness at a particular subcutaneous site may not be a valid measure of total body fatness in an individual.

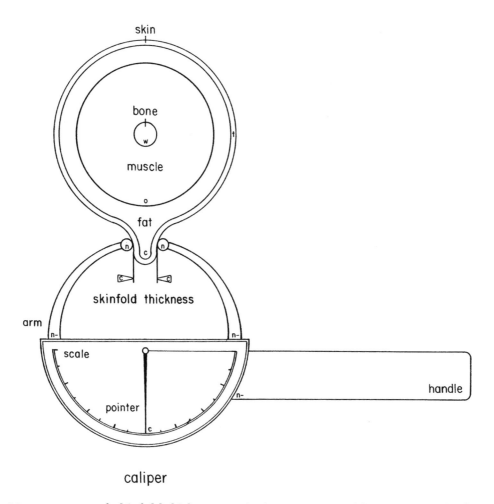

caliper

Figure 11.10 **Measurement of skinfold thickness.** Color the cross section of the upper arm, identifying the bone, muscle, subcutaneous fat, and skin. Color the caliper, noting that the pointer displays the skinfold thickness (distance between the tips of the caliper arms) on a calibrated scale. Observe that the arms of the caliper pinch the fold (double layer) of skin and fat; a thicker skinfold yields a higher measurement. Observe also that muscle is not included in a properly obtained skinfold measurement.

Bioelectrical impedence analysis

Bioelectrical impedance analysis (BIA) is an indirect method for assessing the relative proportions of fat-free mass and fat mass. The method is based on the principle that the electrical conductivity of fat-free mass is greater than that of fat mass because fat-free mass contains a higher concentration of electrolytes and water (Figure 11.11). The technique employs a small portable instrument that delivers a low-amplitude, high-frequency alternating electrical current (~50 µA at a frequency of 50 kHz) to surface electrodes placed on an extremity. The measured value of electrical impedance (a parameter inversely related to electrical conductivity) is substituted into an equation that converts bioelectrical impedance values into numerical values for fat-free body mass. These equations, which are different for men and women, incorporate anthropometric measurements such as weight and height. Thus, fat mass is calculated from the difference between body mass (measured directly) and fat-free mass (estimated from the equation).

The accuracy of this method is influenced by the hydration level of the subject. For example, hyperhydration (too much water in extracellular fluid) decreases the electrolyte concentration in extracellular fluid and increases the measured value of bioelectrical impedance, thereby overestimating the fat mass. Conversely, dehydration (too little water in extracellular fluid) increases the electrolyte concentration in extracellular fluid and decreases the bioelectrical impedance of the body, thereby underestimating the fat mass.

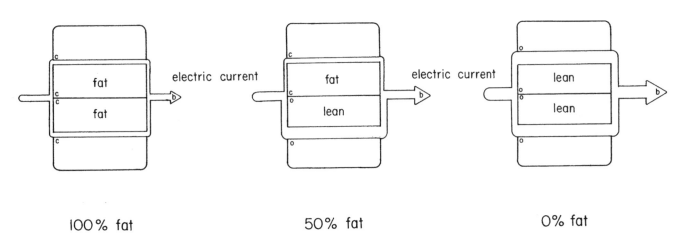

Figure 11.11 Effect of body composition on bioelectrical impedance. Color the panels from left to right, noting that the voltage gradient across the tissue samples is assumed to be the same in all cases. Because the electrical impedance of fat is higher than that of lean (fat-free) tissue, note that less current flows through fat tissue (narrower path) than through lean tissue (wider path). Observe that the total current is small in the left panel (100% fat, 0% lean), intermediate in the middle panel (50% fat, 50% lean) and highest in the right panel (0% fat, 100% lean). This hypothetical example shows that intrinsic differences in the conductivity of fat and fat-free mass can be used to obtain information related to body composition from measurements of electrical impedance.

Other indirect techniques of assessment

A number of other techniques for assessment of body composition are utilized in research settings, including computerized tomography, dual-energy X-ray absorptiometry, and magnetic resonance imaging. The instruments used for these methods are complex and expensive, and operators must be highly skilled. These techniques can provide information on the tissue components of lean body mass or on the sizes of individual fat depots.

Adipose tissue mass and lean body mass can be derived from a series of X-rays using a technique called *computerized tomography* (popularly known as CAT scans). The images are used to produce a three-dimensional representation of adipose tissue in a given anatomical region, thereby enabling the volume of the tissue to be computed and, based on the known density of adipose tissue, used to obtain a value for adipose tissue mass. Lean body mass is then calculated by subtracting adipose tissue mass from total body mass.

Dual-energy X-ray absorptiometry (DXA or DEXA) also utilizes X-rays but at two different energy levels. It not only permits estimation of adipose tissue mass and lean body mass but it also partitions lean body mass into soft tissue and bone.

Magnetic resonance imaging (MRI) also provides images of adipose tissue, bone, and other tissues. Unlike DXA, it does not require X-rays but utilizes nuclear magnetic resonance (NMR). In certain naturally occurring isotopes (e.g., ^{1}H, ^{31}P),

the nuclei align themselves relative to a magnetic field; they are made to rotate within the field and the characteristic energy that they release as they return to their previous state is the signal that is collected. This information on the elemental composition of the region scanned is used to construct an image. The volume and mass of fat depots can be calculated from this image.

Body weight

Although body weight alone does not provide information on fat mass, measurements of body weight and height provide information that can be used to infer risk of morbidity and mortality. Insurance companies have compiled tables of *"desirable body weight"* that list body weights of men and women, arranged according to height and frame size, that are associated with the lowest risk of death. It is a common practice in fitness counseling to utilize these weight-for-height tables to express an individual's body weight as a percent of desirable body weight, i.e.,

$$\text{percent desirable weight} = (\text{actual weight} \cdot 100) \, / \, (\text{desirable weight})$$

Using this method, individuals may be categorized as overweight if their actual weight exceeds their desirable weight by more than 20% (>120% of desirable weight). Given that body weight does not distinguish among the weights of adipose and lean tissue, a person could weigh more than 120% of desirable weight (for height and frame size) because of increased skeletal muscle mass and not excessive fat mass.

Because obesity is defined as an excess of body fatness, the individual would not be obese and would not be at increased risk of morbidity or mortality since it is body fatness that is associated with disease risk. Similarly, an individual who is within 20% of desirable weight, but because of very low physical activity has a low lean body mass and an excess of adipose tissue mass, could be obese. For these reasons, body weight and percent of desirable weight are not reliable indices of obesity, despite their common usage.

Body Mass Index

Despite the shortcomings of weight-for-height measurements in determining obesity, height and weight are often the only measurements available from studies of large populations. A calculated value that is widely used in public health and obesity research to assess body fatness is the *Body Mass Index* (BMI). This value is obtained as follows:

Body Mass Index (kg/m^2) = body mass (kg) / [height (m)]^2

A BMI between 20 and 25 is associated with desirable weight and low disease risk, while a BMI of 30 or more is now generally accepted as denoting obesity (Figure 11.1). Note that body composition is not taken into account so that, for example, a body builder may have an elevated BMI and not be obese.

Changes in body weight

A change in body weight could be due to changes in adipose tissue mass, lean body mass, or water content. Body composition assessments done at two or more times can provide information about changes in body composition that accompany changes in body weight. Increases in both adipose tissue mass and lean body mass are produced by energy intakes that exceed energy expenditures; resistance training can be utilized to selectively increase lean body mass. Decreases in adipose tissue mass and lean body mass are produced by energy expenditures that exceed energy intakes; the relative amounts of adipose tissue mass and lean body mass that are lost depend on the diet and exercise regimen.

Energy balance

Energy balance is a method that compares energy intake with energy output. Positive energy balance is said to occur when energy intake is greater than output, and negative energy balance is said to occur when energy intake is less than output (Figure 11.12). Energy intake is determined by the total physiological fuel value of the food consumed (Figure 3.15). Energy output (total daily energy expenditure, TDEE) is determined by the sum of the basal (BMR) or resting (RMR) metabolic rate, the thermic effect of exercise (TEE), and the thermic effect of feeding (TEF) (Figure 3.26).

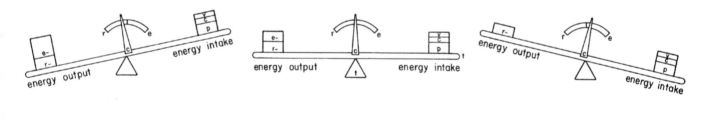

weight loss　　　　weight stable　　　　weight gain

Figure 11.12　Effect of energy balance on body weight. Color the balance, pointer, and weight scale. For each panel, color and compare the rectangles that indicate energy output (left side of balance) and energy intake (right side of balance). Observe that weight loss occurs when energy output exceeds energy intake (left panel), weight is stable when energy output equals energy intake (middle panel), and weight gain occurs when energy intake exceeds energy output (right panel).

Regulation of energy intake

Physiological mechanisms govern the amount and, to some extent, the composition of food consumed. Therefore, eating behavior is modulated by both conscious and unconscious mechanisms. The term "hunger" refers to the physiological drive for food, "satiety" refers to the cessation of that drive, and "appetite" refers to the desire for particular eating experiences, independent of hunger. In order for weight stability to be achieved, energy intake and energy expenditure must be matched, at least in the long term.

Eating is a complex behavior that involves finding, selecting, preparing, and ingesting food. Neural mechanisms, which control the onset and termination of the behavior, determine the frequency of eating and the duration of the period of eating. Information related to ingested food and to body energy stores is supplied to the brain. For example, blood levels of glucose, as well as neural and endocrine signals from the gastrointestinal tract, provide information concerning the composition and amount of ingested food; neural signals from the liver or humoral signals from fat cells provide information on the energy content of the body's fuel stores. The brain uses this information to modulate food intake by controlling eating behavior.

Leptin

A recently discovered humoral signal that conveys information related to body fatness is the hormone leptin, which is a protein synthesized by adipocytes and released into the blood. The concentration of leptin in the blood is proportional to the individual's percent body fat, so that the fatter the person, the higher the blood level of leptin. Receptors for leptin have been located in specific regions of the brain and in other tissues. Leptin inhibits food intake by acting on neural pathways that control feeding. Leptin also increases resting metabolic rate through mechanisms mediated by neural pathways in the brain. Both of these changes favor negative energy balance and therefore promote weight loss (Figure 11.13).

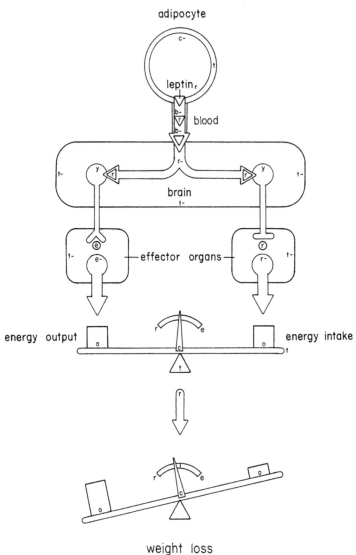

Figure 11.13   Mechanism of leptin action. Color the adipocyte (fat cell) at the top and its release of leptin (triangles) into the blood, noting that blood levels of leptin are related to the amount of adipose tissue in the body. Color the brain and the humoral and neural pathways by which leptin influences effector organs to increase energy output and decrease food intake. Color the balance, the pointer, the scale, and the rectangles that indicate energy output (left side of balance) and energy intake (right side of balance). Color the balance beneath, noting that leptin increases energy output (larger rectangle on left side of balance) and decreases energy intake (smaller rectangle on right side of balance). Observe that these adjustments tip the energy balance in the direction of weight loss. Although this mechanism may help maintain normal levels of body fat in weight-stable, lean individuals, it does not appear to be effective in most obese individuals.

Research in animals has shown that an increase in stored body fat leads to increased blood levels of leptin, which reduce food intake and increase energy expenditure. These changes promote fat loss, which, in turn, leads to lower leptin production and lower blood levels of leptin. Although this mechanism for regulating body fatness may work effectively in weight-stable, lean individuals, it does not appear to be effective in most obese humans, in whom elevated blood levels of leptin do not produce the changes in energy intake and output that would lead to negative energy balance and weight loss. These observations, which suggest that ineffective leptin function is a cause of obesity, raise the possibilities that impaired function of leptin receptors, or of other mechanisms, prevent leptin from regulating energy balance and controlling body fatness in obese people.

Estimation of daily energy requirements

An individual's total daily energy expenditure (TDEE) can be determined by direct calorimetry (Figure 3.16) or indirect calorimetry (Figure 3.19). Alternatively, TDEE can be estimated from the sum of the three components of energy usage, i.e.,

$$TDEE = BMR + TEE + TEF$$

where BMR represents basal metabolic rate, TEE represents the thermic effect of exercise, and TEF represents the thermic effect of feeding (Figure 3.26). Equations have been developed to estimate a person's BMR. For example, the *Harris Benedict Equation* calculates BMR (kcal/ day) in adults from their body weight (in kg), height (in cm), and age (in yr), i.e.,

$$Men: BMR = 66.5 + 13.7 \text{ (weight)} + 5.0 \text{ (height)} - 6.8 \text{ (age)}$$

$$Women: BMR = 655.1 + 9.56 \text{ (weight)} + 1.85 \text{ (height)} - 4.7 \text{ (age)}.$$

Note that BMR increases with body weight and height but decreases with age. The BMR accounts for most of a sedentary person's daily expenditure. Resting metabolic rate (RMR), which is about 10% greater than BMR and more convenient to measure, may also be used in calculating TDEE.

The thermic effect of exercise (TEE) is the most variable component of daily energy expenditure, both among people and within an individual, since it is determined by the amount of physical activity performed in a given day. The energy expended during physical activity depends on the intensity, duration, and nature of exercise, as well as on the individual's body weight, skill, and state of training. Published tables of energy expenditure list the rates of energy expendi-

ture associated with specified activities normalized for body weight [kcal/(kg·min)]. Training can improve skill in a given activity; this results in greater economy of exercise so that less energy will be expended in the performance of the same activity. The magnitude of TEE is approximately 20% of BMR (0.2·BMR) in a sedentary person and 70% of BMR (0.7·BMR) in a person engaged in vigorous endurance training.

The thermic effect of feeding (TEF) is usually estimated as 10% of the energy used for BMR plus TEE, ie., TEF = 0.1·(BMR + TEE). The substitution of these estimates for TEE and TEF into the above equation for TDEE predicts that TDEE ≈ 1.32·BMR (32% above BMR) in sedentary persons and ≈1.87·BMR (87% above BMR) in highly active persons. At a daily kcal intake of these amounts, these individuals would be expected to be in energy balance and would therefore neither gain nor lose weight (assuming no changes in body composition).

Changes in energy balance

Energy balance can be shifted by altering energy input, energy output, or both. That is, changes in food intake relative to total daily energy expenditure can lead to establishment of an energy surplus (positive balance) and weight gain, or an energy deficit (negative balance) and weight loss (Figure 11.12). Note that a person who is obese but who is not gaining weight would have an energy input equal to energy output (zero balance).

In positive energy balance, fuel nutrients consumed in excess of energy output are converted to storage forms, which include a limited amount of glycogen (about 1 kg) and a potentially unlimited amount of triglyceride. These storage forms add to the mass of the body. In addition, an increase in the protein content of muscle can be promoted by resistance training, if the diet provides sufficient amounts of amino acids and energy.

In negative energy balance, fuels are mobilized from their storage forms to compensate for the deficit in energy intake. Glycogen in liver and muscle is broken down to glucose for use as a fuel. Triglyceride in adipose tissue is broken down by lipolysis to fatty acids and glycerol for use as fuels. Lipolysis causes a shrinking of the lipid droplet in the adipocyte so that the cell becomes smaller and adipose tissue mass decreases. Protein in muscle and other tissues is broken down to amino acids for use as a fuel. For these reasons, weight loss generally involves loss of both adipose tissue mass and lean body mass. Changes in body weight, as well as in the relative amounts of adipose tissue and lean tissue, depend on the diet and exercise regimen.

Effect of exercise on weight loss

Increasing energy expenditure by exercise can tip energy balance in the direction of weight loss (Figure 11.12), unless energy intake increases by the same amount. Exercise promotes weight loss by increasing energy output during both the activity and the postexercise period immediately following the activity.

A loss of body weight usually involves a loss of both lean mass and fat mass. This results in a lower level of resting metabolic rate (RMR), because RMR is related to the amount of lean body mass. Regular exercise, particularly resistance training, can prevent or mitigate the loss of lean body mass and, therefore, help preserve RMR (Figure 11.14). This effect is of practical significance because individuals involved in weight reduction programs typically experience diminishing success in weight loss as their lean body mass and RMR (and total daily energy expenditure) decline (Figure 11.15). Total daily energy expenditure also declines with weight loss due to the decrease in energy expenditure of weight-bearing activities, since their energy cost is based on body weight

Figure 11.14   Effect of exercise on composition of weight loss. Color the vertical bars that represent initial and final body weights during a hypothetical weight loss program with (right panel) and without (left panel) supplemental exercise. Observe that both protocols produced the same absolute amount of weight loss (vertical arrows). Observe also that weight loss was accompanied by a loss of lean body mass in the no-exercise condition (downward sloping arrow) but not in the exercise condition (horizontal arrow). These results show that exercise helps preserve lean body mass.

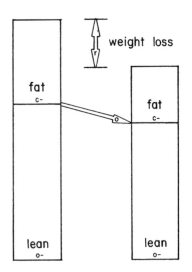

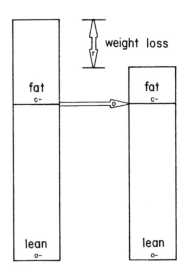

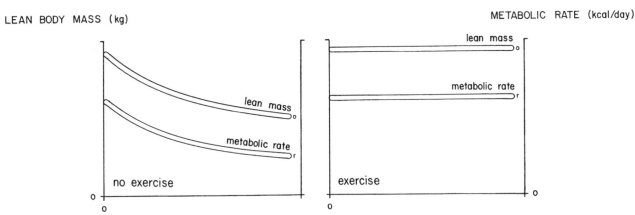

Figure 11.15   Effect of exercise on metabolic rate during weight loss. Color the lines that plot lean body mass and metabolic rate against diet duration during a weight loss program with (right panel) and without (left panel) supplemental exercise. Observe that a loss of lean body mass in the no-exercise condition is accompanied by a decline in metabolic rate (left panel). Observe also that lean body mass and metabolic rate are maintained in the exercise condition (right panel). These results indicate that loss of lean body mass lowers metabolic rate, while preservation of lean body mass with an appropriate exercise regimen can maintain metabolic rate, and thereby promote weight loss by maintaining energy output.

(kcal/kg); an increase in physical activity can offset this effect. Therefore, exercise is an important component of weight loss programs not only because it increases energy output but it also maintains lean body mass and therefore, resting metabolic rate.

Effect of diet on weight loss

Weight reduction diets vary considerably in their nutrient composition and the degree of energy deficit they are designed to produce. These differences affect the rate and composition of weight loss.

Diet composition refers to the percentages of kcal derived from carbohydrate, fat, and protein, respectively. The diet composition recommended for the general population is >50% of kcal as carbohydrate, <30% as fat, and ~20% as protein (Figure 10.5). Nutritionally adequate weight-loss diets generally involve an overall reduction in the number of

kcal, along with a decrease in the percent of kcal from fat; such diets can lead to lifelong improvements in eating habits.

Very low carbohydrate diets

Very low carbohydrate (< 50 g/day) or carbohydrate-free diets initially produce rapid weight loss due to body water loss. Because very low levels of carbohydrate consumption result in lower blood glucose levels, glycogen stores in liver and muscle are broken down to supply glucose to the blood. Under these conditions, weight loss is due to a loss of glycogen and the water associated with it; because each gram of glycogen is hydrated by about 3 g of water, glycogen depletion leads to rapid weight loss (Figure 11.16, left panel). For example, depletion of 500 g of glycogen can result in a 2 kg loss in body weight in the first week of the diet. This weight loss, which is due primarily to water loss, is quickly regained when normal carbohydrate consumption is resumed and glycogen repletion occurs.

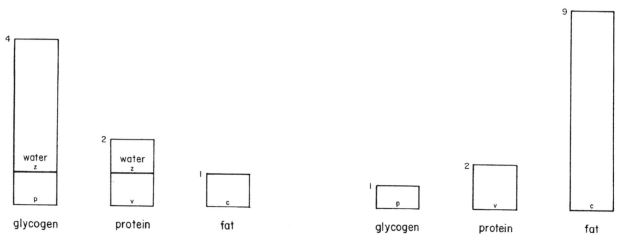

GRAMS BODY MASS PER GRAM FUEL CALORIE EQUIVALENT OF ONE GRAM BODY MASS

Figure 11.16   Composition of weight loss and its calorie equivalent. Color the set of three vertical bars at left depicting the total grams of body mass that are lost for each gram of stored fuel that is depleted during weight loss; observe the relative amounts of the water (top) and fuel (bottom) components for each as well as the fraction of total weight loss that is actually due depletion of the fuel. Color the set of three bars at right depicting the amount of the energy deficit (calorie equivalent) required to produce the loss of one gram of body mass. Observe that a deficit of 1 kcal is needed per g of glycogen that is lost, a deficit of 2 kcal is needed per g of protein that is lost, and a deficit of 9 kcal is needed per g of fat (triglyceride) that is lost. The reasons for these differences are that: (1) the energy equivalents of the fuels themselves differ (glycogen: 4 kcal/g; protein: 4kcal/g; fat: 9kcal/g); and (2) as shown in the left panel, the actual loss in body weight consists of the loss of the mass of fuel plus its associated water. For example, because the loss of 1 g of glycogen is accompanied by the loss of 3 g of water; a 4 kcal deficit brings about a total loss of 4 g of body weight (4 kcal/4g). For these reasons, even with the same energy deficit, the amount of body weight that is lost per kcal of energy deficit depends on the relative amounts of glycogen, protein, and fat that are depleted.

When glycogen stores are depleted, blood glucose concentration is maintained by breaking down body protein to provide amino acids for the pathway of gluconeogenesis. Under these conditions, weight loss is due to a loss of protein and the water associated with it (Figure 11.16, left panel). These considerations explain why very low carbohydrate diets may produce weight loss with little loss of adipose tissue mass. As a consequence, this type of weight loss would not reduce obesity-related disease risk and would be likely to impair performance in activities that are limited by glycogen depletion, such as high-intensity exercise or long-duration exercise.

Effect of energy deficit on weight loss

In general, the more negative the energy balance, the greater the rate of weight loss. The relationship between weight loss and energy deficit may be grossly estimated to be a pound of weight for each 3500 kcal deficit (or about 7700 kcal deficit per kg). This relationship, however, is not constant because it depends on the composition of the weight loss (Figure 11.16). Loss of 1 g of fat requires a greater energy deficit than that needed to lose 1 g of protein or 1 g of carbohydrate (Figure 11.6, right panel). Stated another way, a given amount of weight loss requires a smaller energy deficit when it is comprised of body components other than fat.

An implication of this changing relationship between weight loss and energy deficit is that weight loss during the first week of a weight loss program may occur rapidly if it is comprised mainly of water and glycogen, since weight loss requires a small energy deficit. However, the rate of weight loss tends to decrease as the program continues because more of the weight loss is due to depletion of body fat and a larger energy deficit is required per kg of weight lost (Figure 11.17).

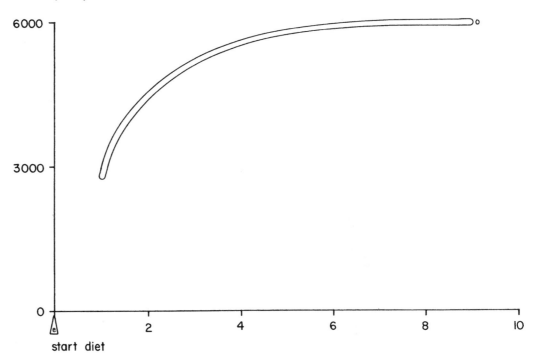

CALORIES PER KILOGRAM (kcal)

DURATION OF DIET (weeks)

Figure 11.17   Temporal changes in the calorie equivalents of weight loss. Color the line that depicts the change in the energy equivalent of a loss of 1 kg of body mass (kcal/kg) with time on a weight loss (negative energy balance) diet. Observe that it initially increases, so that a greater kcal deficit is needed to lose each kg, and then reaches a plateau where the deficit associated with weight loss is essentially constant (note that the relationship applies to healthy individuals). The reason for the change in the energy equivalent for weight loss over time is that the composition of the fuels (body glycogen, protein, and triglyceride) being depleted to compensate for this deficit in energy intake change with time; glycogen stores are depleted early in the weight loss period and increasing amounts of triglyceride are catabolized with time on the diet. The slowing of weight loss that occurs in most individuals on weight loss regimens can be explained, in part, by this declining weight loss for the same calorie deficit. Compare this figure with Figure 11.16.

301

Causes of obesity

In simplest terms, obesity is the result of a prolonged, large positive energy balance; that is, energy intake has exceeded energy output. A combination of genetic, developmental, and environmental factors has been implicated in the development of obesity (Figure 11.18).

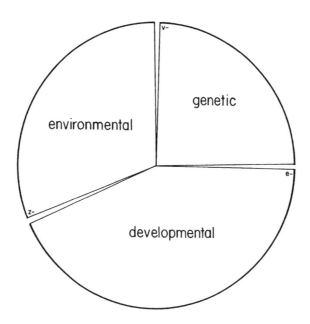

Figure 11.18   Factors that promote obesity. Color the three sections of the circle that represent categories of factors that produce obesity. The relative sizes of the segments represent their relative contributions to obesity in the population; for example, large-scale studies have provided evidence that genetic predisposition accounts for about 25% of the prevalence of obesity. The relative sizes of the other two components are more arbitrary. Environmental factors refer to influences of society and culture, and developmental factors refer to physiological changes (such as fat cell hyperplasia) produced by the state of positive energy balance over the life of the individual. Many factors could be instrumental in producing obesity in a given individual.

Genetic etiology of obesity

Obesity is a familial trait; that is, family members tend to be similar in their body fatness. Obese children are likely to have at least one obese parent. Parental obesity, however, is not a good predictor of children's obesity since people in affluent countries tend to become obese as they get older. Familial association is not proof of genetic inheritance because families also share food preferences, eating habits, and exercise patterns.

There is strong evidence that obesity can be inherited and genes have been identified in animals that confer this trait. For example, there are strains of mice and rats that lack either the gene for leptin or the gene for the brain's receptor for it. There are many other heritable traits that could produce obesity, such as decreased activity of brown adipose tissue (a heat-producing, fuel-wasting tissue) or increased adipose tissue sensitivity to insulin that could promote fat storage.

It has been estimated that parental obesity statistically accounts for about 25% of the prevalence of abdominal fatness. That is, having an obese parent is a significant predictor for the development of excessive abdominal fat.

Developmental origin of obesity

Because greater adipose tissue hyperplasia is associated with lifelong obesity, overfeeding during certain developmental periods may be responsible for adult obesity in some individuals. For example, overfeeding infants can increase the number of their fat cells and theoretically increase their likelihood of obesity throughout life. However, the relationship between infantile "obesity" (generally defined as greater weight-for-height than that of infants of the same age) and adult obesity is not strong; a baby's body weight before one year of age is a better predictor of his or her adult height than it is of the risk of obesity in adulthood. Overfeeding during other developmental periods may be more influential; for example, obesity in teenagers is associated with adult obesity.

All individuals may not be equally susceptible to stimulation of fat cell hyperplasia. It is possible that one way in which a genetic predisposition to obesity exerts its effect is by making a person's fat cells more likely to proliferate under a given set of circumstances, thereby producing a permanent increase in fat cell number.

Environmental causes of obesity

The dramatic rise in the percent of the U.S. population that is obese (from about 23% in 1960 to about 35% in 1990) argues for an increased contribution of nongenetic causes of obesity, since evolution and changes in the gene pool occur too slowly to account for this finding. A large number of environmental influences, or combinations of them, are likely to play a role.

A decrease in the average energy expenditure of individuals, including children, has occurred over the last few decades. This decrease, seen in affluent countries like the United States, is related to decreased energy expenditure on the job, in travel to work or school, and in recreational activities. That this decrease in energy expenditure may influence obesity risk is supported by studies such as those reporting that the amount of television watched by children is predictive of their BMI several years later.

Food availability, snacking patterns, diet composition, and palatability may all influence the amount of food a person ingests. Food availability is increased by lower price and convenience (fast-food restaurants, ready-to-eat products). Snacking itself does not promote weight gain if meals are merely divided into many smaller ones; however, snacks often represent an addition of calories to the diet and may also change eating from a "main event" to a behavior that continues with little attention paid to the amount consumed while the person is engaged in another activity.

Diets high in fat and low in dietary fiber are associated with excessive energy intake. Highly processed foods tend to be higher in fat and lower in fiber than foods in their natural state, particularly foods of plant origin like vegetables, whole grains, and fruits. Popular foods commonly sold in fast-food restaurants are high in fat and low in fiber, as are typical, highly palatable dessert and snack items. Consumption of high-fat, low-fiber foods which have a high energy density (kcal/g) may interfere with normal physiological regulation of food intake.

Additional environmental influences include the social aspects of food, eating, and body weight. Snacking at most times and places has become acceptable, portions of food in the United States are larger than those in many other societies, and obesity among adults has become commonplace.

Underweight

Very low BMI (< 17 kg/m^2) is associated with elevated disease risk. Loss of lean body mass as well as adipose tissue mass occurs. Low body weights could be due to illness, voluntary restriction of eating, and/or high energy expenditure. Nutritional deficiency signs, including anemia, osteoporosis, poor immune function, and amenorrhea are among the problems associated with being underweight.

The eating disorder *anorexia nervosa* is observed mainly (but not only) in female adolescents and young adults. It is typically a highly controlled restriction of food intake associated with the individual's sense that, although she is actually dangerously thin, she is overweight. Anorexia nervosa can lead to death by starvation, so psychological, medical, and nutritional therapies must be instituted.

Recommended Reading

Åstrand, P-O., and K. Rodahl. *Textbook of Work Physiology,* 2nd edition. New York: McGraw Hill, 1977.

Berne, R.M., and M.N. Levy (Eds.). *Physiology,* 4th edition. St. Louis MO: Mosby, 1998.

Björntorp, P., and B.N. Brodoff. *Obesity.* Philadelphia: J.B. Lippincott, 1992.

Brooks, G.A., T.D. Fahey, and T.P. White. *Exercise Physiology: Human Bioenergetics and Its Applications,* 2nd edition. Mountain View, CA: Mayfield, 1996.

Devlin, T.M. (Ed.). *Textbook of Biochemistry with Clinical Correlations,* 4th edition. New York: John Wiley & Sons, 1997.

Guyton, A.C., C.E. Jones, and T.G. Coleman. *Circulatory Physiology: Cardiac Output and Its Regulation.* Philadelphia: W.B. Saunders, 1973.

Guyton. A.C. and J.E. Hall. *Human Physiology and Mechanisms of Disease,* 6th edition. Philadelphia: W.B. Saunders, 1997.

Horton, E.S., and R.L. Terjung (Eds.). *Exercise, Nutrition, and Energy Metabolism.* New York: Macmillan, 1988.

McArdle, W.D., F.I. Katch, and V.L. Katch. *Exercise Physiology: Energy, Nutrition, and Human Performance,* 4th edition. Baltimore: Williams & Wilkins, 1996.

Plowman, S.A., and D.L. Smith. *Exercise Physiology: For Health, Fitness, and Performance.* Boston: Allyn & Bacon, 1997.

Powers, S.K., and E.T. Howley. *Exercise Physiology: Theory and Application to Fitness and Performance.* Dubuque, IA: Brown & Benchmark, 1997.

Robergs, R.A., and S.O. Roberts. *Exercise Physiology: Exercise, Performance, and Clinical Applications.* St. Louis, MO: Mosby-Yearbook, 1997.

Wasserman, K., J.E. Hansen, D.Y. Sue, R. Casaburi, and B.J. Whipp. *Principles of Exercise Testing and Interpretation,* 3rd edition. Baltimore: Lippincott Williams & Wilkins, 1999.

West, J.B. *Respiratory Physiology—The Essentials.* Baltimore: Williams & Wilkins, 1985.

Wilmore, J.H., and D.L. Costill. *Physiology of Sport and Exercise,* 2nd edition. Champaign, IL: Human Kinetics, 1999.

Wolinsky, I. (Ed.). *Nutrition in Exercise and Sport,* 3rd edition. New York: CRC Press, 1998.

About the Authors

Both authors are research scientists as well as teachers.

Kenneth Axen, PhD, is a Clinical Associate Professor of Rehabilitation Medicine at New York University School of Medicine. Since receiving his PhD in biomedical engineering from New York University, Dr. Axen has been conducting basic research on respiratory perception in humans, regulation of breathing in neuromuscular disorders, and rehabilitation of people with respiratory impairments. His numerous research articles in the *Journal of Applied Physiology* have earned him international recognition in the area of regulation of breathing.

He has also taught exercise physiology at the undergraduate and graduate levels to physical therapy students at Long Island University and to health science majors and physical education students at Brooklyn College, CUNY. Dr. Axen is co-editor of *Pulmonary Therapy and Rehabilitation: Principles and Practice* (Williams & Wilkins, 1991), and the illustrator of the *Princeton Review Physiology Coloring Workbook* (Random House, 1997), the *Chronic Bronchitis and Emphysema Handbook* (John Wiley & Sons, 1990), and the *Essential Asthma Book* (Charles Scribners' Sons, 1987).

Kathleen V. Axen, PhD, CDN, is a Full Professor in the Department of Health and Nutrition Sciences at Brooklyn College of the City University of New York where she teaches undergraduate and graduate courses in nutrition and metabolism. Dr. Axen received her PhD in Nutritional Biochemistry from Columbia University, New York. She trained as a post-doctoral fellow in Endocrinology at the Albert Einstein College of Medicine, New York. She is also a New York State Certified Nutritionist. Dr. Axen's research on the regulation of insulin secretion and on the development and treatment of diabetes mellitus in animal models of obesity has been published in the *American Journal of Physiology* and the *Journal of Clinical Investigation.*

They co-authored the *Princeton Review Physiology Coloring Workbook* (Random House 1997), co-presented a symposium entitled "Exercise Training and Nutritional Therapy in Severe Chronic Obstructive Pulmonary Disease" at the National Yang Ming Medical College, Taipei, Taiwan (1993), and currently team-teach a graduate course in Nutrition and Exercise at Brooklyn College, CUNY.